Vaccines against RNA Viruses

Vaccines against RNA Viruses

Editor

Juan Carlos Saiz

MDPI • Basel • Beijing • Wuhan • Barcelona • Belgrade • Manchester • Tokyo • Cluj • Tianjin

Editor
Juan Carlos Saiz
Instituto Nacional de
Investigacion y Tecnologia
Agraria y Alimentaria
Spain

Editorial Office
MDPI
St. Alban-Anlage 66
4052 Basel, Switzerland

This is a reprint of articles from the Special Issue published online in the open access journal *Vaccines* (ISSN 2076-393X) (available at: https://www.mdpi.com/journal/vaccines/special_issues/RNA_Viruse).

For citation purposes, cite each article independently as indicated on the article page online and as indicated below:

LastName, A.A.; LastName, B.B.; LastName, C.C. Article Title. *Journal Name* **Year**, *Article Number*, Page Range.

ISBN 978-3-03943-623-1 (Hbk)
ISBN 978-3-03943-624-8 (PDF)

Contents

About the Editor . . . . **vii**

Juan-Carlos Saiz
Vaccines against RNA Viruses
Reprinted from: *Vaccines* **2020**, *8*, 479, doi:10.3390/vaccines8030479 . . . . **1**

Andrey P. Rudometov, Anton N. Chikaev, Nadezhda B. Rudometova, Denis V. Antonets, Alexander A. Lomzov, Olga N. Kaplina, Alexander A. Ilyichev and Larisa I. Karpenko
Artificial Anti-HIV-1 Immunogen Comprising Epitopes of Broadly Neutralizing Antibodies 2F5, 10E8, and a Peptide Mimic of VRC01 Discontinuous Epitope
Reprinted from: *Vaccines* **2019**, *7*, 83, doi:10.3390/vaccines7030083 . . . . **5**

Ashwin Ramesh, Jiangdi Mao, Shaohua Lei, Erica Twitchell, Ashton Shiraz, Xi Jiang, Ming Tan and Lijuan Yuan
Parenterally Administered P24-VP8* Nanoparticle Vaccine Conferred Strong Protection against Rotavirus Diarrhea and Virus Shedding in Gnotobiotic Pigs
Reprinted from: *Vaccines* **2019**, *7*, 177, doi:10.3390/vaccines7040177 . . . . **23**

Joshua D. Duncan, Richard A. Urbanowicz, Alexander W. Tarr and Jonathan K. Ball
Hepatitis C Virus Vaccine: Challenges and Prospects
Reprinted from: *Vaccines* **2020**, *8*, 90, doi:10.3390/vaccines8010090 . . . . **37**

Junru Cui, Caitlin M. O'Connell, Connor Hagen, Kim Sawicki, Joan A. Smyth, Paulo H. Verardi, Herbert J. Van Kruiningen and Antonio E. Garmendia
Broad Protection of Pigs against Heterologous PRRSV Strains by a GP5-Mosaic DNA Vaccine Prime/GP5-Mosaic rVaccinia (VACV) Vaccine Boost
Reprinted from: *Vaccines* **2020**, *8*, 106, doi:10.3390/vaccines8010106 . . . . **61**

Da Shi, Xiaobo Wang, Hongyan Shi, Jiyu Zhang, Yuru Han, Jianfei Chen, Xin Zhang, Jianbo Liu, Jialin Zhang, Zhaoyang Ji, Zhaoyang Jing and Li Feng
Significant Interference with Porcine Epidemic Diarrhea Virus Pandemic and Classical Strain Replication in Small-Intestine Epithelial Cells Using an shRNA Expression Vector
Reprinted from: *Vaccines* **2019**, *7*, 173, doi:10.3390/vaccines7040173 . . . . **75**

Rodrigo Cañas-Arranz, Mar Forner, Sira Defaus, Patricia de León, María J. Bustos, Elisa Torres, Francisco Sobrino, Esther Blanco and David Andreu
A Single Dose of Dendrimer B_2T Peptide Vaccine Partially Protects Pigs against Foot-and-Mouth Disease Virus Infection
Reprinted from: *Vaccines* **2020**, *8*, 19, doi:10.3390/vaccines8010019 . . . . **87**

Elena López-Gil, Sandra Moreno, Javier Ortego, Belén Borrego, Gema Lorenzo and Alejandro Brun
MVA Vectored Vaccines Encoding Rift Valley Fever Virus Glycoproteins Protect Mice against Lethal Challenge in the Absence of Neutralizing Antibody Responses
Reprinted from: *Vaccines* **2020**, *8*, 82, doi:10.3390/vaccines8010082 . . . . **99**

Blanca Chinchilla, Paloma Encinas, Julio M. Coll and Eduardo Gomez-Casado
Differential Immune Transcriptome and Modulated Signalling Pathways in Rainbow Trout Infected with Viral Haemorrhagic Septicaemia Virus (VHSV) and Its Derivative Non-Virion (NV) Gene Deleted
Reprinted from: *Vaccines* **2020**, *8*, 58, doi:10.3390/vaccines8010058 . . . . **115**

About the Editor

Juan Carlos Saiz received his Ph.D. in Biochemistry and Molecular Biology from Universidad Autónoma de Madrid (U.A.M.), Spain, in 1987. Then, he was trained in Virology as a post-doctoral at the PIADC/ARS in New York (1987-91), at the Instituto Nacional de Investigación Agraria y Alimentaria, INIA, in Madrid (1991-92), and at the Centro de Biología Molecular "Severo Ochoa", CBMSO (1992-96), also in Madrid. From 1996 to 2002 he was in charge of the Laboratory of Viral Hepatitis at the Hospital Clínic (Barcelona). Since 2002, Professor Saiz is the Research Leader of the "ZOOVIR" laboratory at INIA-CSIC, where he was director of the Dpt. Biotechnology (2010-2015). Professor Saiz's group study different aspects of Flavivirus (West Nile, Dengue, Zika, and Usutu viruses) biology, focusing in the prevention and control of these worldwide threatening infectious pathogens. More specifically, the main group's objectives are i) the identification of viral and cellular targets for antiviral intervention; ii) the development of vaccines candidates and its testing in animal model (mice and birds); and iii) the development of new diagnostic systems. Professor Saiz (Researcher ID: L-4638-2014; Orcid: 0000-0001-8269-5544) is co-author over 160 publications with over 3500 citations in more than 2760 articles (h-index 35), and has been granted with 37 national and international open call projects.

vaccines

MDPI

Editorial

Vaccines against RNA Viruses

Juan-Carlos Saiz

ZOOVIR, Department of Biotechnology, Instituto Nacional de Investigaciones Agrarias (INIA), 28040 Madrid, Spain; jcsaiz2012@gmail.com

Received: 25 August 2020; Accepted: 26 August 2020; Published: 27 August 2020

RNA viruses cause animal, human, and zoonotic diseases that affect millions of individuals, as is being exemplified by the devastating ongoing epidemic of the recently identified SARS-Cov-2. For years vaccines have had an enormous impact on overcoming the global burden of diseases. Nowadays, a vast number of different approaches, from purified inactivated and live attenuated viruses, nucleic acid (DNA or RNA) based candidates, virus-like particles, subunit elements, and recombinant viruses are been employed to combat diverse diseases caused by RNA viruses. However, although for some of them efficient vaccines are available, in most instances, and for different reasons (technologic o economic restrictions, etc.), they are scarcely used in the field, and even for many of them no licensed vaccines exist. This will probably change dramatically with the current Covid-19 pandemic, as a vast variety of vaccinology approaches are being tested against it, with hundreds of candidates under development, dozens of them already in clinical trials phase III and IV, a fact that is breaking records in vaccine development and implementation. This is becoming possible thanks to the enormous work carried out during years to have the bases for a quick response, even against unknown pathogens, in an impressive short time.

In this *Vaccines* Special Issue "Vaccines against RNA viruses", results obtained with different vaccine methodological approaches against human, animal, and zoonotic viruses are presented by field experts.

Human Immunodeficiency Virus (HIV), for which no vaccine is available, continues to be a major global public health issue that has already cost almost 33 million lives so far, and with an estimated 38 million people living with it. Even though antiretroviral therapy considerably prolongs the lifespan of patients making the disease a manageable chronic health condition, treatment is expensive and is not available for all infected patients. Thus, vaccines are needed to control HIV spread. So, in this Issue, Rudometov et al. [1] describe the development of a human immunodeficiency virus-1 (HIV-1) immunogen using a polypeptide recombinant non transferrin bound iron (nTBI) protein carrying four T- and five B-cell epitopes from HIV-1 Env and Gag proteins recognized by broadly neutralizing HIV-1 antibodies, combined with Th-epitopes. Immunization of rabbits with this nTBI protein elicited antibodies that recognize HIV-1 proteins, supporting its possible use as immunogen.

Another relevant human virus is the human rotavirus (HRV) that is a leading cause of severe, dehydrating gastroenteritis, mainly in children. Current live rotavirus vaccines are efficient, but costly, and they may present increased risk of intussusception due to vaccine replication in the gut of vaccinated children. Here, Ramesh and coworkers [2] assess the immunogenicity and protective capacity of a novel P24-VP8* nanoparticle vaccine using the gnotobiotic (Gn) pig model of human rotavirus. Three doses (200 μg/dose) of the vaccine candidate intramuscularly administered with $Al(OH)_3$ (600 μg) as an adjuvant conferred significant protection against infection and diarrhea after challenged with virulent heterologous rotavirus strains. Vaccinated animals showed a significant reduction in the mean duration of diarrhea, virus shedding in feces, and significantly lower fecal cumulative consistency scores in comparison with mock immunized control animals. Vaccinated animals also elicited strong VP8*-specific serum neutralizing antibody responses, but, consistent with the methodological approach (immunization route, adjuvant, and lack of replication), no serum or intestinal IgA antibody responses, or strong effector T cell responses, were induced. Authors indicate that their results open the option of the initiation of clinical trials using the new designed P24-VP8* nanoparticle vaccine candidate.

For his part, Duncan and coworkers [3] update the current status of the hepatitis C virus (HCV) vaccination, describing and discussing the different ongoing research in the field, and emphasizing that, despite the great advances in HCV therapeutics achieved lately, treatments sometime fail to prevent reinfection and are quite expensive and, thus, efficient prophylactic HCV vaccines are still needed.

Pigs are one of the main livestock species, comprising 36% of the worldwide meat consumption, with hundreds of tons produced yearly. Pigs can be infected by a wide variety of RNA viruses that cause huge losses for the food industry. In addition, they can serve as bridge between wild host animals and humans. Thereby, availability of efficient vaccines is crucial. Among the viral infections affecting pigs, a very important one is that of the porcine reproductive and respiratory syndrome virus (PRRSV) that causes reproductive failure in pregnant sows and respiratory disease in young pigs, accounting for huge economic losses to industry across the world. One critical drawback for vaccine development against PRRSV is its high genetic diversity. Here, Ciu and coworkers [4] show their results after testing a glycoprotein GP5-Mosaic DNA vaccine and a recombinant GP5-Mosaic vaccinia virus (rGP5-Mosaic VACV) vaccine in pigs, and compare their immunogenicity and protective capacity against heterologous virulent strains (VR2332 or MN184C) with that of a rGP5-wyld-type, WT (VR2332) DNA and a rGP5-WT (VR2332) VACV vaccine, using as controls groups inoculated with empty vector DNA or empty VACV. The authors show that vaccination with the GP5-Mosaic-based vaccines resulted in cellular reactivity and higher levels of neutralizing antibodies to both VR2332 and MN184C PRRSV strains, whilst vaccination with the GP5-WT vaccines only induced response against the heterologous challenging virus (VR2332). After infection with either strain, viral titers in sera and tissues, as well as lung lesions, were lower in the GP5-Mosaic vaccinated pigs. These results indicate that, using a DNA-prime/VACV boost regimen, the developed GP5-Mosaic candidates confer protection in pigs against heterologous viruses and, thus, are feasible vaccine candidates.

Another important disease in pigs is that caused by the porcine epidemic diarrhea virus (PEDV), a coronavirus responsible of highly contagious intestinal infections that may result in the death of newborn piglets and weight loss in pigs of all ages, and that seriously damages the swine industry. From 2010, novel highly virulent PEDV genotype 2 variants have spread through China, resulting in high mortality of newborn piglets and huge economic losses. Current vaccines against the classical CV777 strain of genotype 1 do not provide effective protection against Chinese highly virulent PEDV variant infections. Thus, Shi and colleagues [5] using a RNA interference (RNAi) approach, show that three short hairpin RNA (shRNA) expressing plasmids directed against the viral nucleocapsid (N) present antiviral activities in intestine epithelial cells infected with a both classical CV777 and LNCT2 strains, and that these shRNAs markedly reduce viral replication of both strains upon downregulation of N protein production; thus, these strategies, based on targeting viral processivity factors, may be feasible vaccine alternatives.

By a different approach, Cañas-Arranz et al. [6] deepen their many years of previous research with peptides as vaccine candidates against foot-and mouth disease virus (FMDV). The virus is responsible for a highly contagious transmissible infection of cloven-hoofed animals (mainly pigs and cows) that may cause huge economic impact and whose control relies on efficient vaccination using a conventional chemically inactivated virus. However, these current vaccines present limitations, as the need for a strict maintenance of the cold chain and for a constant update of vaccine strains due to the virus's antigenic diversity, as well as the fact that the manufacturing process poses significant biosafety concerns, as it has been related to occasional escape episodes. Therefore, vaccines incorporating specific outbreak-relevant epitopes capable of eliciting protective and quick responses can become an invaluable emergency resource for FMD containments during outbreaks. With this background, the Spanish group go one step further by testing in pigs a dendrimer B2T peptide with two copies of a B-cell VP1 epitope linked through maleimide units to a T-cell 3A epitope, and show that a single dose of B2T evokes a specific protective immune response with high neutralizing titers, activates the T cell response, induces IFN production, and fully protects 70% of vaccinated pigs that did not present clinical signs of the disease. Their results strengthen the potential of B2T as a safe, cost-effective candidate vaccine, which can be of particular interest in emergency scenarios.

Rift Valley fever virus (RVFV), a mosquito-borne bunyavirus widely distributed in Sub-Saharan countries, Egypt, and the Arabian Peninsula, is another important pathogen causing disease in humans, in which severe cases can end in encephalitis or hemorrhagic fever, and in ruminant livestock, characterized by an increased incidence of abortion or fetal malformation. At present, there are a few veterinary vaccines available for use in endemic areas, but there is no licensed human vaccine. López-Gil and coworkers [7], by using an approach based on the modified vaccinia Ankara (MVA) virus encoding the RVFV glycoproteins (rMVAGnGc), extend their previous observations that a single inoculation was sufficient to induce a protective immune response in mice after a lethal viral challenge, which was related to the presence of glycoprotein specific CD8+ cells and a low-level detection of in vitro neutralizing antibodies. They tested the efficacy and immune response in mice immunized with recombinant MVA viruses expressing either glycoprotein Gn (rMVAGn) or Gc (rMVAGc) and suggest that, in the absence of serum neutralizing antibodies, protection is strain-dependent and mainly due to the activation of the cellular response against Gc epitopes. Even more, their data point to the induction of a suboptimal humoral immune response, since disease was exacerbated upon the virus challenge in the presence of rMVAGnGc or rMVAGn immune serum. These results support that Gc-specific cellular immunity is an important component that contributes to efficient protection against RVFV infection.

The fishing industry is increasingly relevant, and the number of farms has grown exponentially, being a very important source of food. Viral hemorrhagic septicemia virus (VHSV), a novirhabdovirus, is one of the worst viral threats to fish farming. VHSV has been isolated from more than 50 fish species across the world, including farmed and free-living marine species. Detection of even a single positive sample in a farm has to be notified to the Office International des Epizooties, and implies the sacrifice of all the farmed fish, thus leading to serious economic losses. Non-virion (NV) gene-deleted VHSV (dNV-VHSV) has been postulated as an attenuated virus, as its absence leads to lower induced pathogenicity. In the study by Chinchilla et al. [8] the immune transcriptome profiling in trout infected with dNV-VHSV and wt-VHSV and the pathways involved in immune responses were analyzed in the context of infection. The authors show that dNV-VHSV upregulates more trout-signaling immune related genes and pathways, whereas wt-VHSV maintains more non-regulated genes. Therefore, wt-VHSV impairs the activation at short stages of infection of pro-inflammatory, antiviral, proliferation, and apoptosis pathways, delaying innate humoral response and cellular crosstalk, whereas dNV-VHSV promotes the opposite effects, supporting the use of dNV-VHSV as a potential live vaccine candidate.

Finally, Jiménez de Oya and coworkers [9] deeply update current knowledge and available data about the vaccination of birds against the West Nile virus (WNV), the worldwide most distributed mosquito-borne flavivirus. Although humans and equids can sporadically be infected, birds are the natural host of WNV. When clinical signs arise in birds it is due to multi-organ invasion, mainly in the central nervous system, which can lead to death 24–48 h later. Nowadays, vaccines are only available for use in equids; thus, availability of avian vaccines would benefit bird populations, both domestic and wild ones. Such vaccines could be used in endangered species housed in rehabilitation and wildlife reserves, and in animals located at zoos and other recreational installations, but also in farm birds, and in those that are grown for hunting and restocking activities. Even more, controlling WNV infection in birds can also be useful to prevent its spread and limit outbreaks. In their review, Jimenez de Oya and colleagues comprehensively present the results obtained with commercial and experimental vaccines in domestic and wild avian species, and the possible benefits and drawbacks of bird vaccination against WNV are discussed.

The world remains burdened by high morbidity and mortality diseases and, as exemplified by the current devastating pandemic of SARS-Cov-2, and new emerging or re-emerging pathogens are likely to spread in the future. Hereby, a more comprehensive understanding of the current trends in vaccine development and assessment of the molecular mechanisms and immune responses involved in the elicited responses are essential. In this line, the articles in this Issue highlight recent advances in the development of efficient vaccines against RNA viruses infecting animals and humans, some of which are zoonotic. Different approaches are described from attenuated and recombinant viruses, to peptides, and DNA and RNA-based candidates, which hopefully will contribute to a better and quick preparedness against RNA virus infections.

Funding: This research received no external funding.

Conflicts of Interest: The author declares no conflict of interest.

References

1. Rudometov, A.P.; Chikaev, A.N.; Rudometova, N.B.; Antonets, D.V.; Lomzov, A.A.; Kaplina, O.N.; Ilyichev, A.A.; Karpenko, L.I. Artificial anti-HIV-1 immunogen comprising epitopes of broadly neutralizing antibodies 2F5, 10E8, and a peptide mimic of VRC01 discontinuous epitope. *Vaccines* **2019**, *7*, 83. [CrossRef]
2. Ramesh, A.; Mao, J.; Lei, S.; Twitchell, E.; Shiraz, A.; Jiang, X.; Tan, M.; Yuan, L. Parenterally administered P24-VP8* nanoparticle vaccine conferred strong protection against rotavirus diarrhea and virus shedding in gnotobiotic pigs. *Vaccines* **2019**, *7*, 177. [CrossRef]
3. Duncan, J.D.; Urbanowicz, R.A.; Tarr, A.W.; Ball, J.K. Hepatitis C virus vaccine: Challenges and prospects. *Vaccines* **2020**, *8*, 90. [CrossRef]
4. Cui, J.; O'Connell, C.M.; Hagen, C.; Sawicki, K.; Smyth, J.A.; Verard, P.H.; Van Kruiningen, H.J.; Garmendia, E. Broad protection of pigs against heterologous PRRSV strains by a GP5-mosaic DNA vaccine prime/GP5-mosaic rVaccinia (VACV) vaccine boost. *Vaccines* **2020**, *8*, 106. [CrossRef] [PubMed]
5. Shi, D.; Wang, X.; Shi, H.; Zhang, J.; Han, Y.; Chen, J.; Zhang, X.; Liu, J.; Zhang, J.; Ji, Z.; et al. Significant interference with porcine epidemic diarrhea virus pandemic and classical strain replication in small-intestine epithelial cells using an shRNA expression vector. *Vaccines* **2019**, *7*, 173. [CrossRef] [PubMed]
6. Cañas-Arranz, R.; Forner, M.; Defaus, S.; de León, P.; Bustos, M.J.; Torres, E.; Sobrino, F.; Andreu, D.; Blanco, E. A single dose of dendrimer B_2T peptide vaccine partially protects pigs against foot-and-mouth disease virus infection. *Vaccines* **2020**, *8*, 19. [CrossRef] [PubMed]
7. López-Gil, E.; Moreno, S.; Ortego, J.; Borrego, B.; Lorenzo, G.; Brun, A. MVA vectored vaccines encoding rift valley fever virus glycoproteins protect mice against lethal challenge in the absence of neutralizing antibody responses. *Vaccines* **2020**, *8*, 82. [CrossRef] [PubMed]
8. Chinchilla, B.; Encinas, P.; Coll, J.M.; Gomez-Casado, E. Differential immune transcriptome and modulated signalling pathways in rainbow trout infected with Viral Haemorrhagic Septicaemia Virus (VHSV) and its Derivative Non-Virion (NV) gene deleted. *Vaccines* **2020**, *8*, 58. [CrossRef] [PubMed]
9. de Jiménez Oya, N.; Escribano-Romero, E.; Blázquez, A.B.; Martín-Acebes, M.A.; Saiz, J.C. Current progress of avian vaccines against west nile virus. *Vaccines* **2019**, *7*, 126. [CrossRef] [PubMed]

vaccines

MDPI

Article

Artificial Anti-HIV-1 Immunogen Comprising Epitopes of Broadly Neutralizing Antibodies 2F5, 10E8, and a Peptide Mimic of VRC01 Discontinuous Epitope

Andrey P. Rudometov [1,*], Anton N. Chikaev [2,*], Nadezhda B. Rudometova [1], Denis V. Antonets [1], Alexander A. Lomzov [3], Olga N. Kaplina [1], Alexander A. Ilyichev [1] and Larisa I. Karpenko [1,*]

1 State Research Center of Virology and Biotechnology "Vector", Koltsovo, Novosibirsk Region 630559, Russia
2 Institute of Molecular and Cellular Biology of the Siberian Branch of the Russian Academy of Sciences, 8/2 Lavrentiev Avenue Novosibirsk, Novosibirsk 630090, Russia
3 Institute of Chemical Biology and Fundamental Medicine of the Siberian Branch of the Russian Academy of Sciences, 8 Lavrentiev Avenue, Novosibirsk 630090, Russia
* Correspondence: andrei692@mail.ru (A.P.R.); chikaev@mcb.nsc.ru (A.N.C.); lkarpenko@ngs.ru (L.I.K.); Tel.: +7-383-363-47-00 (ext. 2013) (A.P.R.); +7-383-363-90-72 (A.N.C.); Tel.: +7-383-363-47-00 (ext. 2613) (L.I.K.)

Received: 26 June 2019; Accepted: 30 July 2019; Published: 6 August 2019

Abstract: The construction of artificial proteins using conservative B-cell and T-cell epitopes is believed to be a promising approach for a vaccine design against diverse viral infections. This article describes the development of an artificial HIV-1 immunogen using a polyepitope immunogen design strategy. We developed a recombinant protein, referred to as nTBI, that contains epitopes recognized by broadly neutralizing HIV-1 antibodies (bNAbs) combined with Th-epitopes. This is a modified version of a previously designed artificial protein, TBI (T- and B-cell epitopes containing Immunogen), carrying four T- and five B-cell epitopes from HIV-1 Env and Gag proteins. To engineer the nTBI molecule, three B-cell epitopes of the TBI protein were replaced with the epitopes recognized by broadly neutralizing HIV-1 antibodies 10E8, 2F5, and a linear peptide mimic of VRC01 epitope. We showed that immunization of rabbits with the nTBI protein elicited antibodies that recognize HIV-1 proteins and were able to neutralize Env-pseudotyped SF162.LS HIV-1 strain (tier 1). Competition assay revealed that immunization of rabbits with nTBI induced mainly 10E8-like antibodies. Our findings support the use of nTBI protein as an immunogen with predefined favorable antigenic properties.

Keywords: artificial protein; polyepitope B- and T-cell HIV-1 immunogen; epitopes of broadly neutralizing HIV-1 antibodies; peptide mimic of discontinuous epitope; immunogenicity

---

1. Introduction

Although Human Immunodeficiency Virus (HIV-1) is one of the best-characterized viruses, there is no efficient vaccine against this pathogen so far. Giving credit for notable progress in approaches to antiretroviral therapy that considerably prolongs the lifespan of HIV-infected patients, it should be noted that these are only palliative means to control the virus which cannot stop the HIV-1 pandemic [1,2]. For the most effective control of HIV-1 spread, a prophylactic vaccine should be used widely [3,4]. However, vaccine development is associated with particular well-known issues. First of all, HIV-1 genetic and consequent antigenic drift allows for evasion of the protective effects of the immune system. Therefore, traditional vaccine strategies have failed to protect against the virus [5–7].

Development of artificial polyepitope HIV-1 immunogens using a broad range of protective B- and T-cell epitopes from the viral antigens that can induce broadly neutralizing antibodies and responses of cytotoxic (CD8+ CTL) and helper (CD4+ Th) T-lymphocytes is one of the promising strategies for antiviral vaccine design [6,8–13].

There are a number of efforts developing artificial polyepitope T-cell immunogens [10,14–21]. Some of them have proven successful in inducing CD4+ T-cell and CD8+ T-cell responses of much greater breadth and magnitude in non-human primates compared to the vaccines containing full-length HIV protein genes [6,10]. Several polyepitope T-cell vaccine candidates have undergone phase I clinical trials [22–24].

The development of artificial B-cell HIV-immunogens, including those constructed using epitopes of broadly neutralizing HIV-1 antibodies (bNAbs), is the most complicated problem, since the majority of them recognize conformational epitopes and, significantly more rarely, linear epitopes. Furthermore, conformational B-cell epitopes on HIV surface glycoproteins are formed by lipids and glycans and their combinations [25,26], which further complicates the design of immunogens capable of inducing the required B-cell response. This task is believed to be solved using peptide mimics of conformational epitopes that can be obtained using combinatorial biology (the phage display technique) [27].

Concerning studies related to the development of artificial B-cell immunogens, a protein scaffold approach should be mentioned. Such scaffolds can expose one or several epitopes of broadly neutralizing antibodies to provide the most efficient exposure of the desired epitopes to the immune system [28–32]. Epitope scaffolds developed by rational design were able to elicit 4E10 and 2F5-like antibodies in laboratory animals [28,29]. Zhu et al. proposed computationally designed epitopes that mimic carbohydrate-occluded neutralization epitopes (CONEs) of Env through 'epitope transplantation', in which the target region is presented on a carrier protein scaffold. Although a tested anti-CONE serum demonstrated a modest magnitude of inhibitory activity on HIV-1 infectivity, the consistency of the effect against multiple isolates of HIV-1 Env pseudoviruses allows us to suggest that this approach could provide a broad neutralizing antibody response [33].

Another HIV vaccine strategy is based on the use of soluble stabilized Env trimer spikes for inducing broadly neutralizing antibodies. These trimeric antigens are comprised of cleavage products of gp120 and gp41 subunits forming a native-like Env conformation exposing vulnerable sites recognized by bNAbs [3,34–36]. However, as well as scaffolds, trimers could contain undesirable epitopes, diverting the protective humoral immune response [36,37]. To date, several approaches are used to decrease the immunogenicity of such epitopes [38–41].

Considering all of the above, it seems reasonable to create an immunogen which contains only the HIV-specific epitopes crucial for inducing a protective immune response. This approach focuses the immune response specifically on protective antigenic determinants and excludes the undesirable vaccine epitopes that could induce autoreactive antibodies or antibodies intensifying viral infectivity.

The paper represents the results of a study on constructing and investigating immunogenic properties of an artificial nTBI molecule comprising epitopes recognized by bNAbs 2F5, 10E8 [42,43], and a linear peptide mimic of a conformational epitope recognized by VRC01 [44] (Figure 1).

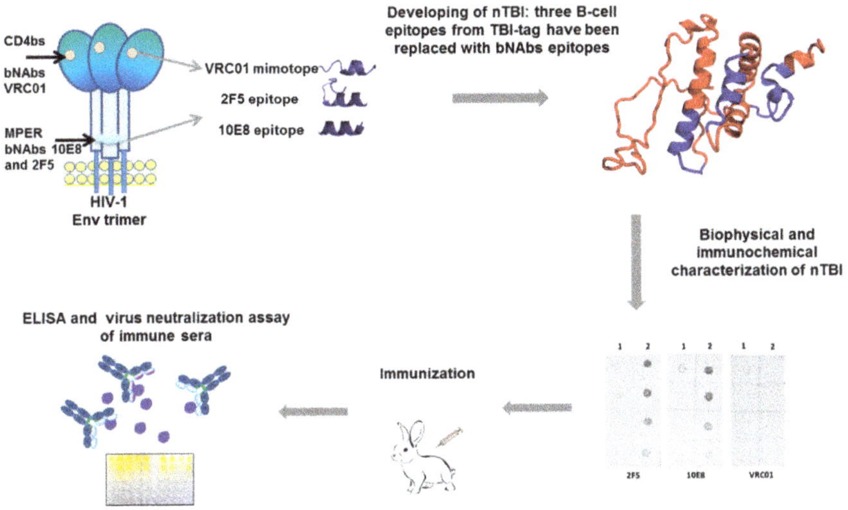

Figure 1. Schematic presentation of the experimental strategy for development of the nTBI protein and studying its immunogenic properties. A spatial model of the nTBI protein structure was obtained using the I-TASSER (Iterative Threading ASSEmbly Refinement) method [45].

2. Materials and Methods

2.1. Monoclonal Antibodies, Peptides, Bacterial Strains, Cell Lines, Plasmids, Media, and Buffers

VRC01, 10E8, and 2F5 monoclonal antibodies were kindly provided by the NIH AIDS Research and Reference Reagent Program (cat. # 12033, 12294, 1475). Murine monoclonal antibody (mAb) 29F2, *E. coli* strain BL21(DE3) pLysS (Invitrogen) and HEK 293T/17 cells (cat. # 103) as well as pTBI plasmid, encoding TBI gene (T- and B-cell containing immunogen) [46,47] were found in the collection of the State Research Center of Virology and Biotechnology Vector (SRC VB Vector, Koltsovo, Russia). TZM-bl cells (cat. # 8129) were also provided by the National Institutes of Health AIDS Research and Reference Reagent Program (USA). Synthesis of *nTBI* and *TBI_tag* genes and further cloning into pET21a expression vector (Novagen) were performed by Evrogen Lab, Ltd. (Moscow, Russia). 10E8 [NWFNITNWLWYIK], 2F5 [NEQELLELDKWASLWNK], and VRC01 [VSWPELYKWTWS] epitope peptides were synthesized by Synpeptide Co., Ltd. (Shanghai, China).

2.2. Expression and Purification of Recombinant Proteins nTBI and TBI_tag

The pET-nTBI and pET-TBI_tag plasmids were maintained and transformed into *E. coli* competent cells, single colonies were picked up and grown overnight in 2xYT medium with ampicillin (100 μg/ml). An overnight culture was diluted to 1:100 and grown at 37°C and 160 rpm until an $OD_{600} = 0.5$. Protein expression was induced with 1 mM isopropyl β-D-1-thiogalactopyranoside (IPTG). Cells were centrifuged at 6000 rpm for five minutes at 4 °C; pellets were resuspended in lysis buffer (0.05% tween 20, 50 mM monosodium phosphate, 300 mM sodium chloride, 30 mM imidazole) and sonicated on ice using Soniprep 150 Plus cell disruptor (16 times per minute at 13.2 μm amplitude). Inclusion bodies were pelleted by centrifugation, washed in Tris-HCl buffer (pH 8.3), and dissolved in 6 M urea for two hours. Insoluble fraction was removed by centrifugation, dissolved fraction was loaded onto a nickel nitrilotriacetic acid (Ni-NTA) column (Qiagen), washed with buffer containing 20 mM Tris-HCl, 0.5 M NaCl, 6 M urea and 20 mM imidazole (pH 7.9), and eluted with the same buffer with an increased concentration of imidazole up to 0.5 M. The proteins were then sequentially dialyzed for five hours at 4 °C against phosphate-buffered saline (PBS) buffer (pH 7.5) containing 6, 4, 2 and 1 M urea, respectively, followed by final dialysis in PBS. Purity and identity of refolded soluble proteins were estimated by SDS-PAGE and Western blotting.

2.3. SDS-PAGE, Western Blot, and New Lav Blot 1 Analysis

Protein samples were analyzed by SDS-PAGE on a 15% gel using Coomassie brilliant blue staining method. Western blot analysis was performed using SNAP i.d. system (Millipore). Proteins were transferred onto a nitrocellulose membrane (Amersham), blocked with 3% BSA for 15 minutes at room temperature, and washed three times with wash buffer (PBS with 0.1% Tween 20). After washing, the membrane was probed with mAbs VRC01, 10E8, 2F5, and 29F2 diluted to 1:10,000 in wash buffer for 10 minutes at room temperature. Antibodies were washed three times with wash buffer. Secondary antibodies (anti-human or anti-mouse) conjugated with alkaline phosphatase were used at 1:10,000, diluted in wash buffer. After 10 minutes, incubation membranes were washed five times. Proteins were visualized using nitro blue tetrazolium/5-bromo-4-chloro-3-indolyl phosphate (NBT/BCIP) substrate solution (Sigma, USA). HIV-1-specific antibodies were detected using a New Lav Blot 1 test kit (Bio-Rad, France), according to the manufacturer's instructions.

2.4. Circular Dichroism

Circular dichroism (CD) assays were carried out at room temperature (25 °C) in normal saline and in 20% trifluoroethanol using a Jasco J-600 spectropolarimeter. Spectra were recorded in the range a 195–260 nm, using a 1 mm path-length quartz cell. Each spectrum was obtained by averaging three scans with 1 nm step and 2 nm spectral bandwidth. The samples TBI_tag and nTBI have the same optical absorption at 214 nm.

The fractions of the secondary structure elements were calculated by minimizing the difference between the theoretical and experimental curves by varying of the impacts of the α-helixes, β-sheets, turns and non-structured forms. Theoretical values at every wavelength were the linear combination of the basis spectra of every type of secondary structure [48].

2.5. Immunization

Male Chinchilla rabbits of four weeks of age (~2 kg body weight) were purchased from Vector's animal breeding facilities and housed in a certified animal facility managed by the Animal Center of SRC VB Vector. All experiments were made to minimize animal suffering and carried out in line with the principles of humanity described in the relevant Guidelines of the European Community and Helsinki Declaration. The protocol was approved by the Institutional Animal Care & Use Committee (IACUC) of the SRC VB Vector (# 03-02.2017).

Animals were randomly divided into two groups (three rabbits per group). The first group was immunized with the nTBI protein, the second with the TBI_tag. Immunization was carried out three times (1, 14, and 28 days). Rabbits were primed with 500 μg of corresponding proteins subcutaneously with complete Freund's adjuvant (Sigma, USA), for the second immunization animals received 500 μg of protein subcutaneously with incomplete Freund's adjuvant. For the third immunization rabbits were injected 500 μg of protein without adjuvant. Serum samples were collected prior to the first immunization (pre-immune) and two weeks after the third immunization.

2.6. Purification of Rabbit IgG

To obtain antigen-specific antibodies and to eliminate non-specific effects of other serum components pooled rabbit sera were purified using protein A chromatography (BioVision, USA). Briefly, samples (9 ml) of rabbit sera were mixed with 9 ml binding buffer (1 × TBS, 0.15 M NaCl, in 50 mM sodium borate, pH 8.0). Diluted serum samples were added to a column containing Protein A agarose equilibrated with binding buffer and passed through a column. The column was washed with 10 volumes of binding buffer. IgG was eluted with 10 ml of 0.1 M citric acid, pH 2.75, and the eluate was immediately neutralized with 1.5 M Tris-HCl, pH 8.8 (150 μl per 1 ml of eluate). For each sample, IgG fractions with the highest protein concentration were pooled and dialyzed three times at 4 °C against 1 × phosphate-buffered saline. IgG purity was assessed by the Coomassie staining of 14% SDS-PAGE gel and was found to be equal to or greater than 90%. The antibody concentrations were quantified by measuring the absorbance at 280 nm using a NanoDrop 2000 Spectrophotometer (Thermo Fisher Scientific, Wilmington, DE, USA), and then stored at – 20°C.

2.7. ELISA

ELISA was used to identify Ab responses of individual rabbits to nTBI and TBI_tag. MaxiSorp 96-well plates (Thermo Fisher Scientific, USA) were coated with 5 μg/ml of nTBI and TBI_tag overnight at 4 °C in PBS. Plates were blocked for two hours with 0.5% casein in PBS at 37 °C and washed three times with 0.05% Tween 20/PBS (PBS-T). Eight serial dilutions of sera samples in PBS-0.1% casein (1/200, 1/1000, 1/5000 … 1/15,625,000) were added to the wells (100 μl per well) and incubated for two hours at 37 °C with shaking. Plates were washed three times with 0.05% PBS-T. Goat anti-rabbit IgG conjugated with alkaline phosphatase (Sigma, USA) were then added to the wells (100 μl/well) at 1:5000 dilution in PBS. Plates were incubated for one hour at room temperature and washed five times with 0.05% PBS-T. To visualize immunogen-specific antibodies BCIP/NBT substrate (Sigma, USA) was added to each well and incubated overnight in the dark at 37 °C. Plates were read at 405 nm (Model 680 Microplate reader, Bio-Rad, USA). Optical density (OD) values were calculated for each group by subtracting two times the average background of pre-immune rabbit serum.

2.8. Production of Env-Pseudoviruses

The reference panel of recombinant plasmids containing full-length Env genes of HIV-1 subtype B [49], HIV-1 Env clone SF162.LS [50], 6535 clone 3 (Cat # 11017), QH0692 (Cat # 11018), TRO.11 (Cat # 11023), PV04 (Cat # 11022), backbone Env-deficient plasmid pSG3Δenv was obtained through the NIH AIDS Reagent Program, Division of AIDS, NIAID, NIH. Plasmids phGPMΔMD-1 encoding GP of Marburg virus were constructed at SRC VB Vector.

HIV-1 Env-pseudotyped were prepared as described in [51]. Briefly, 293T cells in a T-75 culture flask were cotransfected with 10 μg of plasmids encoding heterologous envelope variants and 10 μg of an Env-deficient pSG3 env backbone plasmid using MATra reagent (PromoKine, Germany). Pseudoviruses were collected after a 48-hour incubation, filtered through a 0.45 μm pore size filter (TPP, Switzerland) and stored at –80 °C until use. Lentiviral particles pseudotyped with Marburg envelope glycoprotein (MGP) were used as a specificity control virus in the neutralization assay. The median tissue culture infective doses ($TCID_{50}$) of each pseudovirus was calculated by the Reed and Muench method to be used in a neutralization assay.

2.9. Neutralization Assay

Neutralization activities of immunogen-specific rabbit-derived antibodies were measured in the decrease of Tat-induced *Luc* reporter gene expression after a single round Env-pseudotyped HIV-1 infection of TZM-bl cells, as described previously [14,51]. Briefly, antibodies were serially diluted in a four-fold stepwise manner (initial concentration 4 mg/ml) and mixed with 50 μL of 200 $TCID_{50}$ of pseudovirus in 96-well flat-bottom culture plates (Corning-Costar) in triplicate and incubated for 30 minutes at 37 °C. Purified IgG (initial concentration 4 mg/ml) from the pool of pre-immune sera were used as a negative control. mAbs 4E10, 2F5, and VRC01 (initial concentration 30, 25, and 10 μg/ml, respectively) were used as a positive control. The mixture was transferred to TZM-bl cells (10^4 per well) and incubated for 48 hours at 37 °C. Following a 48-hour incubation, 150 μl of culture medium was removed from each well and replaced with a *Luc* reporter gene assay system reagent. After a two-minute incubation at room temperature to allow cell lysis, 150 μl of cell lysate were transferred to 96-well black solid plates for measurements of luminescence using a LuMate 4400 microplate luminometer (Awareness Technology Inc., Palm City, F L, USA) (expressed as relative luminescence units (RLUs) equivalent). The percentage decrease expressed in RLU (% neutralization) was determined by calculating the difference in average RLU between test wells (cells + sample + virus) and cell control wells (cells only), dividing this result by the difference in average RLU between virus control (cell + virus) and cell control wells, subtracting from 1 and multiplying by 100. To quantify neutralizing activities of rabbit antisera, the concentration of Ab required to obtain 50% neutralization (the IC_{50}) was calculated. All the assays were carried out in triplicate, statistical analysis was performed using GraphPad Prism 6 software (GraphPad, USA) to calculate concentrations of antibodies (µg/ml).

2.10. Competition Neutralization Assay

10E8 [NWFNITNWLWYIK], 2F5 [NEQELLELDKWASLWNK], and VRC01 [VSWPELYKWTWS] peptides were synthesized by Synpeptide Co., Ltd. (Shanghai, China) with >80% purity and tested for their ability to compete with HIV-1 Env-pseudotyped virus SF162 for binding to anti-nTBI IgG, anti-TBI_tag IgG, and mAbs 10E8, 2F5, and VRC01. Competition assay was carried out as described previously [52]. Briefly, serial dilutions of Ab were tested and IC 90 values for SF162 were determined by linear regression. Next, 1:1 (v/v) mixtures of each peptide (2 mg/ml) and corresponding antibodies were incubated for 30 minutes at 37 °C, added to SF162 pseudovirus (200 $TCID_{50}$) and coincubated for one hour at 37 °C. Further, a mix of the peptide, antibodies, and SF162 was added (1:1 v/v) to the TZM-bl indicator cell line. Luciferase activity was detected 48 hours after infection assay reagent II (Promega, USA). To control for nonspecific inhibition of the interaction between SF162 and target cells by the peptides, a neutralization assay was performed in the absence of antibodies (negative control). The inhibiting effect of peptides was detected in regards to $\log_{10}$ RLU data obtained in the neutralization of SF162 pseudovirus with respective antibodies without the addition of peptides and $\log_{10}$ RLU data obtained with the addition of peptides.

2.11. Statistical Analysis

A non-parametric Mann–Whitney U-test was used for multiple comparisons of the interactions between corresponding peptides and antibodies. Multiple testing correction was performed according to the Benjamini–Hochberg procedure (FDR). Statistical analysis and plotting were carried out using R, the open source statistical analysis language and environment (v. 3.3.2) [53].

3. Results

3.1. Design and Construction of Plasmids Encoding Immunogens TBI_tag and nTBI

In order to assemble the polyepitope nTBI protein, previously designed TBI (T- and B-cell immunogen) was used as a frame [46,47]. Several steps were made to improve the immunogenic properties of this modified version. Firstly, to enhance protein expression, the *TBI* gene sequence was codon optimized using the GenScript Rare Codon Analysis Tool [54]. Next, we added an *E. coli infB* gene fragment encoding N-terminal expressivity tag into the *TBI* gene's structure [55]. The codon-optimized and expressivity tag-fused *TBI* gene was cloned into pET21a expression vector in-frame with C-terminal 6x-HIS tag, which allowed the purification of the corresponding protein by Ni-NTA chromatography. The genetic construction modified in this manner was named TBI_tag.

Next, we decided to modify the TBI_tag peptide composition by replacing three B-cell epitopes that have weak capacity to elicit virus neutralizing antibodies (according to the Los Alamos HIV Database) with the epitopes recognized by bNAbs. For this purpose, Env (255–266) and Gag (92–109) epitopes that have a predominantly alpha-helical structure were replaced with the 10E8 bNAb-specific epitopes NWFNITNWLWYIK and NEQELLELDKWASLWNK, recognized by bNAb 2F5. Both of these sequences were predicted as alpha-helical; besides, Env (255–266) and Gag (92–109) epitopes are located at the N- and C- termini of TBI, so we assumed that their replacement would not dramatically disrupt the protein backbone.

The remaining Gag (351–361) epitope had an irregular secondary structure and was surrounded by two alpha-helical regions in the context of TBI protein. Instead of this epitope, we decided to put the phage display-selected linear peptide mimic of the epitope recognized by the VRC01 antibody [52]. Similar to Gag (351–361), this peptide has an irregular structure, therefore it was assumed that incorporation of the peptide between alpha-helical motifs could give it a certain rigidity and the ability to be exposed on the protein's surface.

The proteins' structures were predicted using the I-TASSER [45] and PSSpred [56] prediction tools, proteins models were shown in Figures 1 and 2, respectively. According to modeling data, the constructed immunogens TBI_tag and nTBI have a structure of mainly α-helical regions and flexible interhelical loops.

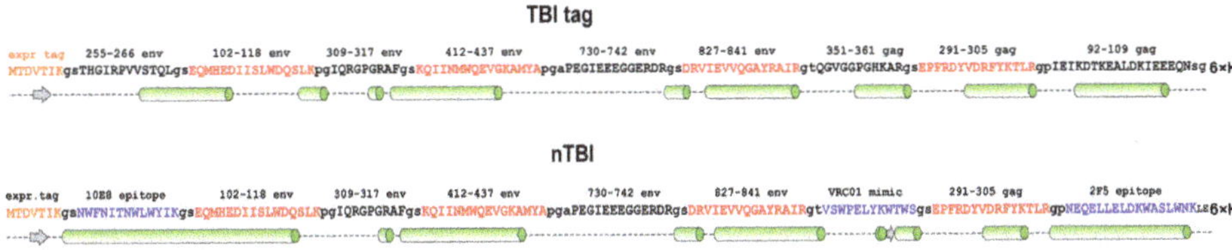

Figure 2. Depicting secondary structure of TBI_tag and nTBI proteins. The structures were predicted using the PSSpred tool available at [56]. bNAbs epitopes that were appended into the nTBI protein are highlighted with blue; T-h epitopes are marked with red; α-strings—light green cylinders; β-coils—grey arrows; unshaped structures—dashed lines. All proteins comprised a C-terminal sequence from histidine amino acid residues.

3.2. Expression, Purification, and Antigenic Properties of Recombinant nTBI and TBI_tag Proteins

The designed and synthesized *TBI_tag* and *nTBI* genes were cloned in plasmid pET21a and expressed in BL21(DE3) pLysS E. coli cells. Expression of recombinant proteins encoded by the cloned genes was characterized by SDS-PAGE, followed by Coomassie blue staining (Figure 3A).

It was revealed that recombinant proteins TBI_tag and nTBI were mainly expressed as inclusion bodies; therefore, we used a purification scheme including the sonication of bacterial cells, solubilizing the inclusion bodies by urea solution, affinity chromatography using Ni-NTA resin and refolding. It was established that the modified TBI_tag can be successfully produced and purified in soluble form, while. nTBI tended to form aggregates after purification step (the solution was opalescent). The of isolated TBI_tag and nTBI proteins were further checked by SDS-PAGE using Coomassie blue staining (Figure 3B).

To ensure that Coomassie-stained bands correspond to the target proteins, Western blot analysis was performed using the mouse monoclonal antibody 29F2 that recognizes the peptide from HIV-1 p24 [EPFRDYVDRFYKTLR], which is a part of both nTBI and TBI-tag. It was demonstrated that both proteins specifically bind to 29F2 (Figure 3C).

To check if all the substituted epitopes retained their antigenic properties in the context of a recombinant protein, we performed Western blot analysis using 10E8, 2F5, and VRC01 mAbs as primary antibodies. It was shown that TBI_tag selectively binds to 29F2 mAb as expected, whereas nTBI reacts with all the mAbs used in screening except for VRC01 (Figure 3C).

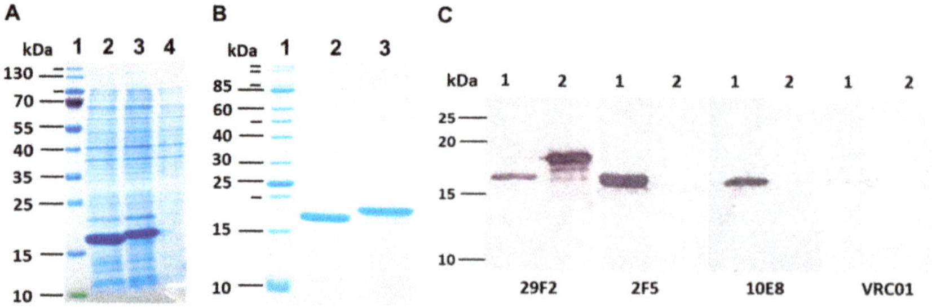

Figure 3. (**A**) SDS PAGE analysis of *E. coli* BL21 (DE3) pLysS cell lysate after IPTG induction. 1) molecular weight marker; 2) lysate of E. coli BL21/pET-nTBI cells; 3) lysate of E. coli BL21/pET-TBI_tag cells; 4) lysate of non-transformed E. coli BL21 cells. (**B**) SDS PAGE analysis of purified samples of nTBI and TBI_tag; 1) molecular weight marker; 2) purified nTBI protein; 3) purified TBI_tag protein. (**C**) Western blot analysis of expressed nTBI and TBI_tag. Purified proteins were separated by SDS-PAGE in 15% gel and transferred onto a nitrocellulose membrane (nTBI at lane 1 and TBI_tag at lane 2). Monoclonal antibodies 29F2, 2F5, 10E8, and VRC01 were used for immunodetection.

3.3. Circular Dichroism

Experimental analysis of the polypeptides' secondary structures was performed using circular dichroism spectroscopy. CD spectra of TBI_tag and nTBI were both registered in saline and in 20% trifluoroethanol in saline (Figure 4). The quantitative analysis of the secondary structure of TBI_tag shown the same fraction of α-helices and β sheets in the saline. Significant increases of α-helices and decreases of β sheets and non-structured forms were observed after the addition of 20% trifluoroethanol, which stabilizes the secondary structure of the protein (Table 1). The CD signal magnitude was close to zero for nTBI in the studied conditions.

Table 1. Circular dichroism spectra of the TBI_tag protein.

Secondary Structures	Saline	20% Trifluoroethanol
α-helices	13%	54%
β-sheets	14%	4%
Turns_I	2%	4%
Unordered structures	70%	37%

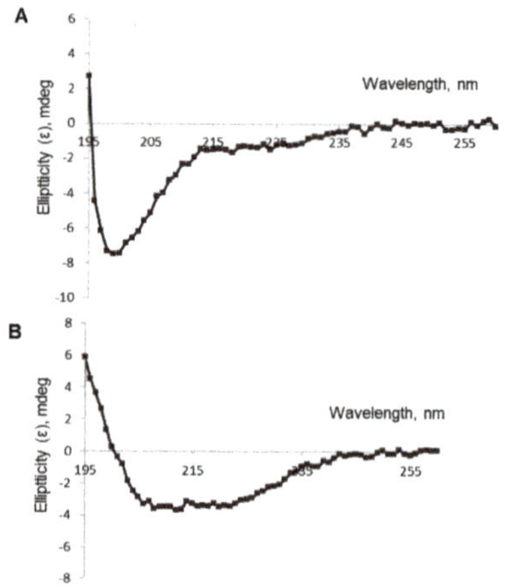

Figure 4. CD spectra of TBI_tag protein: (**A**) saline; (**B**) 20% trifluoroethanol in saline.

3.4. Assessment of Immune Response in Rabbits

To assess the immunogenicity of recombinant proteins, ELISA was performed using sera from immunized rabbits. Pre-immune sera were used as a negative control. It was found that sera from both groups of immunized rabbits contain antigen-specific antibodies. Average antibody titers in both groups of animals immunized with TBI_tag as well as nTBI were more than 1:3,125,000 after the third immunization. Furthermore, there was no significant difference in serum level between rabbits from one group. At the same time, the signal of pre-immune sera in ELISA was no more than the background level.

Further, sera were tested for the presence of antibodies specific to HIV-1 proteins (Figure 5). For the purpose, we used a commercially available test system, New Lav Blot 1 (Bio-Rad), including nitrocellulose stripes coated with HIV-1 proteins. Pre-immune sera were used as a negative control, while inactivated human serum containing anti-HIV-1 antibodies (from the New Lav Blot 1 kit) served as a positive control.

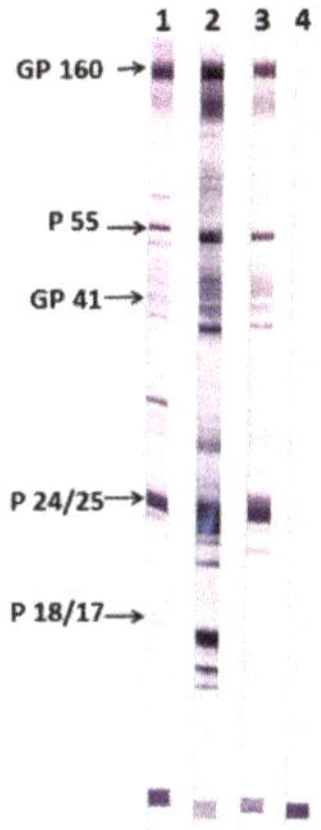

Figure 5. Western blot of sera from animals immunized with TBI_tag and nTBI using the New Lav Blot 1 test system. 1) Positive control from the New Lav Blot kit. 2) Pooled sera of rabbits immunized with TBI_tag. 3) Pooled sera of rabbits immunized with nTBI. 4) A pool of pre-immune sera of rabbits from both groups.

It was shown that antisera raised in nTBI-immunized rabbits contain antibodies against gp120, gp160, gp41, and p24 (p55), whereas TBI_tag-induced antibodies were additionally recognized p17. These results are consistent with our expectations, as nTBI doesn't bear the p17 HIV-1 epitope which was replaced with the 2F5 epitope from the membrane-proximal external region (MPER).

3.5. Neutralizing Activity of Purified Specific Antibodies

IgGs purified from pool sera of rabbits immunized with TBI_tag and nTBI were tested for the capability of neutralizing HIV-1 pseudoviruses. Env-pseudotyped viruses from the global panel of reference Env clones (NIH) were packaged and used to perform a neutralization assay.

At the first step, we used easy-to-neutralize (tier 1) SF162.LS pseudovirus. It was shown that both anti-nTBI and anti-TBI_tag antibodies efficiently neutralized the tier 1 pseudotyped HIV-1 strain, while IgGs from pre-immune sera showed no neutralization activity (Figure 6). In addition, we found out that IC_{50} anti-nTBI antibodies was 0.44 µg/mL, approximately six times lower than the IC_{50} for anti-TBI_tag antibodies (2.76 µg/mL). mAbs 2F5 and VRC01 (Figure 6) were used as positive controls. Next, we performed a neutralization assay using tier 2 and tier 3 Env-pseudotyped HIV strains (6535, QH0692 иPV04). A similar trend was observed for these pseudoviruses with percent neutralization being higher for anti-nTBI IgG compared to the anti-TBI_tag IgG. However, since the mean IC_{50} values were more than 50 μg/mL, we cannot assume virus neutralizing activity relating to the used pseudoviruses.

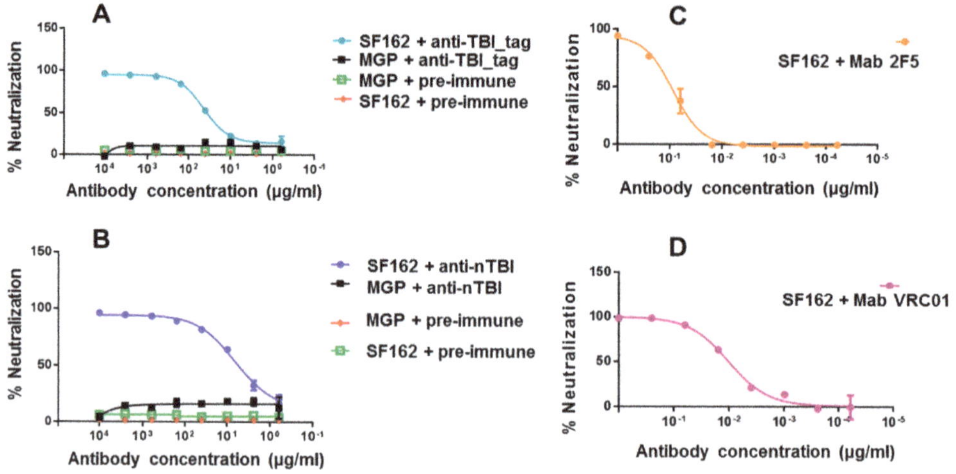

Figure 6. Neutralizing activity of IgGs isolated from sera of immunized animals against SF162.LS pseudovirus. The figure depicts neutralization curves for anti-TBI_tag (**A**), anti-nTBI (**B**) rabbit IgGs, as well as for human mAbs 2F5 (**C**) and VRC01 (**D**). 2F5 and VRC01 were used as positive controls. A pool of IgGs purified from pre-immune sera of rabbits (IgGs-pre-immune) was used as a negative control. Lentiviral particles pseudotyped with Marburg envelope glycoprotein (MGP) were used as a specificity control virus in the neutralization assay.

3.6. Competition Neutralization Assay

Next, we decided to test whether bNAb epitopes that were included into nTBI are able to interfere with the neutralization activity of corresponding antibodies. We carried out competitive inhibition of the neutralization of the Env-pseudotyped SF162.LS HIV strain by 10E8, VRC01 and 2F5 mAbs, and purified IgG from immune sera using synthetic peptides 10E8 [NWFNITNWLWYIK], 2F5 [NEQELLELDKWASLWNK], and VRC01 [VSWPELYKWTWS].

Preliminary experiments revealed that these peptides are non-toxic for TZM-bl cells and induce no non-specific inhibition of the interaction between pseudovirus and target cells.

10E8 peptide showed the inhibition of neutralizing activity of anti-nTBI antibodies against SF162.LS ($p < 0.01$). Additionally, inhibition of neutralization of TBI_tag-specific antibodies by this peptide was not observed (Figure 7A). Predictably, 10E8 peptide epitope blocked neutralization of SF162.LS by 10E8 ($p < 0.01$) (Figure 7A).

A peptide mimic of the VRC01 epitope inhibited neutralization of SF162 by VRC01 ($p < 0.01$), but weakly blocked neutralization of SF162 by anti-nTBI antibodies ($p < 0.20$), and not inhibit TBI_tag-specific antibodies (Figure 7C). As expected, the 2F5 epitope interfered with 2F5 mAb and decreased its neutralizing activity against SF162, whereas we observed no inhibition of neutralizing activity of both anti-nTBI and anti-TBI_tag antibodies (Figure 7B).

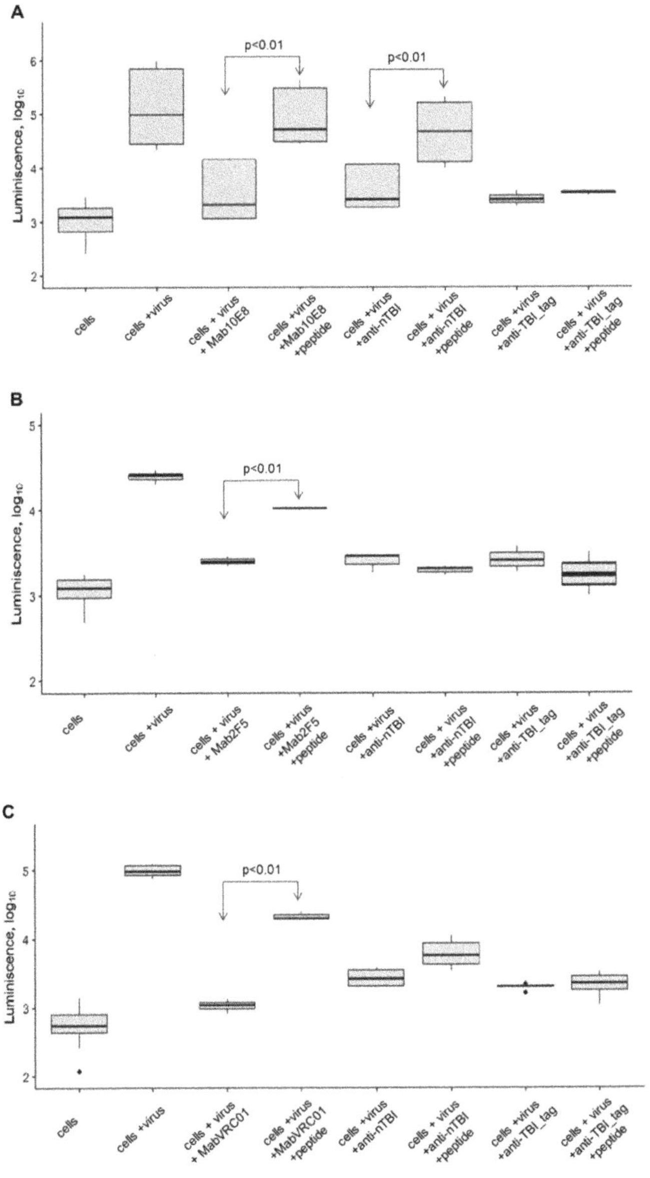

Figure 7. Inhibition of virus-neutralizing activity of antibodies by synthesized peptides: (**A**) 10E8 [NWFNITNWLWYIK], (**B**) 2F5 [NEQELLELDKWASLWNK], (**C**) VRC01 [VSWPELYKWTWS]. The following combinations were tested in the assay: cell + virus; cell + virus + monoclonal mAb 10E8 or 2F5, or VRC01; cell + virus + monoclonal mAb 10E8 or 2F5, or VRC01 + corresponding synthetic peptide; cell + virus + anti-nTBI IgG; cell + virus + anti-nTBI IgG + synthetic peptide; cell + virus + anti-TBItag IgG; cell + virus + anti-TBItag IgG + synthetic peptide. Relative luminescence intensity is indicated on the Y-axis (log10 RLU). Statistical differences between groups cell + virus + mAb 10E8, or 2F5, or VRC01 and cell + virus + mAb 10E8, or 2F5, or VRC01 + synthetic peptide is $p < 0.01$; statistical differences between groups cell + virus + anti-nTBI IgG and cell + virus + anti-nTBI IgG + synthetic peptide is $p < 0.01$.

4. Discussion

Eroshkin et al. have previously designed an artificial polyepitope TBI protein (T- and B-cell epitopes containing immunogen) composed of conservative epitopes from Env and Gag HIV-1 and based on a well-known protein structural motif, i.e., a four-helix bundle [47]. TBI included four Th-cell epitopes (amphipathic α-helix) and five B-cell epitopes (regions with flexible hydrophilic loops) [46,47]. The rationale for the TBI design was that combining T- and B-cell epitopes in one construct would stimulate both proper B-cell and T-cell responses and the necessary interplay between B- and T-cells. The TBI protein had a CD spectra similar to α-helical proteins and showed crystal-yielding capacity, which was demonstrated for the first time in an artificial protein with a predicted tertiary structure [57].

It was shown that TBI induced both cellular and humoral responses to HIV-1 in immunized mice and rhesus macaques, and TBI-induced antibodies showed virus-neutralizing activity to HIV-1 [58]. Lately, TBI was included into the composition of the CombiHIVvac candidate vaccine that had undergone phase I clinical trials [24,58].

Based on its ability to crystallize, we assumed that the TBI protein structure was similar to that of the natural protein. We decided to design a modified protein based on TBI with an enhanced ability to induce HIV-neutralizing antibodies.

First, in order to increase the yield of recombinant protein, we changed the expression vector to pET21a, which led to an increase of gene expression level and allowed the use of the 6xHis/Ni-NTA system for protein purification. Additionally, we added an *E. coli infB* gene fragment encoding an N-terminal expressivity tag to its structure [55]. This protein was referred to as TBI-tag and used for further modifications. At the next step, we replaced three B-cell epitopes from TBI-tag with epitopes recognized by bNAbs. We substituted the Env (255–266), Gag (99–109), and Gag (351–361) epitopes (Figure 2). The first two epitopes were replaced with peptides from the MPER region, i.e., (NEQELLELDKWASLWNK) and (NWFNITNWLWYIK), recognized by bNAbs 2F5 and 10E8, respectively. Instead of Gag (351–361), we added a phage display-selected linear peptide mimic of the epitope recognized by the VRC01 antibody, into the protein structure [52]. According to the PSSpred tool modeling data, the epitopes for 10E8 and 2F5 have retained their peculiar α-helical structure, which was shown to be required for their antigenic and immunogenic properties (Figure 2).

T-helper epitopes and spacer sequences between epitopes remained unchanged, since they form amphipathic α-helices which seem to stabilize protein structure (Figure 2). Significance of the helical amphipathicity of epitopes for the recognition of T-cells is evident, since 70% of T-helper epitopes have an α-helical conformation. Previously, it was shown that TBI elicited HIV-specific T-cell response in mice, which supported the idea that TBI processing as well as presentation of T cell epitopes were adequate [46]. Since antigen-presenting cells present T-cell epitopes as linear peptides after antigen processing, we suppose that the functional activity of T-helper epitopes in the context of nTBI should have remained at about the same level as in TBI.

Modeling the secondary structure enabled us to assume that accomplished modifications didn't significantly affect the recombinant protein organization, since the predicted secondary structures of TBI_tag and nTBI were found to be similar (Figures 1 and 2).

To evaluate the secondary structure of the TBI_tag and nTBI proteins, we used a circular dichroism spectroscopic method. CD spectra analysis of the proteins in a 20% trifluoroethanol solution revealed that TBI_tag contains 54% α-helices and 4% β-sheets, which is consistent with theoretical data predicted with PSSpred; 52% and 2%, respectively. The corresponding predicted values for nTBI were the following: 59% of α-helices and 3% of β-sheets. However, we failed to determine its secondary structure using CD. The probable reason is that the inclusion of the peptide mimic of the VRC01 conformational epitope into an internal area of the molecule TBI_tag resulted in a destabilizing of the protein structure and changing of its physico-chemical properties, since it became prone to aggregation. Western blot analysis revealed that the mAb VRC01 poorly interacted with the peptide mimic as part of nTBI as compared to the same peptide as part of protein p3 of bacteriophage M13 [52]. Two other peptides, 2F5 and 10E8, included in the nTBI molecule are effectively recognized by their corresponding MPER bNAbs (2F5 and 10E8) (Figure 3A).

Antibody titers of rabbits' antisera derived after three-fold immunization with both TBI-tag and nTBI were more than 1:3,125,000, which indicates the high immunogenicity of both proteins. New Lav Blot 1 analysis showed that induced antibodies in rabbits by immunization with TBI_tag and nTBI were capable of binding to HIV-1 proteins (Figure 5). Consequently, both immunogens were able to elicit HIV-specific antibodies.

The analysis of virus neutralizing activity of sera from animals immunized with both TBI_tag and nTBI revealed that both proteins elicit antibodies capable of neutralizing tier 1 SF162.LS. Additionally, anti-nTBI IgG neutralizing activity proved to be higher than that of the antibodies induced with TBI_tag. The IC50 of anti-nTBI antibodies was six times lower than the IC50 for anti-TBI_tag antibodies (Figure 6). To test whether the neutralizing activity of anti-nTBI IgGs from rabbits' immune sera is mediated by the antibodies which were elicited against substituted epitopes, we performed a peptide competition neutralization assay.

The 10E8 peptide was the most immunogenic, since its inhibition capacity of anti-nTBI IgG significantly differed from control (Figure 7A). Thus, enhancement of virus neutralizing activity of antibodies induced by nTBI seems to be connected to the inclusion of peptide 10E8 in the compound of the TBI protein.

VRC01 mimotope VSWPELYKWTWS contributes poorly to the induction of neutralizing antibodies. When immunized with the nTBI protein, the neutralizing activity of the antibodies induced against this mimotope decreased after the addition of the VSWPELYKWTWS peptide; although the difference between the control group was not significant (Figure 7C). Probably, this may be explained by a shielding of the peptide mimic by flanking amino acid sequences in the nTBI compound. Thereby, placing the peptide mimetic of the VRC01 epitope into the internal region of nTBI could alter the immunogenicity of this peptide. Importantly, the peptide mimic of the VRC01 epitope efficiently inhibited the binding of bNAbs VRC01 to the SF162 pseudovirus, which is consistent with the literature [52].

Concerning 2F5 peptide, we failed to demonstrate inhibition of SF162 neutralization by IgGs from rabbits immunized with TBI_tag and nTBI. The epitope recognized by the bNAb 2F5 was designed at the protein C-terminus, and was followed by an additional six histidine residues. Inclusion of this hexahistidine tag helped streamline protein purification, yet it could also affect the structure and accessibility of the adjacent epitope. This could be one of the possible reasons why the 2F5 epitope retained antigenicity in the context of the nTBI, but failed to induce 2F5-like Abs (as shown by the competition analysis using the synthetic 2F5 peptide). It seems that 2F5 epitope heavily relies on its natural environment to expose its immunogenic features [29]. The obtained findings will be considered in the further enhancement of TBI immunogen. It is possible that removing the histidines from the C-terminus of nTBI will result in efficient presentation of the 2F5 peptide.

Another possible explanation of low neutralizing activity of the immune sera could be the animal model that we used for the experiment. Although rabbits can be used for characterization of HIV-1 immunogenicity, they are not a valid model for the analyses of novel immunogens driving an anti-HIV response. One reason is that they are naturally resistant to HIV infection, and more importantly, sequences of their immunoglobulin genes are too diverged from those of primates. In our future experiments testing the elicitation of neutralizing antibodies, common marmosets will be used as the model animals.

5. Conclusions

Approach to the development of artificial proteins constructed using conservative T- and B-cell epitopes and their mimics is believed to be promising for the development of vaccines against variable viruses, including HIV. In such constructs, all of the component helper T cell epitopes may be expected to provide T cell help for antibody production against all of the component B cell epitopes, thus overcoming the limitation of genetic restriction [46]. In theory, this approach makes it possible to evade the antigenic variability of the virus, focus the immune responses on protective determinants, and exclude from the vaccine compound undesired determinants capable of inducing autoantibodies or antibodies increasing virus infectivity.

In this study, we used a polyepitope-based HIV immunogen design strategy to develop an artificial nTBI protein exposing epitopes recognized by bNAbs 2F5, 10E8, and a phage display-selected peptide mimic of the VRC01 discontinuous epitope. Antigenic properties of the incorporated peptides were saved in the compound of nTBI, except for the peptide mimic VRC01. nTBI became less soluble as compared to the initial TBI. This is probably because substitution of the initial TBI B-cell epitopes by new ones negatively affected its conformation, despite the prediction results. However, compared to the initial TBI, nTBI demonstrated a better capacity to induce virus neutralizing antibodies in comparison with the initial TBI, at least for the SF162 pseudovirus the neutralizing activity of nTBI-induced IgGs outperformed that of the TBI_tag-induced IgGs (the IC50 of anti-nTBI antibodies was six times lower than the IC50 of anti-TBI_tag antibodies (Figure 6)). Competition assay revealed that immunization of rabbits with nTBI induced mainly 10E8-like antibodies, whereas no 2F5 epitope and VRC01 mimotope-induced antibodies were detected. We considered several strategies for boosting the antigenicity and immunogenicity of nTBI. The peptide mimetic targeted by VRC01 can be placed at the C- or N- terminus of TBI, which may translate into the induction of neutralizing antibodies. Our earlier results [52] indicate that the peptide mimetic selected using phage display was able to induce neutralizing antibodies, either in the context of the M13 phage or as individual synthetic peptide. Furthermore, following affinity selection, we obtained many more VRC01 mimetics, and these may be considered viable alternatives for future modifications of TBI.

As for the 2F5 epitope, testing whether the C-terminal hexahistidine tag affects its immunogenicity remains an attractive experiment to do. Also, one may think of increasing the spacers between the epitopes, as this may translate into greater accessibility of the epitopes to B-cell receptors. Establishing a broader range of TBI derivatives may therefore be highly productive, as this may help identify the variants showing greater activity. Finally, the lead immunogen should be thoroughly tested in various prime-boost immunization schemes. The ultimate goal of this approach is to obtain an anti-HIV vaccine component that would provide the desired neutralizing immune response. It is possible that such an immunogen will comprise a cocktail of several lead TBI versions.

Author Contributions: Conceptualization, A.P.R., A.N.C., A.A.I., and L.I.K.; Data curation, A.P.R. and N.B.R.; Formal analysis, D.V.A.; Investigation, A.P.R., N.B.R., A.A.L. and O.N.K.; Methodology, A.N.C.; Project administration, L.I.K.; Visualization, A.P.R., A.A.I., and L.I.K.; Writing—Original Draft, A.P.R., A.N.C., A.A.I., and L.I.K.

Funding: The work was supported by RFBR Grant N 18-29-08051 mk and RFBR and the government of the Novosibirsk region of the RF, grant N 18-44-543017.

Acknowledgments: The authors are grateful to Alexey Eroshkin for his helpful advice. The authors also thank Dmitrii Shcherbakov and Nadezhda Shcherbakova for help with discussion the results.

Conflicts of Interest: The authors declare no conflict of interest, financial or otherwise.

References

1. Eisinger, R.W.; Fauci, A.S. Ending the HIV/AIDS Pandemic. *Emerg. Infect. Dis.* **2018**, *24*, 413–416. [CrossRef] [PubMed]
2. Lorenzo-Redondo, R.; Fryer, H.R.; Bedford, T.; Kim, E.Y.; Archer, J.; Pond, S.L.K.; Chung, Y.S.; Penugonda, S.; Chipman, J.G.; Fletcher, C.V.; et al. Persistent HIV-1 replication maintains the tissue reservoir during therapy. *Nature* **2016**, *530*, 51–56. [CrossRef] [PubMed]
3. Haynes, B.F.; Burton, D.R. HIV Developing an HIV vaccine What are the paths and obstacles to a practical vaccine? *Science* **2017**, *355*, 1129–1130. [CrossRef] [PubMed]
4. Fauci, A.S. An HIV Vaccine Is Essential for Ending the HIV/AIDS Pandemic. *JAMA* **2017**, *318*, 1535–1536. [CrossRef] [PubMed]

5. Hsu, D.C.; O'Connell, R.J. Progress in HIV vaccine development. *Hum. Vaccin. Immunother.* **2017**, *13*, 1018–1030. [CrossRef] [PubMed]
6. McMichael, A.J.; Haynes, B.F. Lessons learned from HIV-1 vaccine trials: New priorities and directions. *Nat. Immunol.* **2012**, *13*, 423–427. [CrossRef] [PubMed]
7. Gray, G.E.; Laher, F.; Lazarus, E.; Ensoli, B.; Corey, L. Approaches to preventative and therapeutic HIV vaccines. *Curr. Opin. Virol.* **2016**, *17*, 104–109. [CrossRef]
8. Sahay, B.; Nguyen, C.Q.; Yamamoto, J.K. Conserved HIV Epitopes for an Effective HIV Vaccine. *J. Clin. Cell. Immunol.* **2017**, *8*, 518. [CrossRef]
9. Korber, B.; Hraber, P.; Wagh, K.; Hahn, B.H. Polyvalent vaccine approaches to combat HIV-1 diversity. *Immunol. Rev.* **2017**, *275*, 230–244. [CrossRef]
10. Hanke, T. Conserved immunogens in prime-boost strategies for the next-generation HIV-1 vaccines. *Expert Opin. Biol. Ther.* **2014**, *14*, 601–616. [CrossRef]
11. Karpenko, L.I.; Bazhan, S.I.; Antonets, D.V.; Belyakov, I.M. Novel approaches in polyepitope T-cell vaccine development against HIV-1. *Expert Rev. Vaccines.* **2014**, *13*, 155–173. [CrossRef] [PubMed]
12. Castelli, M.; Cappelletti, F.; Diotti, R.A.; Sautto, G.; Criscuolo, E.; Dal Peraro, M.; Clementi, N. Peptide-Based Vaccinology: Experimental and Computational Approaches to Target Hypervariable Viruses through the Fine Characterization of Protective Epitopes Recognized by Monoclonal Antibodies and the Identification of T-Cell-Activating Peptides. *Clin. Dev. Immunol.* **2013**, *2013*, 521231. [CrossRef] [PubMed]
13. Reche, P.; Flower, D.R.; Fridkis-Hareli, M.; Hoshino, Y. Peptide-Based Immunotherapeutics and Vaccines 2017. *J. Immunol. Res.* **2018**, *2018*, 4568239. [CrossRef] [PubMed]
14. Karpenko, L.I.; Danilenko, A.V.; Bazhan, S.I.; Danilenko, E.D.; Sysoeva, G.M.; Kaplina, O.N.; Volkova, O.Y.; Oreshkova, S.F.; Ilyichev, A.A. Attenuated Salmonella enteritidis E23 as a vehicle for the rectal delivery of DNA vaccine coding for HIV-1 polyepitope CTL immunogen. *Microb. Biotechnol.* **2012**, *5*, 241–250. [CrossRef] [PubMed]
15. Fischer, W.; Perkins, S.; Theiler, J.; Bhattacharya, T.; Yusim, K.; Funkhouser, R.; Kuiken, C.; Haynes, B.; Letvin, N.L.; Walker, B.D.; et al. Polyvalent vaccines for optimal coverage of potential T-cell epitopes in global HIV-1 variants. *Nat. Med.* **2007**, *13*, 100–106. [CrossRef] [PubMed]
16. Borthwick, N.; Ahmed, T.; Ondondo, B.; Hayes, P.; Rose, A.; Ebrahimsa, U.; Hayton, E.J.; Black, A.; Bridgeman, A.; Rosario, M.; et al. Vaccine-elicited Human T Cells Recognizing Conserved Protein Regions Inhibit HIV-1. *Mol. Ther.* **2014**, *22*, 464–475. [CrossRef] [PubMed]
17. Ondondo, B.; Murakoshi, H.; Clutton, G.; Abdul-Jawad, S.; Wee, E.G.T.; Gatanaga, H.; Oka, S.; McMichael, A.J.; Takiguchi, M.; Korber, B.; et al. Novel Conserved-region T-cell Mosaic Vaccine With High Global HIV-1 Coverage Is Recognized by Protective Responses in Untreated Infection. *Mol. Ther.* **2016**, *24*, 832–842. [CrossRef] [PubMed]
18. Bazhan, S.I.; Belavin, P.A.; Seregin, S.V.; Danilyuk, N.K.; Babkina, I.N.; Karpenko, L.I.; Nekrasova, N.A.; Lebedev, L.R.; Ignatyev, G.M.; Agafonov, A.P.; et al. Designing and engineering of DNA-vaccine construction encoding multiple CTL-epitopes of major HIV-1 antigens. *Vaccine* **2004**, *22*, 1672–1682. [CrossRef] [PubMed]
19. Bazhan, S.I.; Karpenko, L.I.; Ilyicheva, T.N.; Belavin, P.A.; Seregin, S.V.; Danilyuk, N.K.; Antonets, D.V.; Ilyichev, A.A. Rational design based synthetic polyepitope DNA vaccine for eliciting HIV-specific CD8+T cell responses. *Mol. Immunol.* **2010**, *47*, 1507–1515. [CrossRef] [PubMed]
20. Reguzova, A.Y.; Karpenko, L.I.; Mechetina, L.V.; Belyakov, I.M. Peptide-MHC multimer-based monitoring of CD8 T-cells in HIV-1 infection and AIDS vaccine development. *Expert Rev. Vaccines* **2015**, *14*, 69–84. [CrossRef] [PubMed]
21. Sandstrom, E.; Nilsson, C.; Hejdeman, B.; Brave, A.; Bratt, G.; Robb, M.; Cox, J.; VanCott, T.; Marovich, M.; Stout, R.; et al. Broad Immunogenicity of a Multigene, Multiclade HIV-1 DNA Vaccine Boosted with Heterologous HIV-1 Recombinant Modified Vaccinia Virus Ankara. *J. Infect. Dis.* **2008**, *198*, 1482–1490. [CrossRef] [PubMed]
22. Afolabi, M.O.; Ndure, J.; Drammeh, A.; Darboe, F.; Mehedi, S.R.; Rowland-Jones, S.L.; Borthwick, N.; Black, A.; Ambler, G.; John-Stewart, G.C.; et al. A Phase I Randomized Clinical Trial of Candidate Human Immunodeficiency Virus type 1 Vaccine MVA. HIVA Administered to Gambian Infants. *PloS ONE* **2013**, *8*, 0078289. [CrossRef] [PubMed]

23. Borthwick, N.; Lin, Z.S.; Akahoshi, T.; Llano, A.; Silva-Arrieta, S.; Ahmed, T.; Dorrell, L.; Brander, C.; Murakoshi, H.; Takiguchi, M.; et al. Novel, in-natural-infection subdominant HIV-1 CD8(+) T-cell epitopes revealed in human recipients of conserved-region T-cell vaccines. *PloS ONE* **2017**, *12*, 0176418. [CrossRef] [PubMed]
24. Karpenko, L.I.; Bazhan, S.I.; Bogryantseva, M.P.; Ryndyuk, N.N.; Ginko, Z.I.; Kuzubov, V.I.; Lebedev, L.R.; Kaplina, O.N.; Reguzova, A.Y.; Ryzhikov, A.B.; et al. Results of phase I clinical trials of a combined vaccine against HIV-1 based on synthetic polyepitope immunogens. *Russ. J. Bioorganic Chem.* **2016**, *42*, 170–182. [CrossRef]
25. Cerutti, N.; Loredo-Varela, J.L.; Caillat, C.; Weissenhorn, W. Antigp41 membrane proximal external region antibodies and the art of using the membrane for neutralization. *Curr. Opin. HIV AIDS* **2017**, *12*, 250–256. [CrossRef]
26. McCoy, L.E.; Burton, D.R. Identification and specificity of broadly neutralizing antibodies against HIV. *Immunol. Rev.* **2017**, *275*, 11–20. [CrossRef] [PubMed]
27. Aghebati-Maleki, L.; Bakhshinejad, B.; Baradaran, B.; Motallebnezhad, M.; Aghebati-Maleki, A.; Nickho, H.; Yousefi, M.; Majidi, J. Phage display as a promising approach for vaccine development. *J. Biomed. Sci.* **2016**, *23*, 66. [CrossRef]
28. Correia, B.E.; Bates, J.T.; Loomis, R.J.; Baneyx, G.; Carrico, C.; Jardine, J.G.; Rupert, P.; Correnti, C.; Kalyuzhniy, O.; Vittal, V.; et al. Proof of principle for epitope-focused vaccine design. *Nature* **2014**, *507*, 201–206. [CrossRef]
29. Ofek, G.; Guenaga, F.J.; Schief, W.R.; Skinner, J.; Baker, D.; Wyatt, R.; Kwong, P.D. Elicitation of structure-specific antibodies by epitope scaffolds. *Proc. Natl. Acad. Sci. USA* **2010**, *107*, 17880–17887. [CrossRef]
30. Habte, H.H.; Banerjee, S.; Shi, H.L.; Qin, Y.L.; Cho, M.W. Immunogenic properties of a trimeric gp41-based immunogen containing an exposed membrane-proximal external region. *Virology* **2015**, *486*, 187–197. [CrossRef]
31. Banerjee, S.; Shi, H.L.; Habte, H.H.; Qin, Y.L.; Cho, M.W. Modulating immunogenic properties of HIV-1 gp41 membrane-proximal external region by destabilizing six-helix bundle structure. *Virology* **2016**, *490*, 17–26. [CrossRef] [PubMed]
32. Xu, K.; Acharya, P.; Kong, R.; Cheng, C.; Chuang, G.Y.; Liu, K.; Louder, M.K.; O'Dell, S.; Rawi, R.; Sastry, M.; et al. Epitope-based vaccine design yields fusion peptide-directed antibodies that neutralize diverse strains of HIV-1. *Nat. Med.* **2018**, *24*, 857–867. [CrossRef] [PubMed]
33. Zhu, C.; Dukhovlinova, E.; Council, O.; Ping, L.; Faison, E.M.; Prabhu, S.S.; Potter, E.L.; Upton, S.L.; Yin, G.; Fay, J.M.; et al. Rationally designed carbohydrate-occluded epitopes elicit HIV-1 Env-specific antibodies. *Nat. Commun.* **2019**, *10*, 948. [CrossRef] [PubMed]
34. Dey, A.K.; Cupo, A.; Ozorowski, G.; Sharma, V.K.; Behrens, A.J.; Go, E.P.; Ketas, T.J.; Yasmeen, A.; Klasse, P.J.; Sayeed, E.; et al. cGMP production and analysis of BG505 SOSIP.664, an extensively glycosylated, trimeric HIV-1 envelope glycoprotein vaccine candidate. *Biotechnol. Bioeng.* **2018**, *115*, 885–899. [CrossRef] [PubMed]
35. Briney, B.; Sok, D.; Jardine, J.G.; Kulp, D.W.; Skog, P.; Menis, S.; Jacak, R.; Kalyuzhniy, O.; de Val, N.; Sesterhenn, F.; et al. Tailored Immunogens Direct affinity maturation toward HIV neutralizing antibodies. *Cell* **2016**, *166*, 1459–1470. [CrossRef] [PubMed]
36. Medina-Ramirez, M.; Sanders, R.W.; Sattentau, Q.J. Stabilized HIV-1 envelope glycoprotein trimers for vaccine use. *Curr. Opin. HIV AIDS* **2017**, *12*, 241–249. [CrossRef] [PubMed]
37. Burton, D.R. Scaffolding to build a rational vaccine design strategy. *Proc. Natl. Acad. Sci. USA* **2010**, *107*, 17859–17860. [CrossRef]
38. Schief, W.R.; Ban, Y.E.A.; Stamatatos, L. Challenges for structure-based HIV vaccine design. *Curr. Opin. HIV AIDS* **2009**, *4*, 431–440. [CrossRef] [PubMed]
39. Crooks, E.T.; Tong, T.; Chakrabarti, B.; Narayan, K.; Georgiev, I.S.; Menis, S.; Huang, X.X.; Kulp, D.; Osawa, K.; Muranaka, J.; et al. Vaccine-Elicited Tier 2 HIV-1 Neutralizing Antibodies Bind to Quaternary Epitopes Involving Glycan-Deficient Patches Proximal to the CD4 Binding Site. *Plos Pathog.* **2015**, *11*, 1004932. [CrossRef]

40. Leaman, D.P.; Lee, J.H.; Ward, A.B.; Zwick, M.B. Immunogenic Display of Purified Chemically Cross-Linked HIV-1 Spikes. *J. Virol.* **2015**, *89*, 6725–6745. [CrossRef]
41. Sanders, R.W.; Derking, R.; Cupo, A.; Julien, J.P.; Yasmeen, A.; de Val, N.; Kim, H.J.; Blattner, C.; de la Pena, A.T.; Korzun, J.; et al. A Next-Generation Cleaved, Soluble HIV-1 Env Trimer, BG505 SOSIP.664 gp140, Expresses Multiple Epitopes for Broadly Neutralizing but Not Non-Neutralizing Antibodies. *Plos Pathog.* **2013**, *9*, 1003618. [CrossRef] [PubMed]
42. Purtscher, M.; Trkola, A.; Gruber, G.; Buchacher, A.; Predl, R.; Steindl, F.; Tauer, C.; Berger, R.; Barrett, N.; Jungbauer, A.; et al. A broadly neutralizing human monoclonal-antibody against gp41 of human-immunodeficiency-virus type-1. *AIDS Res. Hum. Retroviruses* **1994**, *10*, 1651–1658. [CrossRef] [PubMed]
43. Huang, J.H.; Ofek, G.; Laub, L.; Louder, M.K.; Doria-Rose, N.A.; Longo, N.S.; Imamichi, H.; Bailer, R.T.; Chakrabarti, B.; Sharma, S.K.; et al. Broad and potent neutralization of HIV-1 by a gp41-specific human antibody. *Nature* **2012**, *491*, 406–412. [CrossRef] [PubMed]
44. Zhou, T.Q.; Georgiev, I.; Wu, X.L.; Yang, Z.Y.; Dai, K.F.; Finzi, A.; Kwon, Y.D.; Scheid, J.F.; Shi, W.; Xu, L.; et al. Structural Basis for Broad and Potent Neutralization of HIV-1 by Antibody VRC01. *Science* **2010**, *329*, 811–817. [CrossRef] [PubMed]
45. Roy, A.; Kucukural, A.; Zhang, Y. I-TASSER: A unified platform for automated protein structure and function prediction. *Nat. Protoc.* **2010**, *5*, 725–738. [CrossRef]
46. Eroshkin, A.M.; Karginova, E.A.; Gileva, I.P.; Lomakin, A.S.; Lebedev, L.R.; Kamyinina, T.P.; Pereboev, A.V.; Ignatev, G.M. Design of 4-helix bundle protein as a candidate for HIV vaccine. *Protein Eng.* **1995**, *8*, 167–173. [CrossRef]
47. Eroshkin, A.M.; Zhilkin, P.A.; Shamin, V.V.; Koroley, S.; Fedorov, B.B. Artificial protein vaccines with predetermined tertiary structure - application to anti-HIV-1 vaccine design. *Protein Eng.* **1993**, *6*, 997–1001. [CrossRef] [PubMed]
48. Perczel, A.; HollÓsi, M.; TusnÁdy, G.; Fasman, G.D. Convex constraint analysis: A natural deconvolution of circular dichroism curves of proteins. *Protein Eng. Des. Sel.* **1991**, *4*, 669–679. [CrossRef]
49. Li, M.; Gao, F.; Mascola, J.R.; Stamatatos, L.; Polonis, V.R.; Koutsoukos, M.; Voss, G.; Goepfert, P.; Gilbert, P.; Greene, K.M.; et al. Human immunodeficiency virus type 1 env clones from acute and early subtype B infections for standardized assessments of vaccine-elicited neutralizing antibodies. *J. Virol.* **2005**, *79*, 10108–10125. [CrossRef]
50. Stamatatos, L.; Lim, M.; Cheng-Mayer, C. Generation and structural analysis of soluble oligomeric gp140 envelope proteins derived from neutralization-resistant and neutralization-susceptible primary HIV type 1 isolates. *AIDS Res. Hum. Retroviruses* **2000**, *16*, 981–994. [CrossRef]
51. Montefiori, D.C. Measuring HIV neutralization in a luciferase reporter gene assay. *Methods Mol. Biol.* **2009**, *485*, 395–405. [PubMed]
52. Chikaev, A.N.; Bakulina, A.Y.; Burdick, R.C.; Karpenko, L.I.; Pathak, V.K.; Ilyichev, A.A. Selection of Peptide Mimics of HIV-1 Epitope Recognized by Neutralizing Antibody VRC01. *PloS ONE* **2015**, *10*, 0120847. [CrossRef] [PubMed]
53. The R Project for Statistical Computing. Available online: https://www.r-project.org (accessed on 8 October 2018).
54. GenScript Rare Codon Analysis Tool. Available online: https://www.genscript.com/tools/rare-codon-analysis (accessed on 15 September 2017).
55. Hansted, J.G.; Pietikainen, L.; Hog, F.; Sperling-Petersen, H.U.; Mortensen, K.K. Expressivity tag: A novel tool for increased expression in Escherichia coli. *J. Biotechnol.* **2011**, *155*, 275–283. [CrossRef] [PubMed]
56. PSSpred. Available online: https://zhanglab.ccmb.med.umich.edu/PSSpred/ (accessed on 22 October 2017).

57. Mikhailov, A.M.; Loktev, V.B.; Lebedev, L.R.; Eroshkin, A.M.; Kornev, A.N.; Kornilov, V.V.; Vainshtein, B.K. Crystallization and X-ray study of the artificial TBI protein, an experimental multiple-epitope vaccine against type 1 human immunodeficiency virus. *Crystallogr. Rep.* **1999**, *44*, 868–870.
58. Karpenko, L.I.; Ilyichev, A.A.; Eroshkin, A.M.; Lebedev, L.R.; Uzhachenko, R.V.; Nekrasova, N.A.; Plyasunova, O.A.; Belavin, P.A.; Seregin, S.V.; Danilyuk, N.K.; et al. Combined virus-like particle-based polyepitope DNA/protein HIV-1 vaccine - Design, immunogenicity and toxicity studies. *Vaccine* **2007**, *25*, 4312–4323. [CrossRef] [PubMed]

vaccines

MDPI

Article

Parenterally Administered P24-VP8* Nanoparticle Vaccine Conferred Strong Protection against Rotavirus Diarrhea and Virus Shedding in Gnotobiotic Pigs

Ashwin Ramesh [1], Jiangdi Mao [1], Shaohua Lei [1], Erica Twitchell [1], Ashton Shiraz [1], Xi Jiang [2,3], Ming Tan [2,3] and Lijuan Yuan [1,*]

1 Department of Biomedical Sciences and Pathobiology, Virginia-Maryland College of Veterinary Medicine, Virginia Tech, Blacksburg, VA 24060, USA; akramesh@vt.edu (A.R.); jmao2018@vt.edu (J.M.); lsh2013@vt.edu (S.L.); etwitche@vt.edu (E.T.); aks2026@vt.edu (A.S.)
2 Division of Infectious Diseases, Cincinnati Children's Hospital Medical Center, Cincinnati, OH 45229, USA; Jason.Jiang@cchmc.org (X.J.); Ming.Tan@cchmc.org (M.T.)
3 Department of Pediatrics, University of Cincinnati College of Medicine, Cincinnati, OH 45229, USA
* Correspondence: lyuan@vt.edu

Received: 16 August 2019; Accepted: 24 October 2019; Published: 6 November 2019

Abstract: Current live rotavirus vaccines are costly with increased risk of intussusception due to vaccine replication in the gut of vaccinated children. New vaccines with improved safety and cost-effectiveness are needed. In this study, we assessed the immunogenicity and protective efficacy of a novel P24-VP8* nanoparticle vaccine using the gnotobiotic (Gn) pig model of human rotavirus infection and disease. Three doses of P24-VP8* (200 μg/dose) intramuscular vaccine with $Al(OH)_3$ adjuvant (600 μg) conferred significant protection against infection and diarrhea after challenge with virulent Wa strain rotavirus. This was indicated by the significant reduction in the mean duration of diarrhea, virus shedding in feces, and significantly lower fecal cumulative consistency scores in post-challenge day (PCD) 1–7 among vaccinated pigs compared to the mock immunized controls. The P24-VP8* vaccine was highly immunogenic in Gn pigs. It induced strong VP8*-specific serum IgG and Wa-specific virus-neutralizing antibody responses from post-inoculation day 21 to PCD 7, but did not induce serum or intestinal IgA antibody responses or a strong effector T cell response, which are consistent with the immunization route, the adjuvant used, and the nature of the non-replicating vaccine. The findings are highly translatable and thus will facilitate clinical trials of the P24-VP8* nanoparticle vaccine.

Keywords: rotavirus nanoparticle vaccine; gnotobiotic pigs

1. Introduction

Human rotavirus (HRV) is a leading cause of severe, dehydrating gastroenteritis in children under five years of age. Although two live-attenuated oral vaccines, RotaTeq® and Rotarix®, have been implemented as part of national vaccination programs in over 98 different countries [1], their vaccine efficacy was reported to be lower in low- and middle- income countries (LMICs [39%–70%]) compared to that in high-income countries (80%–90%) [2–7]. A combination of factors have been suggested to be responsible for the lower efficacy, which have been reviewed and discussed in detail by Arnold [8] and Desselberger [9]. Both these live vaccines have also been linked to a low risk of intussusception (1–7 cases per 100,000 vaccinated infants) as a result of the vaccine rotavirus (RV) strains replicating in the intestines [10,11], and have remained expensive even after Gavi, the Vaccine Alliance, subsidization [12], particularly in resource-deprived countries. These scenarios have increased the demand for a safer, more cost-effective, and more efficacious vaccine, especially in LMICs that can be easily administered.

Parenteral intramuscular (IM) vaccines have been preferred to oral vaccines due to their increased immunogenicity. They are also not directly affected by microbiome composition or gut enteropathy, both of which have been known to affect the efficacy of oral vaccines in LMICs [13]. Non-replicating rotavirus vaccines (NRRV) have been proposed as safer alternatives to live-attenuated vaccines as they do not lead to intussusception due to their parenteral immunization route [14].

The VP4 region of RV constitutes surface spike proteins that are cleaved by host intestinal proteases into two fragments, VP5* and VP8*. VP8* forms the distal portion of the VP4 spikes, interacting with glycan receptors to facilitate viral attachment and entry [15,16]. VP8* expressed in various culture systems has been explored as an immunogen in rotavirus vaccine development [17–22]. VP8*-containing vaccine candidates have been shown to induce rotavirus-specific neutralizing antibodies and/or protection in mouse, guinea pigs, and gnotobiotic (Gn) pig models [23–28]. Among those, the leading candidate is the P2-VP8 (VP8* fused to a universal tetanus toxin CD4+ T cell epitope P2) vaccine, adsorbed with aluminum hydroxide for IM administration, which has progressed to phase 1/2 human clinical trials [19,29].

The norovirus (NoV) P particle, referred to as the P24 particle, is an octahedral nanoparticle (≈840 kDa) composed of 24 copies of the protrusion (P) domain of the NoV capsid protein. It can be easily produced in large quantities using an *E. coli* expression system. The distal surface of each P domain, corresponding to the outermost surface of the P particle, contains three surface loops, which can tolerate large sequence insertions. Based on this concept, a nanoparticle vaccine was developed by inserting the HRV VP8* antigen into the loop sections of the P domains. The P24-VP8* nanoparticle consists of a 24-valent core of NoV P particle and 24 surface-displayed HRV VP8*s. The P24-VP8* nanoparticle shares the features of the P24 particle in self-formation, easy production, and high stability over a wide range of temperatures [30]. Efficacy studies in mice revealed that the P24-VP8* nanoparticle vaccine is highly immunogenic and capable of inducing a significantly higher VP8* specific antibody response as compared with free VP8* particles even without adjuvant [30].

The main objectives of this study were to assess the immunogenicity and protective efficacy of a novel P24-VP8* nanoparticle vaccine using the gnotobiotic (Gn) pig model of human rotavirus infection and disease. The Gn pig model of HRV (Wa, G1P [8]) infection and diarrhea has been well established and used in the pre-clinical evaluation of HRV vaccine efficacies [31]. No other conventional lab animals develop diarrhea after HRV inoculation [32]. Pigs are genetically, physiologically, anatomically, and immunologically similar to humans [33–35], allowing data from Gn pigs to be translated to humans. The immunogenicity and protective efficacy of the P24-VP8* nanoparticle vaccine were determined using the Gn pig model of HRV infection and disease. High serum IgA, IgG, and virus-neutralizing (VN) antibody titers, as well as HRV-specific IFN-γ producing T cells, have been correlated with protection from HRV infection and disease, and data has been demonstrated to be comparable in Gn pigs and human studies [24,36,37].

2. Materials and Methods

2.1. Human Rotavirus

The virulent HRV (VirHRV) inoculum consisted of a pool composed of intestinal contents collected from the 27th passage in Gn pigs of the Wa strain HRV based on successive passages carried out in Gn pigs. A total of 1×10^5 fluorescent focus-forming units (FFUs) of VirHRV were diluted in 5 mL of Diluent #5 [minimal essential media (MEM, ThermoFisher Scientific); 100 IU of penicillin per mL, 0.1 mg of dihydrostreptomycin per ml; and 1% HEPES] for the inoculation of each Gn pig. The median infectious dose (ID_{50}) and median diarrhea dose (DD_{50}) of the VirHRV in Gn pigs were determined as approximately 1 FFU [38].

The cell culture-adapted HRV Wa strain (AttHRV), derived from the 35th passage in African green monkey kidney cells (MA104, ATCC# CRL-2378.1) [38,39], were used as the positive control for the assessment of RV antigens in feces using enzyme-linked immunosorbent assay (ELISA). The origination and passage history of the VirHRV and AttHRV have been explained by Wentzel et al. [40].

2.2. Vaccine

The P24-VP8* vaccine was comprised of 200 μg of P24-VP8* proteins and 600 μg Aluminum hydrogel ($Al(OH)_3$) adjuvant. The vaccine was stored at 4 °C (up to 8 months) until administered to Gn pigs (Supplementary Figure S1). The dosage of the P24-VP8* vaccine was selected based on a similar VP8* molar amount of the P2-VP8 subunit vaccine used in the clinical trial [19,27,29]. The VP8* region used in this vaccine was designed based on the sequence of Wa HRV. As the negative control, the $Al(OH)_3$ adjuvant (G-Biosciences, St. Louis, MO, USA) was diluted in sterile PBS to form a final concentration of 600 μg/mL and stored at room temperature, as per manufacturer instructions, until administered.

The purified P24-VP8* proteins were used as the detector antigen in ELISA for the detection of serum IgA and IgG antibody responses [41] and as stimulating antigen in the intracellular IFN-γ staining assay [39,42].

2.3. Gn Pigs and Treatments

Pigs (Large white cross breed) used in this study were surgically derived by hysterectomy and maintained in sterile isolators, as described previously [43]. The sterility status of the pigs housed in the gnotobiotic isolators was confirmed by culturing isolator swabs and pig rectal swabs on blood agar plates and in thioglycolate broth first at 3 days after derivation and then repeated once a week until the end of the study. Pigs were fed on a diet that solely consisted of commercial UHT sterile whole cow's milk (The Hershey Company, Hershey, PA, USA) until post-inoculation day (PID) 21, and were switched over to Similac® baby formula (Abbott Laboratories, Chicago, IL, USA) until the end of the study.

A total of 25 pigs were assigned to two groups, and a subset of pigs in each group were euthanized either pre-challenge (PID 28) or at post-challenge day (PCD) 7 (Table 1).

Table 1. Assignment of treatment groups for gnotobiotic (Gn) pigs.

Group	Number of Pigs	Challenge	Time of Euthanasia
Control	3	No	PID 28
Control	7	Yes	PCD 7
P24-VP8* Vaccine	7	No	PID 28
P24-VP8* Vaccine	8	Yes	PCD 7

Pigs were administered IM with an equal volume (1 mL) of either P24-VP8* vaccine formulated with adjuvant or adjuvant alone at 5 days of age (PID 0), followed by two booster doses at PID10 and PID21. The Phase I and Phase II clinical trials carried out to evaluate the effects of P2-VP8* vaccine demonstrated that participants who received a 3-dose vaccination regime shed fewer attenuated rotavirus in feces as compared to trial participants who received two doses [19,29]. Based on this rationale, we opted to use the 3-dose regimen in this current study. The timing of 3 injections in Gn pigs are established in previous studies [27,37] based on the time needed to prime and boost immune responses in Gn pigs. Serum was collected at PID 0, PID 10, PID 21, PID 28, and PCD 7 for the detection of VP8*-specific IgA, IgG, and Wa HRV-specific neutralizing antibody responses.

One subset of pigs (n = 3–7) from each group was euthanized before the challenge at PID 28. Another subset of pigs (n = 7–8) was orally challenged with 1×10^5 FFU of VirHRV Wa strain and monitored from PCD 0 to PCD 7 to assess the protection against virus shedding and diarrhea conferred by the vaccine before euthanasia on PCD 7. The pathogenesis of the Wa VirHRV infection has been studied in detail in Gn pigs; diarrhea and virus shedding persisted between 4 to 7 days post infection [33,38,44,45]. Based on these observations, we limited the study duration to 7 days post-challenge in order to assess the immediate protection conferred by the vaccine against VirWa challenge. Four milliliters of 200 mM $NaHCO_3$ were given orally 15–20 min before the VirHRV challenge to reduce stomach acidity to allow for rotavirus inoculum to pass through the stomach without being degraded due to low pH in the stomach.

At euthanasia, small and large intestinal contents (SIC and LIC) were collected from all pigs and processed, as described [46], for the detection of intestinal antibody responses by ELISA. Ileum, blood, and spleen were collected, and mononuclear cells (MNCs) were isolated from them for the detection of effector T cell responses by flow cytometry as described [42].

2.4. Assessment of Diarrhea and Detection of RV Shedding in Feces by Rotavirus Antigen ELISA and CCIF

The pigs were on a milk-based diet throughout the duration of the study, making their fecal consistency resemble that of a newborn infant. For the assessment of diarrhea, fecal consistency was recorded daily from PCD 0–7 and categorized as follows: 0: normal; 1: pasty; 2: semi-liquid; 3: liquid. The fecal scoring system used here has been well established and used for multiple Gn pigs studies [32,33,38,44,45,47,48]. Pigs were considered to be having diarrhea when their daily fecal consistency scores were recorded to be 2 or greater (≥2).

Rectal swabs were collected daily to monitor virus shedding by ELISA (for the detection of RV antigens) and cell culture immunofluorescence (CCIF; for the detection of infectious virions) from PCD 0–7. Rectal swabs were processed, as reported previously [49]. ELISA and CCIF assays for the detection and titration of VirHRV antigen in rectal swabs were carried out as previously described [33,38,44,45,47,50–52]. CCIF titers [fluorescent focus units (FFU)/mL)] were determined by Equation (1):

$$\frac{ffu}{mL} = \frac{\#\, Plaques\ counted}{d\ x\ V} \tag{1}$$

where d = dilution factor, and V = volume of virus added.

2.5. RV-Specific Serum VN, and VP8*-Specific Serum and Intestinal IgA and IgG Antibody Titration

VN antibody titers in serum samples were determined based on methods described previously [47]. MA104 cells were cultured in 96-well plates until an even monolayer was formed (≈3–4 days). Cells were washed once with sf-EMEM, and enriched with 100 µL of sf-EMEM and incubated at 37 °C for 2 h. The media was then discarded, and the cells were inoculated with trypsin-activated AttHRV (4×10^3 FFU in 10 µg/mL trypsin) in the absence or presence of 4-fold decreasing concentrations of Gn pig serum samples. The inoculum was discarded, and the plates were incubated at 37 °C for 18 h in 5% CO_2 containing fresh sf-EMEM. The remainder of the steps has been described in detail in a previous publication [47]. The VN antibody titer was expressed as the reciprocal of the serum dilution, which reduced the number of fluorescent cell-forming units by >80% compared to the negative control serum. VP8*-specific IgA and IgG antibody titers in serum and intestinal contents were measured by using isotype-specific antibody ELISA with purified P24-VP8* as detector antigen at the plate coating concentration of 6.63 µg/mL, following methods described elsewhere [46,47,53]. When loading the testing samples on ELISA plates, four-fold serial dilutions of each sample started from 1:4 to 1:16384 for IgA, SIC, and LIC and 1:256 to 1:1048576 for IgG.

2.6. Flow Cytometry

Mononuclear cells (MNCs) collected from the ileum, blood, and spleen were diluted to a concentration of 2×10^6 cells/mL and were seeded into 12-well plates and stimulated with 12 µg/mL of P24-VP8* antigen for 17 h at 37 °C in 5% CO_2 as determined previously [42]. CD3+CD4+ and CD3+CD8+ cell surface marker staining and IFN-γ intracellular staining have been described in previous publications [42,47,54,55]. All samples were stored in 0.05 mL of stain buffer and were maintained at 4 °C. A minimum of 100,000 events were acquired using a FACSAria flow cytometer

(BD Biosciences, San Jose, CA, USA). Flow cytometry data were analyzed using FlowJo X software (Tree Star, Ashland, OR, USA).

2.7. Statistical Analysis

Gn pigs were randomly assigned into treatment groups upon derivation regardless of gender and body weight by animal care technicians. Student's *t*-test was used for comparisons of virus shedding and diarrhea data between the treatment groups. One-way analysis of variance (ANOVA) (General linear model) was used to compare rotavirus-specific IgA, IgG, virus-neutralizing (VN) antibody titers between the treatment groups. Tukey-Kramer HSD was used for the comparison of different time points within the same treatment group. Two-way ANOVA, followed by a Multiple *t*-test, was used for comparisons of frequencies of IFN-γ producing T cells between treatment groups. ANOVA analyses were carried out using JMP 14.0 (SAS Institute, Kerry, NC, USA), and all other statistical analyses were performed using GraphPad Prism 7.0 (GraphPad Software, San Diego, CA, USA). A p value lower than 0.05 was accepted to be statistically significant.

3. Results

3.1. Protection against Diarrhea and Virus Shedding upon Challenge with VirHRV

Vaccinated and control Gn pigs were challenged with VirHRV at PID 28 and were monitored daily for clinical signs (diarrhea) and virus shedding from PCD 1 to PCD 7. Gn pigs that were administered with P24-VP8* vaccine had a significantly delayed onset of diarrhea (from 1.6 to 4.4 days), a significantly reduced duration of diarrhea (from 6.0 to 3.3 days), significantly lower mean diarrhea scores on PID 1 and 2, and a significantly lower cumulative fecal consistency score (from 14.3 to 9.1) as compared to the mock-vaccinated control group (Table 2 and Figure 1A). A delayed onset of virus shedding, a reduced peak titer, a reduced cumulative virus titer (presented as the area under the curve, AUC), and a significantly reduced duration (from 5.9 to 2.5 days) of virus shedding were observed in P24-VP8* vaccinated pigs when compared to the control group (Table 2). In addition, the mean daily virus shedding titer in the vaccinated pigs was significantly reduced at PCD 2 (Figure 1B), and the reduction of total virus shed (AUC) was 2.27-fold compared to the control pigs (Table 2). However, the vaccine did not significantly reduce the incidence (%) of diarrhea and virus shedding (Table 2).

Table 2. Diarrhea and rotavirus fecal virus shedding in Gn pigs after the VirHRV challenge.

		Diarrhea				Fecal Virus Shedding				
Treatment	n	**% with Diarrhea** [a]	**Mean Days to Onset** [b]	**Mean Duration Days** [c,§]	**Mean Cumulative Fecal Score** [c,*]	**% Shedding Virus** [a]	**Mean Days to Onset** [b]	**Mean Duration Days** [c,*]	**Mean Peak Titer (FFU/mL)**	**AUC**
P24-VP8*	8	87.5	4.4 (0.5) [d,*]	3.3 (0.75) *	9.1 (1.23) *	75	4.8 (1.0)	2.5 (0.89) *	8500 (2196) *	11,750 (3172)
Control	7	100	1.6 (0.3)	6.0 (0)	14.3 (0.44)	85.7	1.9 (0.14)	5.9 (0.14)	11,492 (4300)	26,664 (10,489)

[a] Gn pigs were orally inoculated with 1×10^5 FFU/mL of VirHRV at post-innoculation day (PID) 28. Rectal swabs were collected daily after the challenge from PCD 1 to PCD 7 to monitor for clinical signs and virus shedding. Pigs with daily fecal scores of ≥ 2 were considered diarrheic. Fecal consistency was scored as follows: 0, normal; 1, pasty; 2, semi-liquid; and 3, liquid. Fecal virus shedding data was determined by ELISA and/or CCIF. [b] An arbitrary designation of Day 8 was assigned to pigs that did not develop diarrhea or shed virus in feces for calculating the mean days to onset. [c] For the purposes of calculating diarrhea and virus shedding duration, if no diarrhea or virus shedding was observed in pigs until euthanasia day (PCD 7), the duration days were recorded as 0. [d] Standard error of the mean. [§] Student's *t*-test was used for comparison between vaccine and control groups. Asterisk indicates statistical significance between the groups ($n = 7$–8; *, $p < 0.05$).

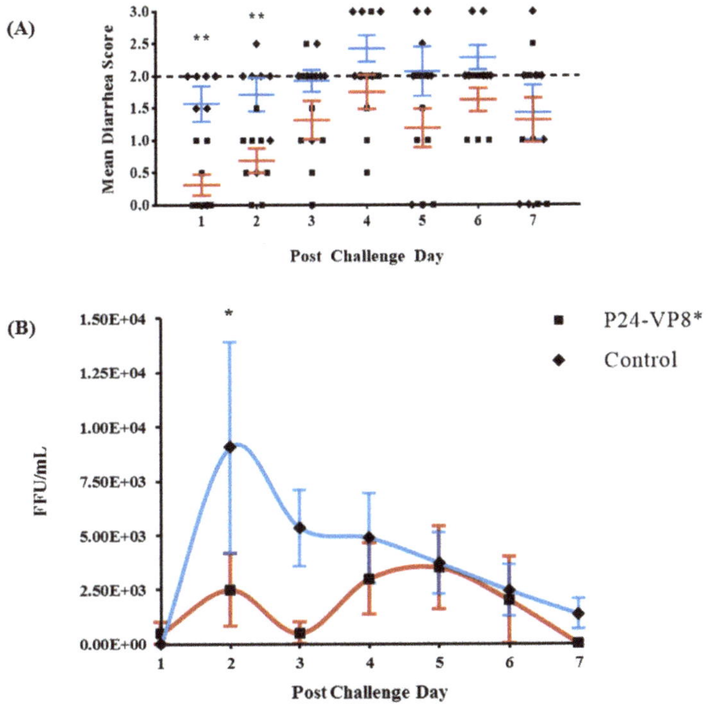

Figure 1. P24-VP8* vaccine protected against VirHRV diarrhea and reduced overall virus shed among vaccinated pigs. Fecal consistency (**A**) and virus shedding (**B**) were monitored daily from post challenge day (PCD) 1 to PCD 7 after the challenge with VirHRV. Fecal consistency scores ≥2 were considered to be diarrheic (dashed line indicates the threshold of diarrhea). Statistical significance between vaccinated and control groups, determined by multiple t tests, are indicated by asterisks (*, $p < 0.05$; **, $p < 0.01$).

3.2. Strong VP8-Specific IgG and Virus Neutralizing, but Lack of IgA, Antibody Responses in Serum*

In order to monitor the development of VP8* specific humoral immunity, serum samples were collected during the time of vaccine administration (PID 0, PID 10, and PID 21) at the VirHRV challenge (PID 28) and upon euthanasia (PCD 7). Serum IgG and IgA antibody responses were quantified using ELISA and depicted in Figures 2A and 2B, respectively. P24-VP8*-specific IgG antibody titers in serum were significantly higher ($p < 0.001$) in vaccinated pigs at PID 10, PID 21, PID 28, and PCD 7 when compared to pigs in the control group (Figure 2A). However, serum IgA titers were only detectable after challenge (PCD 7) with VirHRV (Figure 2B).

HRV neutralizing antibodies were detected in the serum of P24-VP8* vaccinated pigs starting from PID 21 and were observed to increase similarly with VP8*-specific IgG titers until euthanasia at PCD 7. In control pigs, VN antibodies were only detectable after challenge with VirHRV and were at significantly lower levels compared to the vaccinated pigs (Figure 2C).

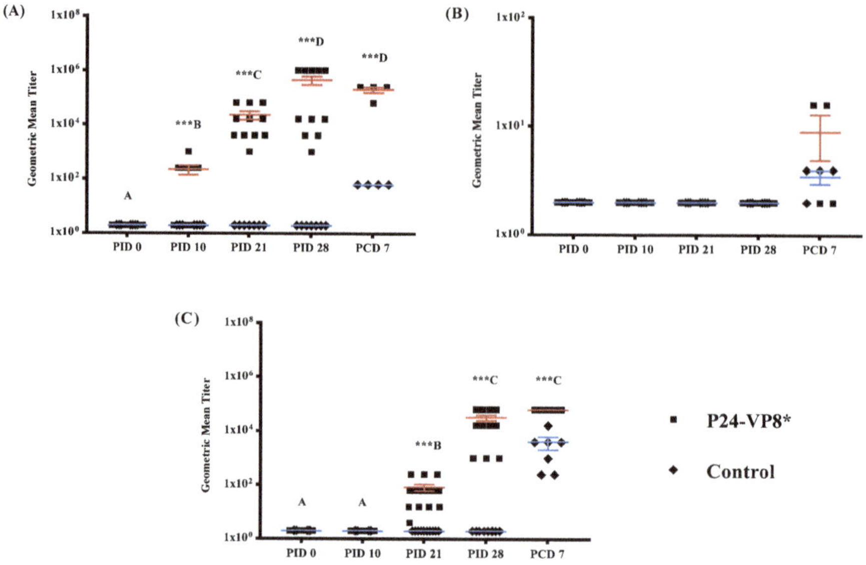

Figure 2. Geometric mean VP8*-specific IgG (**A**) and IgA (**B**) and Wa-HRV neutralizing (**C**) antibody titers in serum collected from Gn pigs at PID 0, 10, 21, 28, and PCD 7. Pigs were vaccinated with P24-VP8* vaccine or $Al(OH)_3$ adjuvant only. Each serum specimen was tested at an initial dilution of 1:4. Negative samples were assigned an arbitrary value of 2 for calculation and graphical illustration purposes. Comparisons between groups at the same time points were carried out using Student's *t*-test and significant differences are identified by *** ($n = 10$–15; $p < 0.001$). Tukey-Kramer HSD was used for the comparison of different time points within the same group, where different capital letters (A, B, C, D) indicate a significant difference, $p < 0.01$, and shared letters indicate no significant difference.

3.3. Lack of P24-VP8* Specific Antibody Responses in the Intestines

P24-VP8*-specific IgA and IgG antibody titers in SIC and LIC, collected at the time of euthanasia (PID 28 and PCD 7), were measured by ELISA. The P24-VP8* vaccine did not induce any detectable intestinal IgA or IgG antibody responses before the challenge at PID 28. After the challenge, among the eight vaccinated and challenged pigs, only VP8*-specific IgG antibodies were detected (ELISA titers ranging from 256 to 1024) in the SIC of three pigs at PCD 7 (Supplementary Figure S2). However, the SIC IgG titers were not associated with the severity of diarrhea or the amount of virus shed in the three pigs throughout the challenge period.

3.4. P24-VP8* Vaccine did not Induce Strong VP8*-Specific Effector T Cell Responses in Intestinal and Systemic Lymphoid Tissues

Frequencies of IFN-γ+CD8+ and IFN-γ+CD4+ T cells in ileum, peripheral blood (PBL), and spleen at PID 28, and PCD 7 are summarized in Figure 3. At PID 28, slightly higher (not statistically significant) IFN-γ producing CD4+ and CD8+ T cell responses to the P24-VP8* antigen was detected in vaccinated pigs as compared to control pigs (Figure 3A). P24-VP8* vaccinated pigs had higher frequencies of IFN-γ+CD4+ T cells in ileum and blood and higher IFN-γ+CD8+ T cells in ileum, blood, and spleen compared to the mock-vaccinated control pigs. Upon the VirHRV challenge, there was still no significant difference in the frequencies of IFN-γ secreting CD4+ and CD8+ T cells between the two groups in the intestinal (ileum) or the systemic tissues (PBL and spleen) (Figure 3B).

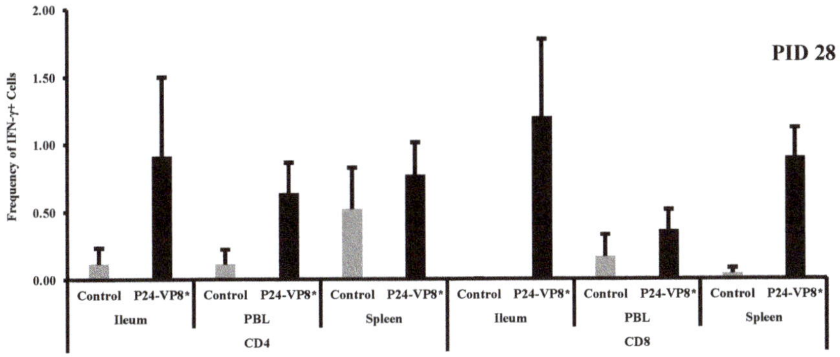

(**A**)

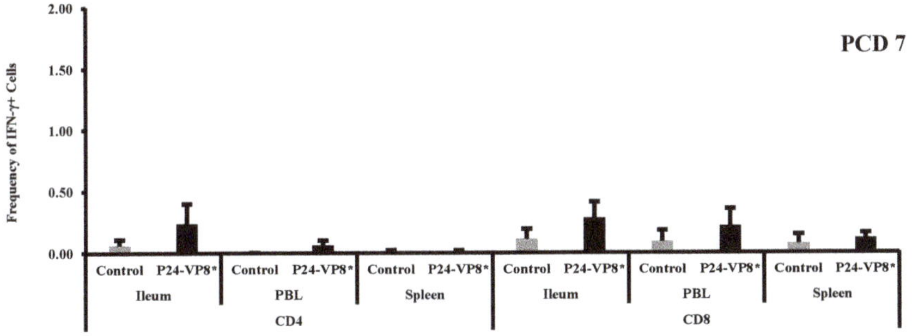

(**B**)

Figure 3. Frequencies of IFN-γ+CD8+ and IFN-γ+CD4+ T cells in ileum, peripheral blood (PBL), and spleen at PID 28 (**A**) and PCD 7 (**B**). Two-way ANOVA followed by Multiple *t*-tests were carried out for comparisons. (n = 3–8; $p < 0.05$). There were no significant differences.

4. Discussion

In this study, the immunogenicity (antibody and T cell responses) and protective efficacy of the P24-VP8* nanoparticle vaccine were evaluated in Gn pigs. We first demonstrated that the IM P24-VP8* vaccine conferred significant protection against infection and diarrhea when challenged with the homotypic virulent strain Wa of HRV. This was indicated by the significant reduction in the mean duration of diarrhea, virus shedding in feces, and significantly lower fecal cumulative consistency scores recorded from PCD 1–7 in vaccinated pigs compared to the controls. However, the vaccine did not significantly reduce the incidence (%) of diarrhea and virus shedding, indicating that there was a lack of protective immune effectors at the site of infection (small intestine) at the time of challenge, which is consistent with the observed intestinal immune responses. The IM P24-VP8* vaccine with $Al(OH)_3$ adjuvant was highly immunogenic in Gn pigs. It induced strong VP8*-specific serum IgG and virus-neutralizing antibody responses from PID 21 to PCD 7 but did not induce serum or intestinal IgA antibody responses or a strong effector T cell response. These results are consistent with the IM immunization route, the $Al(OH)_3$ adjuvant, and the nature of the non-replicating vaccine. Non-replicating vaccines are typically ineffective in inducing effector T cell responses. The $Al(OH)_3$ adjuvant is characteristic for its ability to enhance a Th2 type immune response, promoting strong humoral responses and suppressing effector T cell responses [56].

The observed protection and immune responses data together suggest that the protection conferred by the P24-VP8* vaccine against diarrhea and virus shedding upon challenge with the virulent Wa HRV was mediated by the vaccine-induced antibodies in the serum. Although there were no antibodies present at the lumen of the small intestine, the site of HRV infection, at the time of challenge to totally prevent the initiation of RV infection, the viruses disseminated into blood from the infected small intestinal epithelial cells could have been neutralized by the high titers of VP8*-specific IgG and virus-neutralizing antibodies during the phase of viremia. Such mechanisms can reduce the chance of infection of more epithelial cells by the virus from the basolateral side [45]. Studies showing that passively transferred serum antibodies can suppress or delay viral infection in RV-challenged pigtailed macaques [57], and an inactivated IM HRV vaccine (CDC-9) reduced virus shedding in Gn pigs upon challenge with Wa VirHRV [48] likely share the same protection mechanism with the P24-VP8* vaccine. The serum IgG and virus-neutralizing antibody responses induced by the P24-VP8* IM nanoparticle vaccine had similar dynamics and magnitude as the aluminum phosphate adjuvanted inactivated CDC-9 and P2-VP8* IM vaccines in Gn pigs [27,48]. The P24-VP8* vaccine demonstrated a similar degree of protection against diarrhea but a stronger protection against virus shedding in Gn pigs as compared to the P2-VP8* vaccine [27].

There was a trend of inverse correlation between serum VP8*-specific IgG titers at PID 28 and cumulative diarrhea scores post-challenge in the vaccinated pigs (Pearson's rank correlation, $r = -0.6699$ and $p = 0.0691$), suggesting that vaccinated pigs with higher serum VP8*-specific IgG responses are more likely to be protected against severe diarrhea, which is in agreement with the study of serum IgG antibody in human adults showing that VP4-specific IgG titer was correlated with resistance to HRV infection [58]. The presence of high preexisting IgG titers was also correlated with less severe or shorter duration of diarrhea among children under three years of age [59]. As reviewed by Jiang et al., serum antibodies, if present at critical levels, are either protective themselves or are an important and powerful correlate of protection against rotavirus disease [60].

Additional investigations are required to explore the full potential of P24-VP8* vaccine efficacy. First, P24-VP8* is a candidate dual-vaccine against both NoV and RV, but we only examined the immune responses and protection against HRV, not human norovirus (HuNoV). Further studies in the Gn pig model of HuNoV infection are needed to evaluate its efficacy against NoV. Second, we only examined the protection against challenge with a homotypic HRV, and it remains to be determined whether the P24-VP8* vaccine would be effective in protecting against heterotypic HRV, as the monovalent P[8] HRV vaccine Rotarix showed significant efficacy against P[4] (70.9%) and P[6] (55.2%) HRV associated gastroenteritis in African infants [61]. One of the important potential advantages of the novel P24-VP8* nanoparticle dual vaccine is that the vaccine can be formulated as a cocktail vaccine to cover multiple types of RVs and NoVs for broad protection. Thus far, the Gn pig model of HRV infection and diarrhea has only been evaluated using the P [8] Wa HRV, requiring the need to test the effectiveness of Gn pigs as a suitable model for additional HRV P types to evaluate the broadness of protection of the novel P24-VP8* nanoparticle vaccine.

5. Conclusions

The P24-VP8* vaccine candidate is a typical nanoparticle vaccine with 24 copies of the major RV surface neutralizing antigen VP8* displayed on the self-assembled norovirus P24 particles. The P24-VP8* nanoparticles are easily produced in *E. coli* with a high yield and simple purification procedures at a low cost. Significant enhancement of the immunogenicity of both VP8* and P domain backbone have been demonstrated in mouse immunization studies. In this current study, the usefulness of the P24-VP8* vaccine was assessed in a Gn pig model, followed by the challenge of HRV. Three doses of IM immunization of Gn pigs demonstrated the nanoparticle vaccine's effectiveness to significantly shorten the duration of HRV diarrhea and virus shedding, reduce the severity of diarrhea, and lower the amount of virus shed when challenged. Immune responses associated with protection include high titers of VP8*-specific serum IgG antibodies and virus-neutralizing antibodies induced by the vaccine after the second and third booster doses. These findings will facilitate clinical trials of this vaccine candidate into a useful, safe, non-replicating, parental vaccine against RVs.

Supplementary Materials: The following are available online at http://www.mdpi.com/2076-393X/7/4/177/s1, Figure S1: Negative stain TEM images of P24-VP8* particles. Figure S2: Geometric mean VP8*-specific IgG titers in SIC of Gn pigs.

Author Contributions: Conceptualization, L.Y. and X.J.; Validation, A.R. and L.Y.; Formal Analysis, A.R.; Investigation, A.R., J.M., S.L., E.T. and A.S.; Resources, X.J. and M.T.; Writing – Original Draft Preparation, A.R. and L.Y.; Writing – Review & Editing, A.R., J.M., S.L., E.T., A.S., X.J., M.T. and L.Y.; Visualization, A.R. and L.Y.; Supervision, L.Y.; Project Administration, A.R. and L.Y.; Funding Acquisition, L.Y.

Funding: This research received no external funding.

Acknowledgments: We thank Enqi Huang for preparation of the vaccines, Sherrie Clark-Deener, Kevin Pelzer, Julie Settlage and Amy Rizzo for veterinary services, Karen Hall, Rachel McNeil for animal care. We thank Melissa Makris for flow cytometry service.

Conflicts of Interest: The authors declare that there are no conflicts of interest.

Ethical Approval: All animal experiments were conducted in accordance with protocols approved by the Institutional Animal Care and Use Committee at Virginia Tech (IACUC protocol: 16-214-BIOL).

References

1. IVAC. Current Vaccine Intro Status. Available online: www.view-hub.org (accessed on 11 June 2019).
2. Gilmartin, A.A.; Petri, W.A. Exploring the role of environmental enteropathy in malnutrition, infant development and oral vaccine response. *Philos. Trans. R. Soc. B Biol. Sci.* **2015**, *370*, 20140143. [CrossRef]
3. Boom, J.A.; Tate, J.E.; Sahni, L.C.; Rench, M.A.; Hull, J.J.; Gentsch, J.R.; Patel, M.M.; Baker, C.J.; Parashar, U.D. Effectiveness of Pentavalent Rotavirus Vaccine in a Large Urban Population in the United States. *Pediatrics* **2010**, *125*, 199–207. [CrossRef] [PubMed]
4. Vesikari, T.; Karvonen, A.; Prymula, R.; Schuster, V.; Tejedor, J.C.; Cohen, R.; Meurice, F.; Han, H.; Damaso, S.; Bouckenooghe, A. Efficacy of human rotavirus vaccine against rotavirus gastroenteritis during the first 2 years of life in European infants: Randomised, double-blind controlled study. *Lancet* **2007**, *370*, 1757–1763. [CrossRef]
5. Armah, G.E.; O Sow, S.; Breiman, R.F.; Dallas, M.J.; Tapia, M.D.; Feikin, D.R.; Binka, F.N.; Steele, A.D.; Laserson, K.F.; Ansah, N.A.; et al. Efficacy of pentavalent rotavirus vaccine against severe rotavirus gastroenteritis in infants in developing countries in sub-Saharan Africa: A randomised, double-blind, placebo-controlled trial. *Lancet* **2010**, *376*, 606–614. [CrossRef]
6. Patel, M.M.; Glass, R.; Desai, R.; E Tate, J.; Parashar, U.D. Fulfilling the promise of rotavirus vaccines: How far have we come since licensure? *Lancet Infect. Dis.* **2012**, *12*, 561–570. [CrossRef]
7. Lamberti, L.M.; Ashraf, S.; Walker, C.L.F.; Black, R.E. A Systematic Review of the Effect of Rotavirus Vaccination on Diarrhea Outcomes among Children Younger Than 5 Years. *Pediatr. Infect. Dis. J.* **2016**, *35*, 992–998. [CrossRef]
8. Arnold, M.M. Rotavirus Vaccines: Why Continued Investment in Research Is Necessary. *Curr. Clin. Microbiol. Rep.* **2018**, *5*, 73–81. [CrossRef]
9. Desselberger, U. Differences of Rotavirus Vaccine Effectiveness by Country: Likely Causes and Contributing Factors. *Pathogens* **2017**, *6*, 65. [CrossRef]
10. Aliabadi, N.; Tate, J.; Parashar, U. Potential safety issues and other factors that may affect the introduction and uptake of rotavirus vaccines. *Clin. Microbiol. Infect.* **2016**, *22*, S128–S135. [CrossRef]
11. World Health Organization. Safety of rotavirus vaccines: Postmarketing surveillance in the WHO Region of the Americas. *Relev. Epidemiol. Hebd.* **2011**, *86*, 66–72.
12. Pecenka, C.; Debellut, F.; Bar-Zeev, N.; Anwari, P.; Nonvignon, J.; Shamsuzzaman, M.; Clark, A. Re-evaluating the cost and cost-effectiveness of rotavirus vaccination in Bangladesh, Ghana, and Malawi: A comparison of three rotavirus vaccines. *Vaccine* **2018**, *36*, 7472–7478. [CrossRef] [PubMed]
13. Velasquez, D.E.; Parashar, U.; Jiang, B. Decreased performance of live attenuated, oral rotavirus vaccines in low-income settings: Causes and contributing factors. *Expert Rev. Vaccines* **2018**, *17*, 145–161. [CrossRef] [PubMed]

14. O'Ryan, M.; A Lopman, B. Parenteral protein-based rotavirus vaccine. *Lancet Infect. Dis.* **2017**, *17*, 786–787. [CrossRef]
15. Liu, Y.; Huang, P.; Tan, M.; Liu, Y.; Biesiada, J.; Meller, J.; Castello, A.A.; Jiang, B.; Jiang, X. Rotavirus VP8: Phylogeny, Host Range, and Interaction with Histo-Blood Group Antigens. *J. Virol.* **2012**, *86*, 9899–9910. [CrossRef] [PubMed]
16. Tan, M.; Jiang, X. Histo-blood group antigens: A common niche for norovirus and rotavirus. *Expert Rev. Mol. Med.* **2014**, *16*, e5. [CrossRef] [PubMed]
17. Andres, I.; Rodriguez-Diaz, J.; Buesa, J.; Zueco, J. Yeast expression of the VP8* fragment of the rotavirus spike protein and its use as immunogen in mice. *Biotechnol. Bioeng.* **2006**, *93*, 89–98. [CrossRef]
18. Dunn, S.J.; Fiore, L.; Werner, R.L.; Cross, T.L.; Broome, R.L.; Ruggeri, F.M.; Greenberg, H.B. Immunogenicity, antigenicity, and protection efficacy of baculovirus expressed VP4 trypsin cleavage products, VP5(1) and VP8 from rhesus rotavirus. *Arch. Virol.* **1995**, *140*, 1969–1978. [CrossRef]
19. Fix, A.D.; Harro, C.; McNeal, M.; Dally, L.; Flores, J.; Robertson, G.; Boslego, J.W.; Cryz, S. Safety and immunogenicity of a parenterally administered rotavirus VP8 subunit vaccine in healthy adults. *Vaccine* **2015**, *33*, 3766–3772. [CrossRef]
20. Gil, M.T.; De Souza, C.O.; Asensi, M.; Buesa, J. Homotypic Protection Against Rotavirus-Induced Diarrhea in Infant Mice Breast-Fed by Dams Immunized with the Recombinant VP8 Subunit of the VP4 Capsid Protein. *Viral Immunol.* **2000**, *13*, 187–200. [CrossRef]
21. Marelli, B.; Pérez, A.R.; Banchio, C.; De Mendoza, D.; Magni, C. Oral immunization with live Lactococcus lactis expressing rotavirus VP8* subunit induces specific immune response in mice. *J. Virol. Methods* **2011**, *175*, 28–37. [CrossRef]
22. Rodríguez-Díaz, J.; Montava, R.; Viana, R.; Buesa, J.; Pérez-Martínez, G.; Monedero, V. Oral immunization of mice with Lactococcus lactis expressing the rotavirus VP8* protein. *Biotechnol. Lett.* **2011**, *33*, 1169–1175. [CrossRef]
23. Wen, X.; Cao, D.; Jones, R.W.; Li, J.; Szu, S.; Hoshino, Y. Construction and characterization of human rotavirus recombinant VP8* subunit parenteral vaccine candidates. *Vaccine* **2012**, *30*, 6121–6126. [CrossRef] [PubMed]
24. Wen, X.; Cao, D.; Jones, R.W.; Hoshino, Y.; Yuan, L. Tandem truncated rotavirus VP8* subunit protein with T cell epitope as non-replicating parenteral vaccine is highly immunogenic. *Hum. Vaccines Immunother.* **2015**, *11*, 2483–2489. [CrossRef] [PubMed]
25. Kang, D.K.; Kim, P.H.; Ko, E.J.; Seo, J.Y.; Seong, S.Y.; Kim, Y.H.; Kwon, I.C.; Jeong, S.Y.; Yang, J.M. Peroral immunization of microencapsulated human VP8 in combination with cholera toxin induces intestinal antibody responses. *Mol. Cells* **1999**, *9*, 609–616. [PubMed]
26. Lentz, E.; Mozgovoj, M.; Bellido, D.; Santos, M.D.; Wigdorovitz, A.; Bravo-Almonacid, F. VP8* antigen produced in tobacco transplastomic plants confers protection against bovine rotavirus infection in a suckling mouse model. *J. Biotechnol.* **2011**, *156*, 100–107. [CrossRef] [PubMed]
27. Wen, X.; Wen, K.; Cao, D.; Li, G.; Jones, R.W.; Li, J.; Szu, S.; Hoshino, Y.; Yuan, L. Inclusion of a universal tetanus toxoid CD4(+) T cell epitope P2 significantly enhanced the immunogenicity of recombinant rotavirus DeltaVP8* subunit parenteral vaccines. *Vaccine* **2014**, *32*, 4420–4427. [CrossRef]
28. Xue, M.; Yu, L.; Che, Y.; Lin, H.; Zeng, Y.; Fang, M.; Li, T.; Ge, S.; Xia, N. Characterization and protective efficacy in an animal model of a novel truncated rotavirus VP8 subunit parenteral vaccine candidate. *Vaccine* **2015**, *33*, 2606–2613. [CrossRef]
29. Groome, M.J.; Koen, A.; Fix, A.; Page, N.; Jose, L.; Madhi, S.A.; McNeal, M.; Dally, L.; Cho, I.; Power, M.; et al. Safety and immunogenicity of a parenteral P2-VP8-P[8] subunit rotavirus vaccine in toddlers and infants in South Africa: A randomised, double-blind, placebo-controlled trial. *Lancet Infect. Dis.* **2017**, *17*, 843–853. [CrossRef]
30. Tan, M.; Huang, P.; Xia, M.; Fang, P.A.; Zhong, W.; McNeal, M.; Wei, C.; Jiang, W.; Jiang, X. Norovirus P Particle, a Novel Platform for Vaccine Development and Antibody Production. *J. Virol.* **2011**, *85*, 753–764. [CrossRef]
31. Yuan, L.; Wen, K. Rotavirus. In *Laboratory Models for Foodborne Infections*; Liu, D., Ed.; CRC Press, Taylor & Francis: Boca Raton, FL, USA, 2017; pp. 95–107.
32. Yuan, L.; Saif, L.J. Induction of mucosal immune responses and protection against enteric viruses: Rotavirus infection of gnotobiotic pigs as a model. *Veter. Immunol. Immunopathol.* **2002**, *87*, 147–160. [CrossRef]

33. Saif, L.J.; Ward, L.A.; Yuan, L.; Rosen, B.I.; To, T.L. The gnotobiotic piglet as a model for studies of disease pathogenesis and immunity to human rotaviruses. *Viral Gastroenteritis* **1996**, *12*, 153–161.
34. Birchall, M.A.; Bailey, M.; Barker, E.V.; Rothkötter, H.-J.; Otto, K.; Macchiarini, P. Model for experimental revascularized laryngeal allotransplantation. *BJS* **2002**, *89*, 1470–1475. [CrossRef] [PubMed]
35. Rothkötter, H.J.; Sowa, E.; Pabst, R. The pig as a model of developmental immunology. *Hum. Exp. Toxicol.* **2002**, *21*, 533–536. [CrossRef] [PubMed]
36. Desselberger, U.; Huppertz, H.I. Immune responses to rotavirus infection and vaccination and associated correlates of protection. *J. Infect. Dis.* **2011**, *203*, 188–195. [CrossRef] [PubMed]
37. Yuan, L.; Kang, S.Y.; Ward, L.A.; To, T.L.; Saif, L.J. Antibody-Secreting Cell Responses and Protective Immunity Assessed in Gnotobiotic Pigs Inoculated Orally or Intramuscularly with Inactivated Human Rotavirus. *J. Virol.* **1998**, *72*, 330–338.
38. Ward, L.A.; Rosen, B.I.; Yuan, L.; Saif, L.J. Pathogenesis of an attenuated and a virulent strain of group A human rotavirus in neonatal gnotobiotic pigs. *J. Gen. Virol.* **1996**, *77*, 1431–1441. [CrossRef]
39. Wen, K.; Tin, C.; Wang, H.; Yang, X.; Li, G.; Giri-Rachman, E.; Kocher, J.; Bui, T.; Clark-Deener, S.; Yuan, L. Probiotic Lactobacillus rhamnosus GG Enhanced Th1 Cellular Immunity but Did Not Affect Antibody Responses in a Human Gut Microbiota Transplanted Neonatal Gnotobiotic Pig Model. *PLoS ONE* **2014**, *9*, e94504. [CrossRef]
40. Wentzel, J.F.; Yuan, L.; Rao, S.; Van Dijk, A.A.; O'Neill, H.G. Consensus sequence determination and elucidation of the evolutionary history of a rotavirus Wa variant reveal a close relationship to various Wa variants derived from the original Wa strain. *Infect. Genet. Evol.* **2013**, *20*, 276–283. [CrossRef]
41. Liu, F.; Wen, K.; Li, G.; Yang, X.; Kocher, J.; Bui, T.; Jones, D.; Pelzer, K.; Clark-Deener, S.; Yuan, L. Dual Functions of Lactobacillus acidophilus NCFM at The Intermediate Dose in Protection Against Rotavirus Diarrhea in Gnotobiotic Pigs Vaccinated with a Human Rotavirus Vaccine. *J. Pediatric Gastroenterol. Nutr.* **2014**, *58*, 171. [CrossRef]
42. Yuan, L.; Wen, K.; Azevedo, M.S.; Gonzalez, A.M.; Zhang, W.; Saif, L.J. Virus-specific intestinal IFN-gamma producing T cell responses induced by human rotavirus infection and vaccines are correlated with protection against rotavirus diarrhea in gnotobiotic pigs. *Vaccine* **2008**, *26*, 3322–3331. [CrossRef]
43. Yuan, L.J.; Jobst, P.M.; Weiss, M. Gnotobiotic Pigs: From Establishing Facility to Modeling Human Infectious Diseases. In *Gnotobiotics*; Schoeb, T.R., Eaton, K.A., Eds.; Acamedic Press: Cambridge, MA, USA, 2017; pp. 349–368.
44. Saif, L.; Yuan, L.; Ward, L.; To, T. Comparative Studies of the Pathogenesis, Antibody Immune Responses, and Homologous Protection to Porcine and Human Rotaviruses in Gnotobiotic Piglets. *Adv. Exp. Med. Biol.* **1997**, *412*, 397–403. [PubMed]
45. Azevedo, M.S.; Yuan, L.; Jeong, K.I.; Gonzalez, A.; Nguyen, T.V.; Pouly, S.; Gochnauer, M.; Zhang, W.; Azevedo, A.; Saif, L.J. Viremia and Nasal and Rectal Shedding of Rotavirus in Gnotobiotic Pigs Inoculated with Wa Human Rotavirus. *J. Virol.* **2005**, *79*, 5428–5436. [CrossRef] [PubMed]
46. Parre, V.; Hodgins, D.C.; Saif, L.J.; Yuan, L.; Kang, S.Y.; Yuan, L.; Ward, L.A.; De Arriba, L. Serum and intestinal isotype antibody responses to Wa human rotavirus in gnotobiotic pigs are modulated by maternal antibodies. *J. Gen. Virol.* **1999**, *80*, 1417–1428. [CrossRef] [PubMed]
47. Twitchell, E.L.; Tin, C.; Wen, K.; Zhang, H.; Becker-Dreps, S.; Azcarate-Peril, M.A.; Vilchez, S.; Li, G.; Ramesh, A.; Weiss, M.; et al. Modeling human enteric dysbiosis and rotavirus immunity in gnotobiotic pigs. *Gut Pathog.* **2016**, *8*, 51. [CrossRef] [PubMed]
48. Wang, Y.; Azevedo, M.; Saif, L.J.; Gentsch, J.R.; Glass, R.I.; Jiang, B. Inactivated rotavirus vaccine induces protective immunity in gnotobiotic piglets. *Vaccine* **2010**, *28*, 5432–5436. [CrossRef] [PubMed]
49. Yang, X.; Twitchell, E.; Li, G.; Wen, K.; Weiss, M.; Kocher, J.; Lei, S.; Ramesh, A.; Ryan, E.P.; Yuan, L. High protective efficacy of rice bran against human rotavirus diarrhea via enhancing probiotic growth, gut barrier function, and innate immunity. *Sci. Rep.* **2015**, *5*, 15004. [CrossRef]
50. Liu, F.; Li, G.; Wen, K.; Bui, T.; Cao, D.; Zhang, Y.; Yuan, L. Porcine Small Intestinal Epithelial Cell Line (IPEC-J2) of Rotavirus Infection as a New Model for the Study of Innate Immune Responses to Rotaviruses and Probiotics. *Viral Immunol.* **2010**, *23*, 135–149. [CrossRef]
51. Arnold, M.; Patton, J.T.; McDonald, S.M. Culturing, storage, and quantification of rotaviruses. *Curr. Protoc. Microbiol.* **2009**, *15*, 15C-3.

52. Shao, L.; Fischer, D.D.; Kandasamy, S.; Rauf, A.; Langel, S.N.; Wentworth, D.E.; Stucker, K.M.; Halpin, R.A.; Lam, H.C.; Marthaler, D.; et al. Comparative In Vitro and In Vivo Studies of Porcine Rotavirus G9P[13] and Human Rotavirus Wa G1P. *J. Virol.* **2015**, *90*, 142–151. [CrossRef]
53. Saif, L.J.; Yuan, L.; Ward, L.A. Serum and intestinal isotype antibody responses and correlates of protective immunity to human rotavirus in a gnotobiotic pig model of disease. *J. Gen. Virol.* **1998**, *79*, 2661–2672.
54. Yuan, L.; Ward, L.A.; Rosen, B.I.; To, T.L.; Saif, L.J. Systematic and intestinal antibody-secreting cell responses and correlates of protective immunity to human rotavirus in a gnotobiotic pig model of disease. *J. Virol.* **1996**, *70*, 3075–3083. [PubMed]
55. Lei, S.; Ryu, J.; Wen, K.; Twitchell, E.; Bui, T.; Ramesh, A.; Weiss, M.; Li, G.; Samuel, H.; Clark-Deener, S.; et al. Increased and prolonged human norovirus infection in RAG2/IL2RG deficient gnotobiotic pigs with severe combined immunodeficiency. *Sci. Rep.* **2016**, *6*, 25222. [CrossRef] [PubMed]
56. HogenEsch, H. Mechanism of Immunopotentiation and Safety of Aluminum Adjuvants. *Front. Immunol.* **2013**, *3*, 406. [CrossRef] [PubMed]
57. Westerman, L.E.; McClure, H.M.; Jiang, B.; Almond, J.W.; Glass, R.I. Serum IgG mediates mucosal immunity against rotavirus infection. *Proc. Natl. Acad. Sci. USA* **2005**, *102*, 7268–7273. [CrossRef] [PubMed]
58. Yuan, L.; Honma, S.; Kim, I.; Kapikian, A.Z.; Hoshino, Y. Resistance to rotavirus infection in adult volunteers challenged with a virulent G1P1A[8] virus correlated with serum immunoglobulin G antibodies to homotypic viral proteins 7 and 4. *J. Infect. Dis.* **2009**, *200*, 1443–1451. [CrossRef] [PubMed]
59. Xu, J.; Dennehy, P.; Keyserling, H.; Westerman, L.E.; Wang, Y.; Holman, R.C.; Gentsch, J.R.; Glass, R.I.; Jiang, B. Serum Antibody Responses in Children with Rotavirus Diarrhea Can Serve as Proxy for Protection. *Clin. Diagn. Lab. Immunol.* **2005**, *12*, 273–279. [CrossRef]
60. Jiang, B.; Gentsch, J.R.; Glass, R.I. The Role of Serum Antibodies in the Protection against Rotavirus Disease: An Overview. *Clin. Infect. Dis.* **2002**, *34*, 1351–1361. [CrossRef]
61. Steele, A.D.; Neuzil, K.M.; Cunliffe, N.A.; Madhi, S.A.; Bos, P.; Ngwira, B.; Witte, D.; Todd, S.; Louw, C.; Kirsten, M.; et al. Human rotavirus vaccine Rotarix™ provides protection against diverse circulating rotavirus strains in African infants: A randomized controlled trial. *BMC Infect. Dis.* **2012**, *12*, 213. [CrossRef]

vaccines

MDPI

Review

Hepatitis C Virus Vaccine: Challenges and Prospects

Joshua D. Duncan [1,2,3,*], Richard A. Urbanowicz [1,2,3], Alexander W. Tarr [1,2,3] and Jonathan K. Ball [1,2,3]

1 School of Life Sciences, The University of Nottingham, Nottingham NG7 2UH, UK; richard.urbanowicz@nottingham.ac.uk (R.A.U.); alex.tarr@nottingham.ac.uk (A.W.T.); jonathan.ball@nottingham.ac.uk (J.K.B.)
2 NIHR Nottingham BRC, Nottingham University Hospitals NHS Trust and the University of Nottingham, Nottingham NG7 2UH, UK
3 Nottingham Digestive Diseases Centre, School of Medicine, University of Nottingham, Nottingham NG7 2UH, UK
* Correspondence: joshua.duncan@nottingham.ac.uk

Received: 30 December 2019; Accepted: 4 February 2020; Published: 17 February 2020

Abstract: The hepatitis C virus (HCV) causes both acute and chronic infection and continues to be a global problem despite advances in antiviral therapeutics. Current treatments fail to prevent reinfection and remain expensive, limiting their use to developed countries, and the asymptomatic nature of acute infection can result in individuals not receiving treatment and unknowingly spreading HCV. A prophylactic vaccine is therefore needed to control this virus. Thirty years since the discovery of HCV, there have been major gains in understanding the molecular biology and elucidating the immunological mechanisms that underpin spontaneous viral clearance, aiding rational vaccine design. This review discusses the challenges facing HCV vaccine design and the most recent and promising candidates being investigated.

Keywords: hepatitis C virus; vaccines; neutralising antibodies; animal models; immune responses

1. Introduction

First discovered in 1989 [1], the hepatitis C virus (HCV) is a major global health burden. Current estimates of HCV prevalence state that approximately 1% of the world's population are infected [2]. Chronic infection with HCV leads to cirrhosis of the liver and is associated with the development of hepatocellular carcinoma (HCC). Annually, 400,000 deaths are attributed to HCV and in the US, deaths from HCV have now overtaken those attributed to the human immunodeficiency virus (HIV) [3]. The extensive damage resulting from chronic infection makes this virus the leading cause for liver transplantation, a procedure that ultimately results in reinfection of the transplanted organ [4,5]. In recent years, the growing problem of HCV prompted the World Health Organisation to set a target to eliminate HCV as a public health burden by 2030. However, in the absence of a vaccine against HCV, this will prove challenging.

Therapeutic treatment of HCV has been vastly improved over the past decade due to the development of direct acting antivirals (DAAs). These compounds act as inhibitors of either the NS3/4a serine protease, NS5a or the NS5b RNA-dependent polymerase [6] and can achieve a 95% cure rate [7]. However, there are limitations to this strategy. Firstly, in order to treat an infection, a diagnosis must be made which may not occur in asymptomatic cases. It has recently been reported that the diagnosis rate in 2014 in the United Kingdom was estimated at capturing less than half of infected individuals [8]. Secondly, the cost of these therapeutics limits their use in developed countries, and all but excludes their use in low and middle-income countries with high HCV burdens. Thirdly, the ability of HCV to rapidly respond to selective pressures means that the emergence of DAA-resistant strains is a major risk [9,10]. Indeed, resistance-associated substitutions (RAS) have been detected in circulating HCV strains in treatment naive patients [11,12]. One such example of a RAS that has been reported in treatment-naïve patients is the C316 mutation which has been associated with resistance to non-nucleotide NS5B inhibitors such as Nesbuvir [13]. Another example is the S282T RAS which is associated with sofosbuvir resistance in vitro [14] although at the time of writing this polymorphism is not prevalent in clinical cohorts. The risk of DAA-resistance is mitigated by using combinational therapies of DAAs that target different HCV proteins.

The ability to effectively treat HCV infection has been a major achievement. However, there is growing evidence that HCV can leave lasting impacts upon its host post infection. For example, during infection extensive liver fibrosis can occur, which can persist for several years after viral clearance. Furthermore, persistent hyperfunctional CD8+ T cell phenotype has been reported following successful treatment with DAAs, suggesting continued immunological impairment [15]. There are also conflicting reports about the risk of hepatocellular carcinoma after virus clearance [16,17]. Understanding the long-term effects following virus clearance will take years more research as more data become available from successful cases. However, it is now apparent that therapeutics alone are unlikely to achieve the 2030 elimination target and thus a vaccine is urgently needed.

Modelling based on viral kinetics in reinfected individuals with pre-existing immunity has shown that transmission risk can be greatly reduced when an immune response occurs, despite detectable virus RNA titres [18]. This is of particular importance when considering vaccination of people who inject drugs, a high-risk group for HCV infection and reinfection. This suggests that a successful vaccine could be used to reduce viral titres rather than inducing sterilising immunity. This is a key point as it provides a realistic goal for HCV vaccine research.

2. Host Immune Responses to Hepatitis C Virus

Virus-host interactions determine the outcome of acute HCV infection. This interplay is complex and includes components of both the adaptive and innate host immune system. The most common scenario is progression to chronic infection. However, 25%–40% of individuals undergo spontaneous viral clearance (SVC) [19,20] within 12 months of infection [21,22]. Approximately 80% of these individuals will achieve SVC a second time following reinfection [23] with a marked decrease in viral RNA titres and reduced infection times compared to the first infection [23,24]. This indicates that initial infection can lead to the establishment of an immunological memory which can control subsequent HCV infection. This protective response consists of both humoral and cellular adaptive immune responses that do not result in sterilising immunity but prevent chronic infection. This phenomenon provides a benchmark for HCV vaccine research and thus is vital to elucidate.

2.1. Innate Immune Reponses

Innate immunity provides a first line of defence against viral infection. The liver presents a unique microenvironment that is enriched with cells that participate in this response, namely Kupffer cells, natural killer (NK) cells, hepatic stellate cells (HSCs) and macrophages. Initial innate responses are triggered by HCV-derived pathogen-associated molecular patterns (PAMPs) that are recognised by pattern recognition receptors (PRRs). Virion-associated PAMPs are the E1 and E2 glycoproteins [25,26], while intracellular detection of viral PAMPs, including viral proteins and RNA, is mediated by toll-like receptors (TLRs), nucleotide-binding oligomerisation domain (NOD)-like receptors (NLRs) and retinoic acid-inducible gene-I-like receptors (RLRs) [27,28]. Activation of signalling cascades downstream of these receptors results in the production of proinflammatory cytokines including interleukin-1β (IL-1β), IL-18 and type I and type III interferons (IFNs). These IFNs mediate upregulation of interferon stimulated genes (ISGs) in an autocrine and paracrine manner leading to an antiviral response in the liver [29,30]. However, the HCV viral proteins core, E2, NS3/4a and NS5a all impair the expression of ISGs through disruption of signalling cascades, allowing the virus to overcome the host innate response [31,32]. This results in an innate immune response that is incapable of clearing HCV.

Successful SVC is influenced by the outcome of innate immune responses. A major example is the association of single nucleotide polymorphisms (SNP) rs12979860 present in the type III IFN gene *IFNλ4* with SVC. In this case approximately 50% of individuals with a C/C genotype achieve SVC [33,34]. Additionally, NK inhibitory receptor, killer immunoglobulin receptor 2DL3 (KIR2DL3) and human leukocyte antigen C group 1 (HLA-C1) are associated with SVC [35] due to a reduced inhibition of cytotoxic NK activity [36,37].

2.2. Ceullar Immune Responses

Cellular immunity has long been associated with spontaneous HCV clearance [38] and is mediated through two main T cell subsets, the cytolytic CD8+ T cells and CD4+ helper T cells. CD8+ T cells destroy infected cells in a manner restricted by MHCI presented epitopes [39]. In contrast, recognition by CD4+ helper T cells is MHCII restricted and their role is to aid the function of CD8+ T cells and the establishment of T cell memory through the secretion of cytokines such as IFN-γ [40,41]. CD4+ T cells also aid B cell activation and a CD4+ T cell subset, follicular helper T cells (T_{FH}) are required to establish a long-term antibody response [42,43]. HCV-specific T cells are detectable within the first 12 weeks of infection and target a broad range of HCV epitopes present on both structural and non-structural viral proteins [44]. During the progression to chronicity, the HCV-specific CD4+ T cells display an exhausted phenotype and the population collapses [45,46]. The decrease in CD4+ T cell function leads to a dysregulated CD8+ T cell response in which these cells become exhausted and dysfunctional with reports of continued IFN-γ secretion but an absence of cytolytic activity [47]. The reasons for this reduction in effective cellular responses are incompletely understood. The loss of functional HCV-specific T cells could be the result of host regulation of the immune system since persistent antigen stimulation could lead to the prolonged production of proinflammatory cytokines which in turn contributes to hepatic tissue damage.

The importance of T cells to SVC was first demonstrated in experimentally infected chimpanzee in which HCV persistence was observed in the absence of either a CD4+ or CD8+ T cell response [48,49]. Interestingly, when CD4+ T cells were depleted HCV persisted alongside functional CD8+ T cell responses. HCV-specific CD4+ T cells and CD8+ T cells are detectable during acute infection [45]. This provides strong evidence that the T cell responses have a major role in the outcome of HCV infection. HCV-specific CD4+ T cells are broadly targeting with the most common epitopes being found in the core, E2, NS3, NS4a, NS4b, NS5a and NS5b HCV proteins [44].

2.3. Humoral Immune Responses

Neutralising antibodies (nAbs) in the context of HCV infection were first described by Farci et al. [50], although their role in spontaneous clearance was disputed for many years due to reports of cell mediated clearance in seronegative individuals [51–53], suggesting that nAbs are not essential to achieve SVC. However, analysis of sera from individuals who cleared HCV has shown the presence of nAbs and these are detectable at earlier time points compared to acute infections that proceed to chronicity and are subsequently lost following viral clearance [54] suggesting that a rapid, short-lived humoral response is required for clearance [55–58]. It has recently been shown that nAbs generated within the first 100 days of infection often have a narrow neutralising capacity directed towards the founder virus [58]. The selective pressure exerted by nAbs upon the circulating strains can also drive the evolution of HCV towards escape mutations that compromise viral fitness further aiding clearance of the infection [59,60]. The delayed appearance of cross-reactive nAb responses are apparent in chronically infected individuals as isolated sera can neutralise circulating strains from previous infection time points with greater potency than the current dominant virus [56] and cross-reactive nAbs have been isolated from chronically infected individuals [61–64]. Although these nAbs cannot clear the infection, they have been associated with reduced liver fibrosis [65] and patients that experience hypogammaglobulinemia have a more severe disease progression [66].

Further insight into the humoral response has been obtained through characterising nAbs derived from patients. Bailey et al. [67] sequenced cross-reactive nAbs isolated from two individuals that cleared HCV and showed these nAbs shared >90% similarity with germline heavy chain variable (VH) genes and >92% similarity with germline light chain gene sequences revealing that generation of cross-reactive nAbs required limited somatic hypermutation. A common feature of these nAbs was the *VH1-69* gene which is found in potent cross-reactive nAbs that target antigenic region 3 (AR3) and is also present in nAbs targeting HIV and Influenza [68–71]. Structural investigation has also shown that cross-neutralising activity is a result of long complementarity-determining region H3 (CDRH3), typically 18–22 residues, that forms a β-hairpin structure that is stabilized by a disulphide bond allowing for interaction with conserved E2 epitopes [72,73]. This level of insight into how potent nAbs work can inform rational design of B-cell immunogens to favour the production of these types of antibodies in the host.

3. Hepatitis C Virus Envelope Proteins as Vaccine Targets

The HCV envelope glycoproteins, E1 and E2, are located at residues 192–746 of the polyprotein and are the targets of the humoral immune response, making them an attractive vaccine target [74] (Figure 1A). Both E1 and E2 are type I transmembrane proteins that form an intracellular non-covalent heterodimer that form higher order covalent structures on the mature virion [75,76]. The E2 ectodomain contains an immunoglobulin-like β-sandwich that is flanked by α-helices which form a front and back layer [77,78]. There are also regions that exhibit high levels of variability which are referred to as hypervariable regions (HVRs) 1 and 2, and a third intergenotypic variable region (IgVR; Figure 1A). The E1 protein is smaller, more conserved than E2 and less well characterized with partial crystal structures resolved for fragments encompassing residues 192-271 [79] and 314–324 [80].

The E1E2 heterodimer mediates entry into the hepatocytes through interactions with four essential host receptors, CD81 [81,82], scavenger receptor B1 (SRB1) [83], claudin [84] and occludin [85,86]. The first step in viral entry is the interaction between SRB1 and the HVR1 (Figure 1A) located at the N-terminus of E2 which induces a conformational change that exposes the conserved E2 core region and the CD81 binding loop (residues 519–535) [77]. The interaction between E2 and CD81 results in recruitment of claudin to CD81 which leads to clathrin-mediated endocytosis [87]. Membrane fusion occurs in low pH endosomes, which is thought to induce a conformational change in the E1E2 heterodimer [88]. This leads to membrane fusion, possibly mediated by E1 via the action of a putative fusion peptide located at residues 272–285 (Figure 1A) [89].

Antibody-mediated neutralisation of HCV is achieved through targeting the E1E2 heterodimer on the surface of the virus. To date, most characterized nAbs target the E2 protein. The are several linear and discontinuous regions of E2 that are targeted by Abs and these have varying nomenclature, being referred to as ARs1-5 [69], Epitopes I-III (Figure 1) [90], or domains A-E [91]. Importantly, AR4 and 5 are reliant on the presence of the E1E2 heterodimer for binding [69]. The epitope I, II and AR3 regions form the neutralising face of E2 which is targeted by some of the most potent cross-reactive nAbs described to date [92] arguing for their inclusion in a nAb-eliciting vaccine.

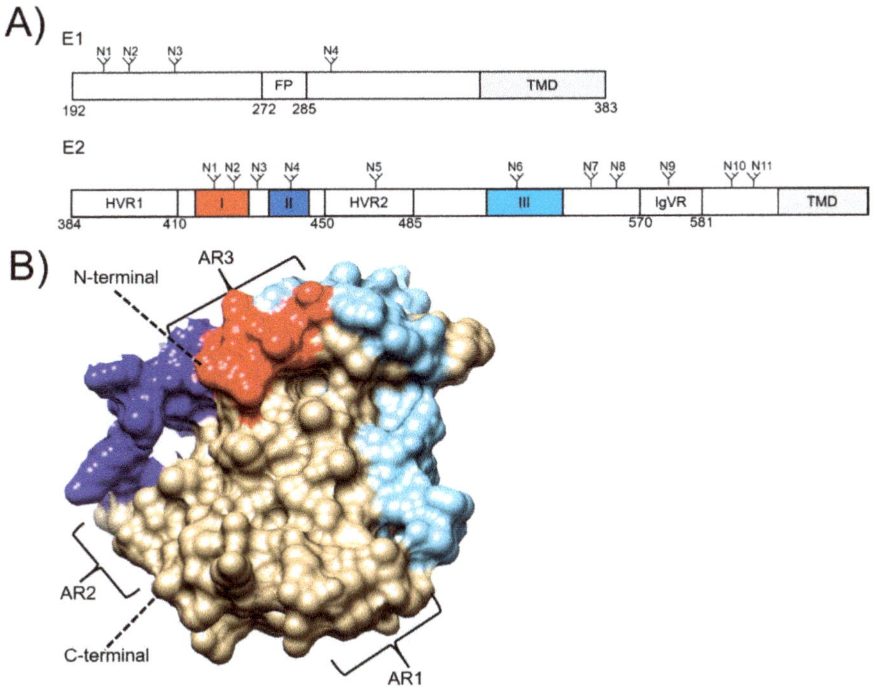

Figure 1. (**A**) Schematic diagrams of the hepatitis C virus envelope glycoproteins E1 and E2, showing N-linked glycosylation sites (N), transmembrane domains (TMDs), and the E1 fusion peptide (FP). E2 hypervariable regions (HVRs) 1 and 2, and the intergentypic variable region (IgVR) are also depicted. Linear epitopes I, II and III are highlighted in red, dark blue and light blue, respectively. (**B**) E2 structure (PDB: 6MEH). Linear epitopes I, II and III are highlighted in the corresponding schematic. Antigenic regions (ARs) are also shown.

4. Challenges to Hepatitis C Virus Vaccine Design

4.1. Genetic Diversity

As a species, HCV exhibits extensive genetic diversity is driven by a mutation rate in the order of 10^{-4} substitutions per site of the genome [93,94]. Mutations are acquired through the activity of the error prone NS5b RNA-dependent RNA polymerase and this coupled with high levels of virus production and selective pressures exerted by the host immune response has driven the diversification of HCV. There are currently eight genotypes (Gt1-8) reported which are defined by 30% difference in nucleotide sequence [95]. Gt1 HCV isolates have the highest prevalence, accounting for 49% of diagnosed cases globally followed by Gt3 accounting for 17.9% of cases [96], and are more prevalent in developed countries [96]. In contrast, Gt4 and Gt5 isolates are more prevalent in lower income countries in Africa and the Middle Eastern regions [96]. Genotypes are further classified into subtypes of which there are currently 90 confirmed groups. These exhibit a 15% variation in nucleotide sequence [95]. Gt1-7 contain multiple subtypes. However, the recently reported Gt8 group currently contains a single subtype isolated from four individuals [97]. Rapid evolution of HCV during the course of an infection leads to the establishment of a heterogeneous population [98]. The diversification of this population is driven by host immune selective pressure and the degree to which variation occurs in acute infection correlates with a progression to chronicity [99].

The extent of genetic diversity gives rise to genotype-specific immune responses. The E1E2 sequence shows the greatest level of variation as a result of the selective pressure exerted by the host immune response [100], leading to humoral responses that can have reduced heterologous neutralising activity [101]. However, cross-reactive nAbs that are capable of targeting isolates from different genotypes have been described in several studies [102], thus highlighting that this challenge can be overcome. Epitope variability also leads to genotype-specific cellular responses for example Luxenburger et al. [103] have recently shown CD8+ T cells from individuals chronically infected with a Gt4 HCV isolate failed to recognize Gt1 derived epitopes. Limited intergenotypic cross-reactivity of Gt3 HCV-specific T cells has also been reported in patients that successfully cleared Gt3 infections [104]. Limited cross-reactive immune responses to distantly related HCV isolates will be a key challenge to produce an effective vaccine

4.2. Evading the Host Adaptive Immune Response

The ability of HCV to establish a chronic infection highlights the efficiency in which this virus can subvert the host immune response. This is achieved through multiple strategies. Firstly, immunodominant epitopes such as the HVR1 of E2 elicit a response of non-neutralising antibodies. Currently it is thought that HVR1 acts as a shield of the more conserved epitopes in the E2 core that contain CD81 binding residues, since removal of HVR1 increases virus susceptibility to neutralisation [105,106]. Evidence also shows that HVR1 induces greater homologous nAbs and deletion induces broader heterologous nAbs [107].

Epitope masking is also achieved through the glycosylation of envelope proteins to form a glycan shield [108]. This mechanism diminishes the binding of nAbs and is used by other viruses such as HIV and Influenza although by comparison, HCV exhibits a reduced variability in the position of each glycan group. The E1 and E2 proteins contain 4 and 11 N-linked glycosylation sites which are highly conserved across different genotypes (Figure 1A) [109]. Deletion of E2 glycosylation sites increases HCV susceptibility to nAbs showing that glycosylation acts via steric hinderance to nAbs [109,110]. Interestingly, removal of E2 glycan sites or expression of this protein in systems that use smaller, less complex glycan groups enhance the immunogenicity compared to mammalian expressed E2 [111–113]. Another mechanism in which nAb resistance can be mediated through glycosylation is glycan shift. This arises through non-synonymous mutations that result in the deletion of a glycosylation site and the appearance of a new glycosylation site in a different position in the protein. Pantua et al. [114] reported this phenomenon after incubating cell cultured HCV (HCVcc) with the murine nAb, AP33 which targets residues within the E2 epitope I region [115]. After 5 days of incubation with AP33, escape mutants could be detected which contained either N417S or N417T residue variations coupled with a new glycosylation site at position 415 [114].

The evasion of nAbs can also be attributed to the presence of host derived factors. One such factor is high-density lipoproteins which are present in human serum and has been shown to increase HCV infectivity via SR-BI interactions which in turn decreases the time available for nAbs to bind to their target [116,117]. Additionally, the presence of host derived apolipoprotein E on the mature HCV virion has been shown to have a role in epitope masking the E2 protein abrogating nAb activity [118]. Another evasion method is through the use of decoys. Recently it has been reported that in a HCVcc system, infected cells produce lipid droplets coated with the E2 protein [119]. This may also be a strategy to subvert the immune system by using these E2-coated droplets to interact with nAbs, thereby reducing the availability of nAbs to target E2 present on the surface of the virus particle. Finally, evasion from nAbs has recently been shown to be associated with resistance to antiviral interferon-induced transmembrane (IFITM) proteins [120] showing that the innate immune response can also be a driving force for nAb evasion.

4.3. Models for Hepatitis C Virus Infection

4.3.1. In Vitro Models

Since the discovery of HCV, research was hampered by the lack of infection models both in vivo and in vitro. The use of models in vaccine research is essential for the assessment of sera and monoclonal antibodies arising from natural infection, experimental immunizations or vaccine trials. In the case of in vitro models, the key challenge was generating a cell culture-based system that could produce infectious HCV at titres suitable for further experimentation. This problem was solved with the discovery of two Gt2a isolates, JFH1 and J6 which produce high titres of infectious HCV from cultured Huh 7.5 cells [121]. Following this, it was found that intergenotypic recombinant viruses consisting of core-NS2 of an isolate of interest fused to NS3-NS5b of JFH-1 could produce viable chimeric viruses [121]. The developments in HCVcc techniques have allowed panels with representatives of the seven major genotypes to be set up [122–124]. Our group has recently described a method in which E1E2 patient derived sequences could be incorporated into chimeric HCVcc expression vectors [125,126], further aiding the ability to characterize isolates that have different neutralisation phenotypes.

Viral pseudotyping has also been used to study the entry mechanism of HCV. This approach utilizes the ability of retroviral gag/pol proteins to self-assemble into enveloped virus particles. Simultaneous expression of foreign viral envelope proteins in the same cells leads to the incorporation on to the surface of the retroviral particle whose entry properties are dictated by the envelope glycoprotein. Infectivity can be measured by the incorporation of a reporter gene, usually luciferase, which is introduced into target cells and expressed. Methods to generate HCV pseudoparticles (HCVpps) commonly use murine leukemia virus or HIV derived vectors [127,128]. Our group and others have utilized these systems to characterize extensive panels of patient-derived E1E2 sequences allowing important characterisation of these unique isolates [57,129–131]. These studies have shown that neutralisation sensitivity of patient derived isolates to both sera and monoclonal nAbs is markedly varied and not associated with genotype but is isolate dependent. Furthermore, it has been shown that the HCV reference isolate H77, a Gt1a isolate that was first adopted due to its ability to infect and cause disease in chimpanzees [132–134], is more susceptible to antibody-mediated neutralisation than many patient-derived isolates [102]. This finding is of significance since H77 neutralisation has been used to validate multiple vaccine candidates and therefore these data provide limited insight into how effective a candidate may be towards clinically relevant isolates. H77 has also been used in the design of immunogens with moderate success, although it could be argued that immunogen design based on more nAb-resistant isolates may elicit more potent nAbs.

The ability to generate both HCVcc and HCVpp provide essential tools for the in vitro study of HCV and assessing the neutralising breadth of sera and monoclonal nAbs. The importance of isolate panels for the validation of vaccine candidates is exemplified in the field of HIV vaccine research, in which candidates have been tested against an extensive panel of 109 isolates developed by Seaman et al. [135], which are grouped based on neutralisation susceptibility. In this way humoral responses following vaccination can be assessed in a standardized manner allowing for relevant comparisons between candidates and vaccines that induce responses capable of neutralising the most resistant isolates can be identified for further development. At the time of writing a consensus panel of isolates is yet to be widely adopted but doing so will greatly enhance our understanding of which candidates are promising and those that are not.

4.3.2. In Vivo Models

Humans are the natural host of HCV, and therefore it is imperative that suitable in vivo models are used in order to test the efficacy and safety of preclinical vaccine candidates. Arguably, the most successful model has been the chimpanzee, which is permissive to HCV infection under experimental conditions. However, ethical concerns over the use of this species has led to a ban on its use in experimental research. An alternative has been the use of chimeric humanized or transgenic mouse models which have humanized livers such as Alb-uPA/SCID mice [136,137] or those engineered to express human CD81 and occludin [138,139]. There are limitations to using chimeric mouse models, most notably that they do not exhibit cirrhosis or HCC, and are technically difficult to produce [140].

In light of the limited options available for the in vivo modelling of HCV, there has been increasing interest in other members of the *Hepacivirus* genus for use as analogues. At the time of writing there are two species of particular interest, the Rodent Hepacivirus (RHV) and the Equine Hepacivirus (EqHV). RHV was initially discovered in the species *Rattus norvegicus* in 2014 [141]. Experimental infection of different lab rat breeds leads to the establishment of permanent infection with features observed during HCV infection in humans such as hepatic fibrosis, steatosis and evidence of SVC in the Holtzman rat strain [142]. There are key contrasts between RHV and HCV infections, notably the lack of IFN-γ+ CD8+ T cell responses during RHV infection [143].

EqHV was initially discovered in canines and subsequent serology testing identified equines as the natural host [144,145]. This virus is the closest relative of HCV and there are shared features of both species such as similar levels of glycosylation of the E1E2 proteins and a conserved seed site in the 5′-UTR for the liver-specific microRNA-122 (miR-122) which contributes to stability, translation, and replication of the viral RNA [146]. Seroprevalence of EqHV is in the region of 30% of surveyed horses, with approximately 3% testing positive for viral RNA [147]. This discrepancy between serology and viral RNA may be indicative of a high viral clearance rate. Despite this potential high clearance rate, EqHV acute infection may proceed to chronicity after 6 months [148], further validating the relevancy of this virus as a model for HCV.

The use of analogous Hepacivirus species will allow for the testing of vaccine strategies and the experimental challenge in the natural host of that species, a feat that cannot currently be achieved for HCV. Whilst these approaches are likely to prove highly valuable to the field of HCV vaccine research it is important to acknowledge the differences in mammalian immune systems and how this will impact on our interpretation of experimental data. For example, the *IgVH 1-69* gene with an extended CDRH3 region has previously been described as a feature of anti-HCV specific nAbs that are elicited in SVC and therefore it is logical that a vaccine candidate could be assessed based on its ability to elicit these types of nAbs. With this in mind it is worth considering how comparable the antibodies of animal model species are to those of humans. One such difference is the length of the CDRH3 regions which are typically 16 residues long [149], however these are reduced to an average of 12 to 14 residues in rodent [149] and equine species [150], respectively. The CDRH3 region can be critical for the formation of the antigen-antibody complex and extended CDRH3 loops are effective at penetrating the glycan shield of viral envelope proteins, a favorable characteristic of anti-HCV nAbs. This raises an important question about the relevance and suitability of current animal models as predictors of the human antibody response. Similarly, the paradigm of vaccine research has been to test novel candidates in small animals followed by larger animal species before clinical testing in humans. This approach enables evaluation of immunogenicity and safety prior to exposure of an immunogen in humans. However, questions should be asked as to whether this approach has hindered the progress of at least some HCV vaccine candidates because of differences between the model and human antibody repertoires.

4.4. Rational Design of Immunogens to Elicit Cross-Reactive Neutralising Antibodies

The informed, rational design of immunogens will be vital in order to produce a successful HCV vaccine. As advances in the analysis of antibody repertoires are allowing deeper insight into the types of nAbs that are associated with SVC, there is potential to use this information to develop immunogens that favour the production of these types of antibodies. An example of this can be seen with the E2 epitope I region or antigenic site 412 (AS412). This linear epitope is structurally flexible and when in complex with nAbs and adopts three distinct conformations. Firstly epitope I forms an extended conformation in complex with the rat nAb 3/11, a β-hairpin conformation is observed when bound to AP33 or the human nAb HCV-1, and an intermediate conformation occurs when in complex with the human nAb HC33.1 [151]. As previously discussed, HCV may escape epitope I targeting nAbs by the mechanism of glycan shift. However, this mechanism does not abrogate and instead enhances the potency of HC33.1 [152]. With this in mind, rational design of an immunogen could strive to present the epitope I region in an intermediate conformation to bias the humoral response to elicit HC33.1-like nAbs. To date this has not been investigated however, efforts have been undertaken to present epitope I in the β-hairpin conformation using cyclic peptides based on θ-defensin which adopts a similar conformation [153]. This approach induced nAb responses when tested in mice however these were lower compared to mice immunized with E2 [153]. The rational design of HCV epitopes in this way is technically challenging and is limited to targeting linear epitopes. Additionally, delivery of cyclic peptides will require further development in order to enhance the immunogenicity and stimulate greater titers of nAbs.

5. Vaccine Prospects

Despite the challenges faced in HCV vaccine design, there have been a variety of different vaccine approaches investigated with a small number of these candidates reaching human trials (summarized in Table 1). Currently, DNA and peptide-based vaccine candidates are actively being investigated in murine models [154–158]. One recently reported peptide candidate consisted of overlapping peptides derived from the p7 protein which induced antigen-specific CD4+ T cells and cytotoxic CD8+ T cells capable of targeting p7 expressing hepatocytes in vivo [154]. This study has been the first to show the immunogenicity of p7 when used as the sole target in a vaccine. Additionally, a DNA-based vaccine has been shown to induce CD4+ T cell and CD8+ T cell responses and elicit T cell memory in mice; however, a non-neutralising Ab response was also observed [156]. These vaccine candidates are in an early stage of development and therefore the following sections will discuss candidates that have been more extensively studied.

5.1. Recombinant Subunit Vaccines

Recombinant subunit vaccines are an attractive technology as they have previously been utilized for a variety of pathogens [159] and are economical to produce on a commercial scale. In the field of HCV vaccine research, attempts to generate a subunit vaccine have focused exclusively on targeting the HCV E proteins. The most successful candidate has been the recombinant E1E2 protein (rE1E2) derived from a Gt1a isolate. Initially, HCV-1 derived rE1E2 was used to vaccinate seven chimpanzees which resulted in a humoral response [160]. Following homologous HCV challenge, five out of seven vaccinated chimpanzees exhibited sterilising immunity with the remaining two developing acute infections that were subsequently cleared [160,161]. This was further validated in small animal models and that immunisation rE1E2 derived from a single isolate could induce cross-reactive nAbs [161]. Following this work, a phase I human trial was performed in which rE1E2 derived from the Gt1a HCV-1 isolate was administered at different doses (4 μg, 20 μg and 100 μg of rE1E2) with the MF59 adjuvant to healthy volunteers [162]. Importantly this study showed that rE1E2 can be safely tolerated in humans, a finding of significance given that a successful HCV vaccine candidate will likely require these proteins or derivatives of them. Polyfunctional CD4+ T cell responses were detected and the magnitude of this response was inversely related to dosage. Humoral responses and nAbs were initially reported [162,163] and further testing using a diverse HCVcc panel with isolates from Gt1-7 showed that 3/16 volunteers had elicited cross reactive nAbs [164]. Additionally, post vaccination sera from 5 volunteers competed with nAbs AP33, AR3B, AR4A, AR5A and IGH526, showing that the humoral response targeted both E1, E2 and the E1E2 heterodimer [165]. The ability for rE1E2 from a single isolate to induce nAbs in humans is significant and encouraging although work should be undertaken to enhance the efficacy at which nAbs are generated. A key issue with rE1E2 was purification which relied on lectin-based affinity methods that were low affinity and non-specific [166]. Furthermore, efforts to improve rE1E2 production were made by removing the transmembrane domains of the E protein. However, this truncated E1E2 was found to be a weak immunogen that elicited low levels of nAbs [167]. In light of these issues, both flag-tagged and Fc-tagged rE1E2 have been investigated and elicit nAbs in mice at comparable levels to wild type rE1E2 [166,168].

Another subunit vaccine approach has been the use of truncated soluble E2 (sE2) which results in a secreted form of the E2 ectodomain. A candidate of particular note is the H77 derived sE2384-661 construct with deleted HVR1, HVR2 and IgVR ($sE2_{\Delta123}$) which can be expressed in a correct conformation which interacts with CD81 and conformation sensitive antibodies [169–171]. Vietheer et al. [170] reported that the expression of $sE2_{\Delta123}$ in mammalian cells results in biochemically and immunogenically distinct isoforms of this protein that exist as monomeric, dimeric, pentameric and a high molecular weight aggregate (HMW1; estimated at 51 protomers). Immunisation of guinea pigs with different isoforms showed that HMW1 elicited greater titres of cross-reactive nAbs that could neutralise isolates from Gt2a, 4a, 5a, 6a and 7a expressed in a HVCcc system [170]. Additionally, HMW1 had exhibited a reduced activity with non-neutralising antibodies, suggesting that this aggregate focuses the humoral immune response away from these epitopes, allowing for greater focusing to nAb epitopes [170]. Whilst this initial report is promising, it was noted that $sE2_{\Delta123}$ reduced homologous neutralisation activity, a likely result of the removal of HVR1 which was also observed by Law and colleagues [172].

5.2. *Virus-Like Particles*

Virus-like particles (VLPs) are a promising area of vaccine research and have been investigated extensively to design a HCV vaccine [173]. To date, there are two widely used commercial vaccines that utilize VLP technology, the hepatitis B virus (HBV) and human papilloma virus vaccines. VLPs are formed when the structural proteins of a virus assemble in a genome-independent manner to produce a particle that resembles the native virus whilst lacking the ability to replicate and are more immunogenic than soluble protein due to their repetitive structure and ability to drain into tissue lymph nodes [107,174].

HCV-LPs were first described by Baumert et al. [175] in which VLPs were expressed in the insect cell line Sf9 following transduction with a recombinant baculovirus containing the core E1 and E2 HCV structural proteins. These HCV-LPs elicited HCV-specific IgG production, IFN-γ secreting CD8+ T cell and CD4+ T cell mediated cellular responses in mice and baboons [176–178]. Immunisation of four chimpanzees with four doses of HCV-LPs resulted in CD4+ and CD8+ T cell responses in all animals [179]. Subsequent challenge with homologous HCV resulted in a reduced viremia in vaccinated animals compared to controls with two animals testing negative for HCV two years post challenge [179]. Interestingly, humoral responses in chimpanzees were not detectable in three of these animals and appear to have been absent during the reduction of viremia. Further work on this candidate has not been progressed since this first study in chimpanzees. However, it is an important example for future HCV vaccine work, as it showed that viral clearance can be achieved using an experimental VLP vaccine candidate. Despite work on this candidate ceasing, HCV-LPs continued to be investigated. Recently, a HCV-LP system has been established through the transduction of the human hepatoma cell line Huh 7 with recombinant adenovirus encoding the structural genes of HCV [180]. Initially designed using the H77 isolate, further development has expanded by generating HCV-LPs using the structural sequences of different isolates representing Gt1b, 2a and 3a subtypes to produce HCV-LPs with a conformation close to that the wild type virus [180–183]. Trials of this candidate in mice showed the induction of nAbs and activation of both CD4+ and CD8+ T cell responses and this has recently been reported in a vaccinated Landrace pigs [184]. To date, assessment of the humoral response has demonstrated that this vaccine elicits nAbs with activity towards homologous strains. Heterologous neutralisation data have not been reported for this candidate. Testing the sera from animals immunized with this quadrivalent vaccine against a diverse panel of HCV isolates would be of particular interest not only for this candidate but to inform future vaccine design.

5.3. Viral Vector Vaccines

Viral vectors have the capacity to induce high level cellular immune responses [185], making them an attractive approach for HCV candidates. Viral vectors of particular interest are human adenovirus 6 (HuAd6), chimpanzees Ad 3 (ChAd3) and modified vaccinia ankara (MVA) [186]. The only HCV vaccine candidates to be tested in phase I and phase I/II human trials has been ChAd3 and MVA which each encoded HCV NS3, NS4a, NS4b, NS5a and inactivated NS5b (NSmut) derived from the Gt1b BK isolate [187,188]. These candidates were tested together in a heterologous primer/boost strategy in which healthy human volunteers were primed with ChAd3-NSmut and boosted with MVA-NSmut 8 weeks later [188]. The results of this phase I study showed that prime/boost ChAd3/MVA-NSmut induced both CD4+ T cell and CD8+ T cell responses directed towards epitopes on all five HCV non-structural proteins, importantly the effect of the MVA-NSmut enhanced the T cell responses and these were detectable at week 70 [188]. Given the promising cellular responses observed in the phase I trial, this approach was tested in patients with chronic HCV infections although this was unable to reverse T cell exhaustion [189], ruling out the use of ChAd3/MVA-NSmut as a therapeutic vaccine. Recently ChAd3/MVA-NSmut was tested in a large phase I/II trial involving 548 high risk individuals was concluded (clinicaltrials.gov identifier: NCT01436357). At the time of writing, this trial has concluded, and data have yet to be published. However, a press release statement from the National Institute of Allergy and Infectious Disease stated that 14 vaccinated individuals became chronically infected with HCV, suggesting that this candidate does not provide protection against HCV infection [190]. Understanding the reasons for this failure will be vital to inform our understanding of vaccine design. Given that the ChAd3/MVA-NSmut candidate exclusively targeted T-cell epitopes, the failure of this vaccine candidate could further emphasize the need for both humoral and cellular immune responses in clearance of acute infections.

Table 1. Summary of recent hepatitis C virus vaccine candidates. Subunit, virus-like particle (VLP), viral vector, peptide and DNA vaccine approaches are listed with the vaccine target, genotype (Gt) and isolate from which the candidate was derived, tested species and the humoral and cellular immune responses were reported.

Vaccine Type	HCV Target	HCV Strain	Tested Species	Antibody Response *	CD4+ T Cell Response †	CD8+ T Cell Response †	Ref.
Subunit							
HCV-1 rE1E2	E1E2	Gt1a HCV-1	humans	homologous and heterologous	yes	N.D	[162,164]
H77 sE2$_{\Delta 123}$	E2core	Gt1a H77	guinea pigs	homologous and heterologous	N.D	N.D	[170]
Virus-Like particles							
core, E1, E2 from Gt1a, 1b, 2a and 3a	core, E1, E2	Gt1a H77, Gt1b BK, Gt2a JFH1, Gt3a	mice, pigs	homologous neutralising antibodies	yes	yes	[181,184]
HBV/HCV-LPs	E1, E2	Gt1a H77	rabbit	homologous, heterologous activity towards Gt1a and 1b, reduced activity towards Gt2a and 3a isolates.	N.D	N.D	[191]
HBV/HCV-LPs	linear E1 and E2 epitopes	not stated	mice	heterologous towards Gt1a, 1b and 2a	N.D	N.D	[192]
murine leukaemia VLP-HCVE1E2	E1, E2	Gt1a H77	mice, macaques	homologous, heterologous towards Gt1b, 2a, 2b and 4c	yes	N.D	[193]
Viral vector							
ChAd3/MVA-Nsmut	NS3, NS4a, NS4b, NS5a, NS5b	Gt1a BK	humans	N/A	yes	yes	[188]
Peptide							
p7	p7	Gt1b J4	mice	N/A	yes	yes	[154]
HCVp6-MAP	E1, E2, NS4b, NS5a, NS5b	Gt4a ED43	mice	homologous, heterologous towards JFH1	yes	yes	[155]
DNA							
pVax-sE1E2-IMX313P	E1, E2	Gt1b	mice	homologous, heterologous towards Gt1a, 1b, 2a, 2b, 3a, 4a, 5, 6	yes	N.D	[158]
DREP-HCV/MVA-HCV	core, E1, E1, p7, NS2, NS3	Gt1a H77	mice	non-neutralising IgG	yes	yes	[156]
pVax-N3-NS5b	NS3, NS4, NS5b	Gt1b, Gt3a	mice	N/A	yes	yes	[157]

* N/A (not applicable) for vaccine candidates that are not designed to elicit HCV-specific B cell responses. † N.D (not determined) in the study.

6. Conclusions

In the 30 years since the discovery of HCV, it has been apparent that this virus is highly complex and presents a major public health challenge. Encouragingly, efforts toward a vaccine continue and investigation into a range of approaches have yielded interesting results. The vast improvements in in vitro analysis of HCV have greatly aided our understanding of how nAbs work, informing rational vaccine design. In this review, we have highlighted the potential advantages of adopting reference panels of patient-derived E1E2 sequences in order to assess vaccine candidates for their potential to induce nAbs capable of targeting circulating HCV strains. Adopting this approach will provide a more rigorous tool for evaluating the nAb response produced by novel HCV vaccine candidates a characteristic that will likely be essential in a successful HCV vaccine.

Author Contributions: Writing—original draft preparation, J.D.D.; review and editing, R.A.U., A.W.T. and J.K.B.; funding acquisition, J.K.B. All authors have read and agreed to the published version of the manuscript.

Funding: This research was supported by the Medical Research Council [grant number MR/R010307/1]; and the NIHR Nottingham Biomedical Research Centre. The views expressed are those of the authors and not necessarily those of the NHS, the NIHR or the Department of Health and Social Care.

Conflicts of Interest: The authors declare no conflict of interest.

References

1. Choo, Q.L.; Kuo, G.; Weiner, A.J.; Overby, L.R.; Bradley, D.W.; Houghton, M. Isolation of a cDNA clone derived from a blood-borne non-A, non-B viral hepatitis genome. *Science* **1989**, *244*, 359–362. [CrossRef]
2. Collaborators, H. Global prevalence and genotype distribution of hepatitis C virus infection in 2015: A modelling study. *Lancet Gastroenterol. Hepatol.* **2017**, *2*, 161–176. [CrossRef]
3. Ly, K.N.; Xing, J.; Klevens, R.M.; Jiles, R.B.; Holmberg, S.D. Causes of death and characteristics of decedents with viral hepatitis, United States, 2010. *Clin. Infect. Dis.* **2014**, *58*, 40–49. [CrossRef]
4. Joshi, D.; Pinzani, M.; Carey, I.; Agarwal, K. Recurrent HCV after liver transplantation-mechanisms, assessment and therapy. *Nat. Rev. Gastroenterol. Hepatol.* **2014**, *11*, 710–721. [CrossRef] [PubMed]
5. Mitchell, O.; Gurakar, A. Management of Hepatitis C Post-liver Transplantation: A Comprehensive Review. *J. Clin. Transl. Hepatol.* **2015**, *3*, 140–148. [CrossRef] [PubMed]
6. Liang, T.J.; Ghany, M.G. Current and future therapies for hepatitis C virus infection. *N. Engl. J. Med.* **2013**, *368*, 1907–1917. [CrossRef] [PubMed]
7. Falade-Nwulia, O.; Suarez-Cuervo, C.; Nelson, D.R.; Fried, M.W.; Segal, J.B.; Sulkowski, M.S. Oral Direct-Acting Agent Therapy for Hepatitis C Virus Infection: A Systematic Review. *Ann. Intern. Med.* **2017**, *166*, 637–648. [CrossRef] [PubMed]
8. Chen, Q.; Ayer, T.; Bethea, E.; Kanwal, F.; Wang, X.; Roberts, M.; Zhuo, Y.; Fagiuoli, S.; Petersen, J.; Chhatwal, J. Changes in hepatitis C burden and treatment trends in Europe during the era of direct-acting antivirals: A modelling study. *BMJ Open* **2019**, *9*, e026726. [CrossRef]
9. Rong, L.; Dahari, H.; Ribeiro, R.M.; Perelson, A.S. Rapid emergence of protease inhibitor resistance in hepatitis C virus. *Sci. Transl. Med.* **2010**, *2*, 30–32. [CrossRef]
10. Bagaglio, S.; Uberti-Foppa, C.; Morsica, G. Resistance Mechanisms in Hepatitis C Virus: Implications for Direct-Acting Antiviral Use. *Drugs* **2017**, *77*, 1043–1055. [CrossRef]
11. Raj, V.S.; Hundie, G.B.; Schurch, A.C.; Smits, S.L.; Pas, S.D.; Le Pogam, S.; Janssen, H.L.A.; de Knegt, R.J.; Osterhaus, A.; Najera, I.; et al. Identification of HCV Resistant Variants against Direct Acting Antivirals in Plasma and Liver of Treatment Naive Patients. *Sci. Rep.* **2017**, *7*, 4688. [CrossRef]
12. Sarrazin, C.; Zeuzem, S. Resistance to direct antiviral agents in patients with hepatitis C virus infection. *Gastroenterology* **2010**, *138*, 447–462. [CrossRef]
13. McCown, M.F.; Rajyaguru, S.; Kular, S.; Cammack, N.; Najera, I. GT-1a or GT-1b subtype-specific resistance profiles for hepatitis C virus inhibitors telaprevir and HCV-796. *Antimicrob. Agents Chemother.* **2009**, *53*, 2129–2132. [CrossRef] [PubMed]

14. Svarovskaia, E.S.; Dvory-Sobol, H.; Parkin, N.; Hebner, C.; Gontcharova, V.; Martin, R.; Ouyang, W.; Han, B.; Xu, S.; Ku, K.; et al. Infrequent development of resistance in genotype 1-6 hepatitis C virus-infected subjects treated with sofosbuvir in phase 2 and 3 clinical trials. *Clin. Infect. Dis.* **2014**, *59*, 1666–1674. [CrossRef] [PubMed]
15. Vranjkovic, A.; Deonarine, F.; Kaka, S.; Angel, J.B.; Cooper, C.L.; Crawley, A.M. Direct-Acting Antiviral Treatment of HCV Infection Does Not Resolve the Dysfunction of Circulating CD8(+) T-Cells in Advanced Liver Disease. *Front. Immunol.* **2019**, *10*, 1926. [CrossRef]
16. Conti, F.; Buonfiglioli, F.; Scuteri, A.; Crespi, C.; Bolondi, L.; Caraceni, P.; Foschi, F.G.; Lenzi, M.; Mazzella, G.; Verucchi, G.; et al. Early occurrence and recurrence of hepatocellular carcinoma in HCV-related cirrhosis treated with direct-acting antivirals. *J. Hepatol.* **2016**, *65*, 727–733. [CrossRef]
17. Kanwal, F.; Kramer, J.; Asch, S.M.; Chayanupatkul, M.; Cao, Y.; El-Serag, H.B. Risk of Hepatocellular Cancer in HCV Patients Treated With Direct-Acting Antiviral Agents. *Gastroenterology* **2017**, *153*, 996–1005.e1001. [CrossRef]
18. Major, M.; Gutfraind, A.; Shekhtman, L.; Cui, Q.; Kachko, A.; Cotler, S.J.; Hajarizadeh, B.; Sacks-Davis, R.; Page, K.; Boodram, B.; et al. Modeling of patient virus titers suggests that availability of a vaccine could reduce hepatitis C virus transmission among injecting drug users. *Sci. Transl. Med.* **2018**, *10*. [CrossRef]
19. Micallef, J.M.; Kaldor, J.M.; Dore, G.J. Spontaneous viral clearance following acute hepatitis C infection: A systematic review of longitudinal studies. *J. Viral. Hepat.* **2006**, *13*, 34–41. [CrossRef]
20. Poustchi, H.; Esmaili, S.; Mohamadkhani, A.; Nikmahzar, A.; Pourshams, A.; Sepanlou, S.G.; Merat, S.; Malekzadeh, R. The impact of illicit drug use on spontaneous hepatitis C clearance: Experience from a large cohort population study. *PLoS ONE* **2011**, *6*, e23830. [CrossRef]
21. Mosley, J.W.; Operskalski, E.A.; Tobler, L.H.; Buskell, Z.J.; Andrews, W.W.; Phelps, B.; Dockter, J.; Giachetti, C.; Seeff, L.B.; Busch, M.P. The course of hepatitis C viraemia in transfusion recipients prior to availability of antiviral therapy. *J. Viral. Hepat.* **2008**, *15*, 120–128. [CrossRef] [PubMed]
22. Page, K.; Hahn, J.A.; Evans, J.; Shiboski, S.; Lum, P.; Delwart, E.; Tobler, L.; Andrews, W.; Avanesyan, L.; Cooper, S.; et al. Acute hepatitis C virus infection in young adult injection drug users: A prospective study of incident infection, resolution, and reinfection. *J. Infect. Dis.* **2009**, *200*, 1216–1226. [CrossRef] [PubMed]
23. Osburn, W.O.; Fisher, B.E.; Dowd, K.A.; Urban, G.; Liu, L.; Ray, S.C.; Thomas, D.L.; Cox, A.L. Spontaneous control of primary hepatitis C virus infection and immunity against persistent reinfection. *Gastroenterology* **2010**, *138*, 315–324. [CrossRef]
24. Sacks-Davis, R.; Aitken, C.K.; Higgs, P.; Spelman, T.; Pedrana, A.E.; Bowden, S.; Bharadwaj, M.; Nivarthi, U.K.; Suppiah, V.; George, J.; et al. High rates of hepatitis C virus reinfection and spontaneous clearance of reinfection in people who inject drugs: A prospective cohort study. *PLoS ONE* **2013**, *8*, e80216. [CrossRef] [PubMed]
25. Brown, K.S.; Keogh, M.J.; Owsianka, A.M.; Adair, R.; Patel, A.H.; Arnold, J.N.; Ball, J.K.; Sim, R.B.; Tarr, A.W.; Hickling, T.P. Specific interaction of hepatitis C virus glycoproteins with mannan binding lectin inhibits virus entry. *Protein Cell* **2010**, *1*, 664–674. [CrossRef] [PubMed]
26. Hamed, M.R.; Brown, R.J.; Zothner, C.; Urbanowicz, R.A.; Mason, C.P.; Krarup, A.; McClure, C.P.; Irving, W.L.; Ball, J.K.; Harris, M.; et al. Recombinant human L-ficolin directly neutralizes hepatitis C virus entry. *J. Innate Immun.* **2014**, *6*, 676–684. [CrossRef] [PubMed]
27. Xu, Y.; Zhong, J. Innate immunity against hepatitis C virus. *Curr. Opin. Immunol.* **2016**, *42*, 98–104. [CrossRef]
28. Chigbu, D.I.; Loonawat, R.; Sehgal, M.; Patel, D.; Jain, P. Hepatitis C Virus Infection: Host(-)Virus Interaction and Mechanisms of Viral Persistence. *Cells* **2019**, *8*, 376. [CrossRef]
29. Wong, M.T.; Chen, S.S. Emerging roles of interferon-stimulated genes in the innate immune response to hepatitis C virus infection. *Cell Mol. Immunol.* **2016**, *13*, 11–35. [CrossRef] [PubMed]
30. Schoggins, J.W.; Wilson, S.J.; Panis, M.; Murphy, M.Y.; Jones, C.T.; Bieniasz, P.; Rice, C.M. A diverse range of gene products are effectors of the type I interferon antiviral response. *Nature* **2011**, *472*, 481–485. [CrossRef]
31. Patra, T.; Ray, R.B.; Ray, R. Strategies to Circumvent Host Innate Immune Response by Hepatitis C Virus. *Cells* **2019**, *8*, 274. [CrossRef] [PubMed]
32. Heim, M.H. Innate immunity and HCV. *J. Hepatol.* **2013**, *58*, 564–574. [CrossRef] [PubMed]
33. Thomas, D.L.; Thio, C.L.; Martin, M.P.; Qi, Y.; Ge, D.; O'Huigin, C.; Kidd, J.; Kidd, K.; Khakoo, S.I.; Alexander, G.; et al. Genetic variation in IL28B and spontaneous clearance of hepatitis C virus. *Nature* **2009**, *461*, 798–801. [CrossRef] [PubMed]

34. Ge, D.; Fellay, J.; Thompson, A.J.; Simon, J.S.; Shianna, K.V.; Urban, T.J.; Heinzen, E.L.; Qiu, P.; Bertelsen, A.H.; Muir, A.J.; et al. Genetic variation in IL28B predicts hepatitis C treatment-induced viral clearance. *Nature* **2009**, *461*, 399–401. [CrossRef] [PubMed]
35. Khakoo, S.I.; Thio, C.L.; Martin, M.P.; Brooks, C.R.; Gao, X.; Astemborski, J.; Cheng, J.; Goedert, J.J.; Vlahov, D.; Hilgartner, M.; et al. HLA and NK cell inhibitory receptor genes in resolving hepatitis C virus infection. *Science* **2004**, *305*, 872–874. [CrossRef]
36. Amadei, B.; Urbani, S.; Cazaly, A.; Fisicaro, P.; Zerbini, A.; Ahmed, P.; Missale, G.; Ferrari, C.; Khakoo, S.I. Activation of natural killer cells during acute infection with hepatitis C virus. *Gastroenterology* **2010**, *138*, 1536–1545. [CrossRef]
37. Yoon, J.C.; Yang, C.M.; Song, Y.; Lee, J.M. Natural killer cells in hepatitis C: Current progress. *World J. Gastroenterol.* **2016**, *22*, 1449–1460. [CrossRef]
38. Missale, G.; Bertoni, R.; Lamonaca, V.; Valli, A.; Massari, M.; Mori, C.; Rumi, M.G.; Houghton, M.; Fiaccadori, F.; Ferrari, C. Different clinical behaviors of acute hepatitis C virus infection are associated with different vigor of the anti-viral cell-mediated immune response. *J. Clin. Investig.* **1996**, *98*, 706–714. [CrossRef]
39. Mittrucker, H.W.; Visekruna, A.; Huber, M. Heterogeneity in the differentiation and function of CD8(+) T cells. *Arch. Immunol. Ther. Exp. (Warsz)* **2014**, *62*, 449–458. [CrossRef]
40. Luckheeram, R.V.; Zhou, R.; Verma, A.D.; Xia, B. CD4(+)T cells: Differentiation and functions. *Clin. Dev. Immunol.* **2012**, *2012*, 925135. [CrossRef]
41. Laidlaw, B.J.; Craft, J.E.; Kaech, S.M. The multifaceted role of CD4(+) T cells in CD8(+) T cell memory. *Nat. Rev. Immunol.* **2016**, *16*, 102–111. [CrossRef] [PubMed]
42. Swain, S.L.; McKinstry, K.K.; Strutt, T.M. Expanding roles for CD4(+) T cells in immunity to viruses. *Nat. Rev. Immunol.* **2012**, *12*, 136–148. [CrossRef] [PubMed]
43. Zhang, J.; Liu, W.; Wen, B.; Xie, T.; Tang, P.; Hu, Y.; Huang, L.; Jin, K.; Zhang, P.; Liu, Z.; et al. Circulating CXCR3(+) Tfh cells positively correlate with neutralizing antibody responses in HCV-infected patients. *Sci. Rep.* **2019**, *9*, 10090. [CrossRef] [PubMed]
44. Semmo, N.; Klenerman, P. CD4+ T cell responses in hepatitis C virus infection. *World J. Gastroenterol.* **2007**, *13*, 4831–4838. [CrossRef]
45. Schulze Zur Wiesch, J.; Ciuffreda, D.; Lewis-Ximenez, L.; Kasprowicz, V.; Nolan, B.E.; Streeck, H.; Aneja, J.; Reyor, L.L.; Allen, T.M.; Lohse, A.W.; et al. Broadly directed virus-specific CD4+ T cell responses are primed during acute hepatitis C infection, but rapidly disappear from human blood with viral persistence. *J. Exp. Med.* **2012**, *209*, 61–75. [CrossRef]
46. Ulsenheimer, A.; Gerlach, J.T.; Gruener, N.H.; Jung, M.C.; Schirren, C.A.; Schraut, W.; Zachoval, R.; Pape, G.R.; Diepolder, H.M. Detection of functionally altered hepatitis C virus-specific CD4 T cells in acute and chronic hepatitis C. *Hepatology* **2003**, *37*, 1189–1198. [CrossRef]
47. Dustin, L.B. Innate and Adaptive Immune Responses in Chronic HCV Infection. *Curr. Drug Targets* **2017**, *18*, 826–843. [CrossRef]
48. Grakoui, A.; Shoukry, N.H.; Woollard, D.J.; Han, J.H.; Hanson, H.L.; Ghrayeb, J.; Murthy, K.K.; Rice, C.M.; Walker, C.M. HCV persistence and immune evasion in the absence of memory T cell help. *Science* **2003**, *302*, 659–662. [CrossRef]
49. Shoukry, N.H.; Grakoui, A.; Houghton, M.; Chien, D.Y.; Ghrayeb, J.; Reimann, K.A.; Walker, C.M. Memory CD8+ T cells are required for protection from persistent hepatitis C virus infection. *J. Exp. Med.* **2003**, *197*, 1645–1655. [CrossRef]
50. Farci, P.; Alter, H.J.; Wong, D.C.; Miller, R.H.; Govindarajan, S.; Engle, R.; Shapiro, M.; Purcell, R.H. Prevention of hepatitis C virus infection in chimpanzees after antibody-mediated in vitro neutralization. *Proc. Natl. Acad. Sci. USA* **1994**, *91*, 7792–7796. [CrossRef]
51. Grebely, J.; Prins, M.; Hellard, M.; Cox, A.L.; Osburn, W.O.; Lauer, G.; Page, K.; Lloyd, A.R.; Dore, G.J. Hepatitis C virus clearance, reinfection, and persistence, with insights from studies of injecting drug users: Towards a vaccine. *Lancet Infect. Dis.* **2012**, *12*, 408–414. [CrossRef]
52. Zeremski, M.; Shu, M.A.; Brown, Q.; Wu, Y.; Des Jarlais, D.C.; Busch, M.P.; Talal, A.H.; Edlin, B.R. Hepatitis C virus-specific T-cell immune responses in seronegative injection drug users. *J. Viral. Hepat.* **2009**, *16*, 10–20. [CrossRef] [PubMed]

53. Post, J.J.; Pan, Y.; Freeman, A.J.; Harvey, C.E.; White, P.A.; Palladinetti, P.; Haber, P.S.; Marinos, G.; Levy, M.H.; Kaldor, J.M.; et al. Clearance of hepatitis C viremia associated with cellular immunity in the absence of seroconversion in the hepatitis C incidence and transmission in prisons study cohort. *J. Infect. Dis.* **2004**, *189*, 1846–1855. [CrossRef]
54. Strasak, A.M.; Kim, A.Y.; Lauer, G.M.; de Sousa, P.S.; Ginuino, C.F.; Fernandes, C.A.; Velloso, C.E.; de Almeida, A.J.; de Oliveira, J.M.; Yoshida, C.F.; et al. Antibody dynamics and spontaneous viral clearance in patients with acute hepatitis C infection in Rio de Janeiro, Brazil. *BMC Infect. Dis.* **2011**, *11*, 15. [CrossRef] [PubMed]
55. Pestka, J.M.; Zeisel, M.B.; Bläser, E.; Schürmann, P.; Bartosch, B.; Cosset, F.L.; Patel, A.H.; Meisel, H.; Baumert, J.; Viazov, S.; et al. Rapid induction of virus-neutralizing antibodies and viral clearance in a single-source outbreak of hepatitis C. *Proc. Natl. Acad. Sci. USA* **2007**, *104*, 6025–6030. [CrossRef] [PubMed]
56. Dowd, K.A.; Netski, D.M.; Wang, X.H.; Cox, A.L.; Ray, S.C. Selection pressure from neutralizing antibodies drives sequence evolution during acute infection with hepatitis C virus. *Gastroenterology* **2009**, *136*, 2377–2386. [CrossRef]
57. Osburn, W.O.; Snider, A.E.; Wells, B.L.; Latanich, R.; Bailey, J.R.; Thomas, D.L.; Cox, A.L.; Ray, S.C. Clearance of hepatitis C infection is associated with the early appearance of broad neutralizing antibody responses. *Hepatology* **2014**, *59*, 2140–2151. [CrossRef]
58. Walker, M.R.; Leung, P.; Eltahla, A.A.; Underwood, A.; Abayasingam, A.; Brasher, N.A.; Li, H.; Wu, B.R.; Maher, L.; Luciani, F.; et al. Clearance of hepatitis C virus is associated with early and potent but narrowly-directed, Envelope-specific antibodies. *Sci. Rep.* **2019**, *9*, 13300. [CrossRef]
59. Kinchen, V.J.; Zahid, M.N.; Flyak, A.I.; Soliman, M.G.; Learn, G.H.; Wang, S.; Davidson, E.; Doranz, B.J.; Ray, S.C.; Cox, A.L.; et al. Broadly Neutralizing Antibody Mediated Clearance of Human Hepatitis C Virus Infection. *Cell Host Microbe* **2018**, *24*, 717–730.e715. [CrossRef]
60. Gu, J.; Hardy, J.; Boo, I.; Vietheer, P.; McCaffrey, K.; Alhammad, Y.; Chopra, A.; Gaudieri, S.; Poumbourios, P.; Coulibaly, F.; et al. Escape of Hepatitis C Virus from Epitope I Neutralization Increases Sensitivity of Other Neutralization Epitopes. *J. Virol.* **2018**, *92*. [CrossRef]
61. Hadlock, K.G.; Lanford, R.E.; Perkins, S.; Rowe, J.; Yang, Q.; Levy, S.; Pileri, P.; Abrignani, S.; Foung, S.K. Human monoclonal antibodies that inhibit binding of hepatitis C virus E2 protein to CD81 and recognize conserved conformational epitopes. *J. Virol.* **2000**, *74*, 10407–10416. [CrossRef] [PubMed]
62. Allander, T.; Drakenberg, K.; Beyene, A.; Rosa, D.; Abrignani, S.; Houghton, M.; Widell, A.; Grillner, L.; Persson, M.A. Recombinant human monoclonal antibodies against different conformational epitopes of the E2 envelope glycoprotein of hepatitis C virus that inhibit its interaction with CD81. *J. Gen. Virol.* **2000**, *81*, 2451–2459. [CrossRef] [PubMed]
63. Johansson, D.X.; Voisset, C.; Tarr, A.W.; Aung, M.; Ball, J.K.; Dubuisson, J.; Persson, M.A. Human combinatorial libraries yield rare antibodies that broadly neutralize hepatitis C virus. *Proc. Natl. Acad. Sci. USA* **2007**, *104*, 16269–16274. [CrossRef] [PubMed]
64. Law, M.; Maruyama, T.; Lewis, J.; Giang, E.; Tarr, A.W.; Stamataki, Z.; Gastaminza, P.; Chisari, F.V.; Jones, I.M.; Fox, R.I.; et al. Broadly neutralizing antibodies protect against hepatitis C virus quasispecies challenge. *Nat. Med.* **2008**, *14*, 25–27. [CrossRef] [PubMed]
65. Swann, R.E.; Cowton, V.M.; Robinson, M.W.; Cole, S.J.; Barclay, S.T.; Mills, P.R.; Thomson, E.C.; McLauchlan, J.; Patel, A.H. Broad Anti-Hepatitis C Virus (HCV) Antibody Responses Are Associated with Improved Clinical Disease Parameters in Chronic HCV Infection. *J. Virol.* **2016**, *90*, 4530–4543. [CrossRef]
66. Bjoro, K.; Froland, S.S.; Yun, Z.; Samdal, H.H.; Haaland, T. Hepatitis C infection in patients with primary hypogammaglobulinemia after treatment with contaminated immune globulin. *N. Engl. J. Med.* **1994**, *331*, 1607–1611. [CrossRef]
67. Bailey, J.R.; Flyak, A.I.; Cohen, V.J.; Li, H.; Wasilewski, L.N.; Snider, A.E.; Wang, S.; Learn, G.H.; Kose, N.; Loerinc, L.; et al. Broadly neutralizing antibodies with few somatic mutations and hepatitis C virus clearance. *JCI Insight* **2017**, *2*. [CrossRef]
68. Chan, C.H.; Hadlock, K.G.; Foung, S.K.; Levy, S. V(H)1-69 gene is preferentially used by hepatitis C virus-associated B cell lymphomas and by normal B cells responding to the E2 viral antigen. *Blood* **2001**, *97*, 1023–1026. [CrossRef]

69. Giang, E.; Dorner, M.; Prentoe, J.C.; Dreux, M.; Evans, M.J.; Bukh, J.; Rice, C.M.; Ploss, A.; Burton, D.R.; Law, M. Human broadly neutralizing antibodies to the envelope glycoprotein complex of hepatitis C virus. *Proc. Natl. Acad. Sci. USA* **2012**, *109*, 6205–6210. [CrossRef]
70. Chen, F.; Tzarum, N.; Wilson, I.A.; Law, M. VH1-69 antiviral broadly neutralizing antibodies: Genetics, structures, and relevance to rational vaccine design. *Curr. Opin. Virol.* **2019**, *34*, 149–159. [CrossRef]
71. Merat, S.J.; Bru, C.; van de Berg, D.; Molenkamp, R.; Tarr, A.W.; Koekkoek, S.; Kootstra, N.A.; Prins, M.; Ball, J.K.; Bakker, A.Q.; et al. Cross-genotype AR3-specific neutralizing antibodies confer long-term protection in injecting drug users after HCV clearance. *J. Hepatol.* **2019**, *71*, 14–24. [CrossRef] [PubMed]
72. Flyak, A.I.; Ruiz, S.; Colbert, M.D.; Luong, T.; Crowe, J.E., Jr.; Bailey, J.R.; Bjorkman, P.J. HCV Broadly Neutralizing Antibodies Use a CDRH3 Disulfide Motif to Recognize an E2 Glycoprotein Site that Can Be Targeted for Vaccine Design. *Cell Host Microbe* **2018**, *24*, 703–716.e703. [CrossRef] [PubMed]
73. Tzarum, N.; Giang, E.; Kong, L.; He, L.; Prentoe, J.; Augestad, E.; Hua, Y.; Castillo, S.; Lauer, G.M.; Bukh, J.; et al. Genetic and structural insights into broad neutralization of hepatitis C virus by human VH1-69 antibodies. *Sci. Adv.* **2019**, *5*, eaav1882. [CrossRef] [PubMed]
74. Ball, J.K.; Tarr, A.W.; McKeating, J.A. The past, present and future of neutralizing antibodies for hepatitis C virus. *Antiviral Res.* **2014**, *105*, 100–111. [CrossRef]
75. Vieyres, G.; Thomas, X.; Descamps, V.; Duverlie, G.; Patel, A.H.; Dubuisson, J. Characterization of the envelope glycoproteins associated with infectious hepatitis C virus. *J. Virol.* **2010**, *84*, 10159–10168. [CrossRef]
76. Vieyres, G.; Dubuisson, J.; Pietschmann, T. Incorporation of hepatitis C virus E1 and E2 glycoproteins: The keystones on a peculiar virion. *Viruses* **2014**, *6*, 1149–1187. [CrossRef]
77. Kong, L.; Giang, E.; Nieusma, T.; Kadam, R.U.; Cogburn, K.E.; Hua, Y.; Dai, X.; Stanfield, R.L.; Burton, D.R.; Ward, A.B.; et al. Hepatitis C virus E2 envelope glycoprotein core structure. *Science* **2013**, *342*, 1090–1094. [CrossRef]
78. Khan, A.G.; Whidby, J.; Miller, M.T.; Scarborough, H.; Zatorski, A.V.; Cygan, A.; Price, A.A.; Yost, S.A.; Bohannon, C.D.; Jacob, J.; et al. Structure of the core ectodomain of the hepatitis C virus envelope glycoprotein 2. *Nature* **2014**, *509*, 381–384. [CrossRef]
79. El Omari, K.; Iourin, O.; Kadlec, J.; Sutton, G.; Harlos, K.; Grimes, J.M.; Stuart, D.I. Unexpected structure for the N-terminal domain of hepatitis C virus envelope glycoprotein E1. *Nat. Commun.* **2014**, *5*, 4874. [CrossRef]
80. Kong, L.; Kadam, R.U.; Giang, E.; Ruwona, T.B.; Nieusma, T.; Culhane, J.C.; Stanfield, R.L.; Dawson, P.E.; Wilson, I.A.; Law, M. Structure of Hepatitis C Virus Envelope Glycoprotein E1 Antigenic Site 314–324 in Complex with Antibody IGH526. *J. Mol. Biol.* **2015**, *427*, 2617–2628. [CrossRef]
81. Bartosch, B.; Vitelli, A.; Granier, C.; Goujon, C.; Dubuisson, J.; Pascale, S.; Scarselli, E.; Cortese, R.; Nicosia, A.; Cosset, F.L. Cell entry of hepatitis C virus requires a set of co-receptors that include the CD81 tetraspanin and the SR-B1 scavenger receptor. *J. Biol. Chem.* **2003**, *278*, 41624–41630. [CrossRef]
82. Pileri, P.; Uematsu, Y.; Campagnoli, S.; Galli, G.; Falugi, F.; Petracca, R.; Weiner, A.J.; Houghton, M.; Rosa, D.; Grandi, G.; et al. Binding of hepatitis C virus to CD81. *Science* **1998**, *282*, 938–941. [CrossRef] [PubMed]
83. Scarselli, E.; Ansuini, H.; Cerino, R.; Roccasecca, R.M.; Acali, S.; Filocamo, G.; Traboni, C.; Nicosia, A.; Cortese, R.; Vitelli, A. The human scavenger receptor class B type I is a novel candidate receptor for the hepatitis C virus. *Embo J.* **2002**, *21*, 5017–5025. [CrossRef] [PubMed]
84. Evans, M.J.; von Hahn, T.; Tscherne, D.M.; Syder, A.J.; Panis, M.; Wolk, B.; Hatziioannou, T.; McKeating, J.A.; Bieniasz, P.D.; Rice, C.M. Claudin-1 is a hepatitis C virus co-receptor required for a late step in entry. *Nature* **2007**, *446*, 801–805. [CrossRef] [PubMed]
85. Ploss, A.; Evans, M.J.; Gaysinskaya, V.A.; Panis, M.; You, H.; de Jong, Y.P.; Rice, C.M. Human occludin is a hepatitis C virus entry factor required for infection of mouse cells. *Nature* **2009**, *457*, 882–886. [CrossRef] [PubMed]
86. Liu, S.; Yang, W.; Shen, L.; Turner, J.R.; Coyne, C.B.; Wang, T. Tight junction proteins claudin-1 and occludin control hepatitis C virus entry and are downregulated during infection to prevent superinfection. *J. Virol.* **2009**, *83*, 2011–2014. [CrossRef]
87. Dubuisson, J.; Cosset, F.L. Virology and cell biology of the hepatitis C virus life cycle: An update. *J. Hepatol.* **2014**, *61*, S3–S13. [CrossRef]
88. Tscherne, D.M.; Jones, C.T.; Evans, M.J.; Lindenbach, B.D.; McKeating, J.A.; Rice, C.M. Time- and temperature-dependent activation of hepatitis C virus for low-pH-triggered entry. *J. Virol.* **2006**, *80*, 1734–1741. [CrossRef]

89. Tong, Y.; Lavillette, D.; Li, Q.; Zhong, J. Role of Hepatitis C Virus Envelope Glycoprotein E1 in Virus Entry and Assembly. *Front. Immunol.* **2018**, *9*, 1411. [CrossRef]
90. Drummer, H.E. Challenges to the development of vaccines to hepatitis C virus that elicit neutralizing antibodies. *Front. Microbiol.* **2014**, *5*, 329. [CrossRef]
91. Keck, Z.; Wang, W.; Wang, Y.; Lau, P.; Carlsen, T.H.; Prentoe, J.; Xia, J.; Patel, A.H.; Bukh, J.; Foung, S.K. Cooperativity in virus neutralization by human monoclonal antibodies to two adjacent regions located at the amino terminus of hepatitis C virus E2 glycoprotein. *J. Virol.* **2013**, *87*, 37–51. [CrossRef] [PubMed]
92. Tzarum, N.; Wilson, I.A.; Law, M. The Neutralizing Face of Hepatitis C Virus E2 Envelope Glycoprotein. *Front. Immunol.* **2018**, *9*, 1315. [CrossRef] [PubMed]
93. Cuevas, J.M.; Gonzalez-Candelas, F.; Moya, A.; Sanjuan, R. Effect of ribavirin on the mutation rate and spectrum of hepatitis C virus in vivo. *J. Virol.* **2009**, *83*, 5760–5764. [CrossRef] [PubMed]
94. Echeverria, N.; Moratorio, G.; Cristina, J.; Moreno, P. Hepatitis C virus genetic variability and evolution. *World J. Hepatol.* **2015**, *7*, 831–845. [CrossRef]
95. Smith, D.B.; Bukh, J.; Kuiken, C.; Muerhoff, A.S.; Rice, C.M.; Stapleton, J.T.; Simmonds, P. Expanded classification of hepatitis C virus into 7 genotypes and 67 subtypes: Updated criteria and genotype assignment web resource. *Hepatology* **2014**, *59*, 318–327. [CrossRef]
96. Petruzziello, A.; Marigliano, S.; Loquercio, G.; Cozzolino, A.; Cacciapuoti, C. Global epidemiology of hepatitis C virus infection: An up-date of the distribution and circulation of hepatitis C virus genotypes. *World J. Gastroenterol.* **2016**, *22*, 7824–7840. [CrossRef]
97. Borgia, S.M.; Hedskog, C.; Parhy, B.; Hyland, R.H.; Stamm, L.M.; Brainard, D.M.; Subramanian, M.G.; McHutchison, J.G.; Mo, H.; Svarovskaia, E.; et al. Identification of a Novel Hepatitis C Virus Genotype From Punjab, India: Expanding Classification of Hepatitis C Virus Into 8 Genotypes. *J. Infect. Dis.* **2018**, *218*, 1722–1729. [CrossRef]
98. Forns, X.; Purcell, R.H.; Bukh, J. Quasispecies in viral persistence and pathogenesis of hepatitis C virus. *Trends Microbiol.* **1999**, *7*, 402–410. [CrossRef]
99. Farci, P.; Shimoda, A.; Coiana, A.; Diaz, G.; Peddis, G.; Melpolder, J.C.; Strazzera, A.; Chien, D.Y.; Munoz, S.J.; Balestrieri, A.; et al. The outcome of acute hepatitis C predicted by the evolution of the viral quasispecies. *Science* **2000**, *288*, 339–344. [CrossRef]
100. Liu, L.; Fisher, B.E.; Dowd, K.A.; Astemborski, J.; Cox, A.L.; Ray, S.C. Acceleration of hepatitis C virus envelope evolution in humans is consistent with progressive humoral immune selection during the transition from acute to chronic infection. *J. Virol.* **2010**, *84*, 5067–5077. [CrossRef]
101. Islam, N.; Krajden, M.; Shoveller, J.; Gustafson, P.; Gilbert, M.; Wong, J.; Tyndall, M.W.; Janjua, N.Z. Hepatitis C cross-genotype immunity and implications for vaccine development. *Sci. Rep.* **2017**, *7*, 12326. [CrossRef] [PubMed]
102. Tarr, A.W.; Urbanowicz, R.A.; Hamed, M.R.; Albecka, A.; McClure, C.P.; Brown, R.J.; Irving, W.L.; Dubuisson, J.; Ball, J.K. Hepatitis C patient-derived glycoproteins exhibit marked differences in susceptibility to serum neutralizing antibodies: Genetic subtype defines antigenic but not neutralization serotype. *J. Virol.* **2011**, *85*, 4246–4257. [CrossRef] [PubMed]
103. Luxenburger, H.; Grass, F.; Baermann, J.; Boettler, T.; Marget, M.; Emmerich, F.; Panning, M.; Thimme, R.; Nitschke, K.; Neumann-Haefelin, C. Differential virus-specific CD8(+) T-cell epitope repertoire in hepatitis C virus genotype 1 versus 4. *J. Viral. Hepat.* **2018**, *25*, 779–790. [CrossRef] [PubMed]
104. Von Delft, A.; Humphreys, I.S.; Brown, A.; Pfafferott, K.; Lucas, M.; Klenerman, P.; Lauer, G.M.; Cox, A.L.; Gaudieri, S.; Barnes, E. The broad assessment of HCV genotypes 1 and 3 antigenic targets reveals limited cross-reactivity with implications for vaccine design. *Gut* **2016**, *65*, 112–123. [CrossRef]
105. Bankwitz, D.; Steinmann, E.; Bitzegeio, J.; Ciesek, S.; Friesland, M.; Herrmann, E.; Zeisel, M.B.; Baumert, T.F.; Keck, Z.Y.; Foung, S.K.; et al. Hepatitis C virus hypervariable region 1 modulates receptor interactions, conceals the CD81 binding site, and protects conserved neutralizing epitopes. *J. Virol.* **2010**, *84*, 5751–5763. [CrossRef]
106. Prentoe, J.; Jensen, T.B.; Meuleman, P.; Serre, S.B.; Scheel, T.K.; Leroux-Roels, G.; Gottwein, J.M.; Bukh, J. Hypervariable region 1 differentially impacts viability of hepatitis C virus strains of genotypes 1 to 6 and impairs virus neutralization. *J. Virol.* **2011**, *85*, 2224–2234. [CrossRef]

107. Bazzill, J.D.; Ochyl, L.J.; Giang, E.; Castillo, S.; Law, M.; Moon, J.J. Interrogation of Antigen Display on Individual Vaccine Nanoparticles for Achieving Neutralizing Antibody Responses against Hepatitis C Virus. *Nano. Lett.* **2018**, *18*, 7832–7838. [CrossRef]
108. Lavie, M.; Hanoulle, X.; Dubuisson, J. Glycan Shielding and Modulation of Hepatitis C Virus Neutralizing Antibodies. *Front. Immunol.* **2018**, *9*, 910. [CrossRef]
109. Helle, F.; Goffard, A.; Morel, V.; Duverlie, G.; McKeating, J.; Keck, Z.Y.; Foung, S.; Penin, F.; Dubuisson, J.; Voisset, C. The neutralizing activity of anti-hepatitis C virus antibodies is modulated by specific glycans on the E2 envelope protein. *J. Virol.* **2007**, *81*, 8101–8111. [CrossRef]
110. Helle, F.; Vieyres, G.; Elkrief, L.; Popescu, C.I.; Wychowski, C.; Descamps, V.; Castelain, S.; Roingeard, P.; Duverlie, G.; Dubuisson, J. Role of N-linked glycans in the functions of hepatitis C virus envelope proteins incorporated into infectious virions. *J. Virol.* **2010**, *84*, 11905–11915. [CrossRef]
111. Li, D.; von Schaewen, M.; Wang, X.; Tao, W.; Zhang, Y.; Li, L.; Heller, B.; Hrebikova, G.; Deng, Q.; Ploss, A.; et al. Altered Glycosylation Patterns Increase Immunogenicity of a Subunit Hepatitis C Virus Vaccine, Inducing Neutralizing Antibodies Which Confer Protection in Mice. *J. Virol.* **2016**, *90*, 10486–10498. [CrossRef] [PubMed]
112. Ren, Y.; Min, Y.Q.; Liu, M.; Chi, L.; Zhao, P.; Zhang, X.L. N-glycosylation-mutated HCV envelope glycoprotein complex enhances antigen-presenting activity and cellular and neutralizing antibody responses. *Biochim. Biophys. Acta* **2016**, *1860*, 1764–1775. [CrossRef] [PubMed]
113. Urbanowicz, R.A.; Wang, R.; Schiel, J.E.; Keck, Z.Y.; Kerzic, M.C.; Lau, P.; Rangarajan, S.; Garagusi, K.J.; Tan, L.; Guest, J.D.; et al. Antigenicity and Immunogenicity of Differentially Glycosylated Hepatitis C Virus E2 Envelope Proteins Expressed in Mammalian and Insect Cells. *J. Virol.* **2019**, *93*. [CrossRef] [PubMed]
114. Pantua, H.; Diao, J.; Ultsch, M.; Hazen, M.; Mathieu, M.; McCutcheon, K.; Takeda, K.; Date, S.; Cheung, T.K.; Phung, Q.; et al. Glycan shifting on hepatitis C virus (HCV) E2 glycoprotein is a mechanism for escape from broadly neutralizing antibodies. *J. Mol. Biol.* **2013**, *425*, 1899–1914. [CrossRef]
115. Owsianka, A.; Tarr, A.W.; Juttla, V.S.; Lavillette, D.; Bartosch, B.; Cosset, F.L.; Ball, J.K.; Patel, A.H. Monoclonal antibody AP33 defines a broadly neutralizing epitope on the hepatitis C virus E2 envelope glycoprotein. *J. Virol.* **2005**, *79*, 11095–11104. [CrossRef]
116. Voisset, C.; Op de Beeck, A.; Horellou, P.; Dreux, M.; Gustot, T.; Duverlie, G.; Cosset, F.L.; Vu-Dac, N.; Dubuisson, J. High-density lipoproteins reduce the neutralizing effect of hepatitis C virus (HCV)-infected patient antibodies by promoting HCV entry. *J. Gen. Virol.* **2006**, *87*, 2577–2581. [CrossRef]
117. Dreux, M.; Pietschmann, T.; Granier, C.; Voisset, C.; Ricard-Blum, S.; Mangeot, P.E.; Keck, Z.; Foung, S.; Vu-Dac, N.; Dubuisson, J.; et al. High density lipoprotein inhibits hepatitis C virus-neutralizing antibodies by stimulating cell entry via activation of the scavenger receptor BI. *J. Biol. Chem.* **2006**, *281*, 18285–18295. [CrossRef]
118. Fauvelle, C.; Felmlee, D.J.; Crouchet, E.; Lee, J.; Heydmann, L.; Lefevre, M.; Magri, A.; Hiet, M.S.; Fofana, I.; Habersetzer, F.; et al. Apolipoprotein E Mediates Evasion From Hepatitis C Virus Neutralizing Antibodies. *Gastroenterology* **2016**, *150*, 206–217.e204. [CrossRef]
119. Deng, L.; Jiang, W.; Wang, X.; Merz, A.; Hiet, M.S.; Chen, Y.; Pan, X.; Jiu, Y.; Yang, Y.; Yu, B.; et al. Syntenin regulates hepatitis C virus sensitivity to neutralizing antibody by promoting E2 secretion through exosomes. *J. Hepatol.* **2019**, *71*, 52–61. [CrossRef]
120. Wrensch, F.; Ligat, G.; Heydmann, L.; Schuster, C.; Zeisel, M.B.; Pessaux, P.; Habersetzer, F.; King, B.J.; Tarr, A.W.; Ball, J.K.; et al. Interferon-Induced Transmembrane Proteins Mediate Viral Evasion in Acute and Chronic Hepatitis C Virus Infection. *Hepatology* **2019**, *70*, 1506–1520. [CrossRef]
121. Lohmann, V.; Bartenschlager, R. On the history of hepatitis C virus cell culture systems. *J. Med. Chem.* **2014**, *57*, 1627–1642. [CrossRef] [PubMed]
122. Pietschmann, T.; Kaul, A.; Koutsoudakis, G.; Shavinskaya, A.; Kallis, S.; Steinmann, E.; Abid, K.; Negro, F.; Dreux, M.; Cosset, F.L.; et al. Construction and characterization of infectious intragenotypic and intergenotypic hepatitis C virus chimeras. *Proc. Natl. Acad. Sci. USA* **2006**, *103*, 7408–7413. [CrossRef] [PubMed]
123. Gottwein, J.M.; Scheel, T.K.; Jensen, T.B.; Lademann, J.B.; Prentoe, J.C.; Knudsen, M.L.; Hoegh, A.M.; Bukh, J. Development and characterization of hepatitis C virus genotype 1-7 cell culture systems: Role of CD81 and scavenger receptor class B type I and effect of antiviral drugs. *Hepatology* **2009**, *49*, 364–377. [CrossRef] [PubMed]

124. Carlsen, T.H.; Pedersen, J.; Prentoe, J.C.; Giang, E.; Keck, Z.Y.; Mikkelsen, L.S.; Law, M.; Foung, S.K.; Bukh, J. Breadth of neutralization and synergy of clinically relevant human monoclonal antibodies against HCV genotypes 1a, 1b, 2a, 2b, 2c, and 3a. *Hepatology* **2014**, *60*, 1551–1562. [CrossRef] [PubMed]
125. McClure, C.P.; Urbanowicz, R.A.; King, B.J.; Cano-Crespo, S.; Tarr, A.W.; Ball, J.K. Flexible and rapid construction of viral chimeras applied to hepatitis C virus. *J. Gen. Virol.* **2016**, *97*, 2187–2193. [CrossRef]
126. King, B.; Urbanowicz, R.; Tarr, A.W.; Ball, J.K.; McClure, C.P. InFusion Cloning for the Generation of Biologically Relevant HCV Chimeric Molecular Clones. *Methods Mol. Biol. (Clifton N.J.)* **2019**, *1911*, 93–104.
127. Bartosch, B.; Dubuisson, J.; Cosset, F.L. Infectious hepatitis C virus pseudo-particles containing functional E1-E2 envelope protein complexes. *J. Exp. Med.* **2003**, *197*, 633–642. [CrossRef]
128. Flint, M.; Logvinoff, C.; Rice, C.M.; McKeating, J.A. Characterization of infectious retroviral pseudotype particles bearing hepatitis C virus glycoproteins. *J. Virol.* **2004**, *78*, 6875–6882. [CrossRef]
129. Urbanowicz, R.A.; McClure, C.P.; Brown, R.J.P.; Tsoleridis, T.; Persson, M.A.A.; Krey, T.; Irving, W.L.; Ball, J.K.; Tarr, A.W. A Diverse Panel of Hepatitis C Virus Glycoproteins for Use in Vaccine Research Reveals Extremes of Monoclonal Antibody Neutralization Resistance. *J. Virol.* **2016**, *90*, 3288–3301. [CrossRef]
130. Urbanowicz, R.A.; McClure, C.P.; King, B.; Mason, C.P.; Ball, J.K.; Tarr, A.W. Novel functional hepatitis C virus glycoprotein isolates identified using an optimized viral pseudotype entry assay. *J. Gen. Virol.* **2016**, *97*, 2265–2279. [CrossRef]
131. Bailey, J.R.; Wasilewski, L.N.; Snider, A.E.; El-Diwany, R.; Osburn, W.O.; Keck, Z.; Foung, S.K.; Ray, S.C. Naturally selected hepatitis C virus polymorphisms confer broad neutralizing antibody resistance. *J. Clin. Investig.* **2015**, *125*, 437–447. [CrossRef] [PubMed]
132. Kolykhalov, A.A.; Agapov, E.V.; Blight, K.J.; Mihalik, K.; Feinstone, S.M.; Rice, C.M. Transmission of hepatitis C by intrahepatic inoculation with transcribed RNA. *Science* **1997**, *277*, 570–574. [CrossRef]
133. Feinstone, S.M.; Alter, H.J.; Dienes, H.P.; Shimizu, Y.; Popper, H.; Blackmore, D.; Sly, D.; London, W.T.; Purcell, R.H. Non-A, non-B hepatitis in chimpanzees and marmosets. *J. Infect. Dis.* **1981**, *144*, 588–598. [CrossRef] [PubMed]
134. Yanagi, M.; Purcell, R.H.; Emerson, S.U.; Bukh, J. Transcripts from a single full-length cDNA clone of hepatitis C virus are infectious when directly transfected into the liver of a chimpanzee. *Proc. Natl. Acad. Sci. USA* **1997**, *94*, 8738–8743. [CrossRef]
135. Seaman, M.S.; Janes, H.; Hawkins, N.; Grandpre, L.E.; Devoy, C.; Giri, A.; Coffey, R.T.; Harris, L.; Wood, B.; Daniels, M.G.; et al. Tiered categorization of a diverse panel of HIV-1 Env pseudoviruses for assessment of neutralizing antibodies. *J. Virol.* **2010**, *84*, 1439–1452. [CrossRef]
136. Mercer, D.F.; Schiller, D.E.; Elliott, J.F.; Douglas, D.N.; Hao, C.; Rinfret, A.; Addison, W.R.; Fischer, K.P.; Churchill, T.A.; Lakey, J.R.; et al. Hepatitis C virus replication in mice with chimeric human livers. *Nat. Med.* **2001**, *7*, 927–933. [CrossRef] [PubMed]
137. Meuleman, P.; Libbrecht, L.; De Vos, R.; de Hemptinne, B.; Gevaert, K.; Vandekerckhove, J.; Roskams, T.; Leroux-Roels, G. Morphological and biochemical characterization of a human liver in a uPA-SCID mouse chimera. *Hepatology* **2005**, *41*, 847–856. [CrossRef]
138. Chen, J.; Zhao, Y.; Zhang, C.; Chen, H.; Feng, J.; Chi, X.; Pan, Y.; Du, J.; Guo, M.; Cao, H.; et al. Persistent hepatitis C virus infections and hepatopathological manifestations in immune-competent humanized mice. *Cell Res.* **2014**, *24*, 1050–1066. [CrossRef]
139. Ding, Q.; von Schaewen, M.; Hrebikova, G.; Heller, B.; Sandmann, L.; Plaas, M.; Ploss, A. Mice Expressing Minimally Humanized CD81 and Occludin Genes Support Hepatitis C Virus Uptake In Vivo. *J. Virol.* **2017**, *91*. [CrossRef]
140. Yong, K.S.M.; Her, Z.; Chen, Q. Humanized Mouse Models for the Study of Hepatitis C and Host Interactions. *Cells* **2019**, *8*, 604. [CrossRef]
141. Firth, C.; Bhat, M.; Firth, M.A.; Williams, S.H.; Frye, M.J.; Simmonds, P.; Conte, J.M.; Ng, J.; Garcia, J.; Bhuva, N.P.; et al. Detection of zoonotic pathogens and characterization of novel viruses carried by commensal Rattus norvegicus in New York City. *Mbio* **2014**, *5*, e01933-14. [CrossRef]
142. Trivedi, S.; Murthy, S.; Sharma, H.; Hartlage, A.S.; Kumar, A.; Gadi, S.V.; Simmonds, P.; Chauhan, L.V.; Scheel, T.K.H.; Billerbeck, E.; et al. Viral persistence, liver disease, and host response in a hepatitis C-like virus rat model. *Hepatology* **2018**, *68*, 435–448. [CrossRef] [PubMed]

143. Atcheson, E.; Li, W.; Bliss, C.M.; Chinnakannan, S.; Heim, K.; Sharpe, H.; Hutchings, C.; Dietrich, I.; Nguyen, D.; Kapoor, A.; et al. Use of an outbred rat hepacivirus challenge model for design and evaluation of efficacy of different immunisation strategies for HCV. *Hepatology* **2019**. [CrossRef] [PubMed]
144. Kapoor, A.; Simmonds, P.; Gerold, G.; Qaisar, N.; Jain, K.; Henriquez, J.A.; Firth, C.; Hirschberg, D.L.; Rice, C.M.; Shields, S.; et al. Characterization of a canine homolog of hepatitis C virus. *Proc. Natl. Acad. Sci. USA* **2011**, *108*, 11608–11613. [CrossRef] [PubMed]
145. Burbelo, P.D.; Dubovi, E.J.; Simmonds, P.; Medina, J.L.; Henriquez, J.A.; Mishra, N.; Wagner, J.; Tokarz, R.; Cullen, J.M.; Iadarola, M.J.; et al. Serology-enabled discovery of genetically diverse hepaciviruses in a new host. *J. Virol.* **2012**, *86*, 6171–6178. [CrossRef]
146. Pfaender, S.; Brown, R.J.; Pietschmann, T.; Steinmann, E. Natural reservoirs for homologs of hepatitis C virus. *Emerg. Microbes Infect.* **2014**, *3*, e21. [CrossRef]
147. Pfaender, S.; Cavalleri, J.M.; Walter, S.; Doerrbecker, J.; Campana, B.; Brown, R.J.; Burbelo, P.D.; Postel, A.; Hahn, K.; Anggakusuma; et al. Clinical course of infection and viral tissue tropism of hepatitis C virus-like nonprimate hepaciviruses in horses. *Hepatology* **2015**, *61*, 447–459. [CrossRef]
148. Tegtmeyer, B.; Echelmeyer, J.; Pfankuche, V.M.; Puff, C.; Todt, D.; Fischer, N.; Durham, A.; Feige, K.; Baumgartner, W.; Steinmann, E.; et al. Chronic equine hepacivirus infection in an adult gelding with severe hepatopathy. *Vet. Med. Sci.* **2019**, *5*, 372–378. [CrossRef]
149. Shi, B.; Ma, L.; He, X.; Wang, X.; Wang, P.; Zhou, L.; Yao, X. Comparative analysis of human and mouse immunoglobulin variable heavy regions from IMGT/LIGM-DB with IMGT/HighV-QUEST. *Theor. Biol. Med. Model.* **2014**, *11*, 30. [CrossRef]
150. Manso, T.C.; Groenner-Penna, M.; Minozzo, J.C.; Antunes, B.C.; Ippolito, G.C.; Molina, F.; Felicori, L.F. Next-generation sequencing reveals new insights about gene usage and CDR-H3 composition in the horse antibody repertoire. *Mol. Immunol.* **2019**, *105*, 251–259. [CrossRef]
151. Li, Y.; Pierce, B.G.; Wang, Q.; Keck, Z.Y.; Fuerst, T.R.; Foung, S.K.; Mariuzza, R.A. Structural basis for penetration of the glycan shield of hepatitis C virus E2 glycoprotein by a broadly neutralizing human antibody. *J. Biol. Chem.* **2015**, *290*, 10117–10125. [CrossRef] [PubMed]
152. Keck, Z.Y.; Angus, A.G.; Wang, W.; Lau, P.; Wang, Y.; Gatherer, D.; Patel, A.H.; Foung, S.K. Non-random escape pathways from a broadly neutralizing human monoclonal antibody map to a highly conserved region on the hepatitis C virus E2 glycoprotein encompassing amino acids 412–423. *PLoS Pathog.* **2014**, *10*, e1004297. [CrossRef] [PubMed]
153. Pierce, B.G.; Boucher, E.N.; Piepenbrink, K.H.; Ejemel, M.; Rapp, C.A.; Thomas, W.D., Jr.; Sundberg, E.J.; Weng, Z.; Wang, Y. Structure-Based Design of Hepatitis C Virus Vaccines That Elicit Neutralizing Antibody Responses to a Conserved Epitope. *J. Virol.* **2017**, *91*. [CrossRef] [PubMed]
154. Filskov, J.; Andersen, P.; Agger, E.M.; Bukh, J. HCV p7 as a novel vaccine-target inducing multifunctional CD4(+) and CD8(+) T-cells targeting liver cells expressing the viral antigen. *Sci. Rep.* **2019**, *9*, 14085. [CrossRef] [PubMed]
155. Dawood, R.M.; Moustafa, R.I.; Abdelhafez, T.H.; El-Shenawy, R.; El-Abd, Y.; Bader El Din, N.G.; Dubuisson, J.; El Awady, M.K. A multiepitope peptide vaccine against HCV stimulates neutralizing humoral and persistent cellular responses in mice. *BMC Infect. Dis.* **2019**, *19*, 932. [CrossRef] [PubMed]
156. Marin, M.Q.; Perez, P.; Ljungberg, K.; Sorzano, C.O.S.; Gomez, C.E.; Liljestrom, P.; Esteban, M.; Garcia-Arriaza, J. Potent Anti-hepatitis C Virus (HCV) T Cell Immune Responses Induced in Mice Vaccinated with DNA-Launched RNA Replicons and Modified Vaccinia Virus Ankara-HCV. *J. Virol.* **2019**, *93*. [CrossRef]
157. Wijesundara, D.K.; Gummow, J.; Li, Y.; Yu, W.; Quah, B.J.; Ranasinghe, C.; Torresi, J.; Gowans, E.J.; Grubor-Bauk, B. Induction of Genotype Cross-Reactive, Hepatitis C Virus-Specific, Cell-Mediated Immunity in DNA-Vaccinated Mice. *J. Virol.* **2018**, *92*. [CrossRef]
158. Masavuli, M.G.; Wijesundara, D.K.; Underwood, A.; Christiansen, D.; Earnest-Silveira, L.; Bull, R.; Torresi, J.; Gowans, E.J.; Grubor-Bauk, B. A Hepatitis C Virus DNA Vaccine Encoding a Secreted, Oligomerized Form of Envelope Proteins Is Highly Immunogenic and Elicits Neutralizing Antibodies in Vaccinated Mice. *Front. Immunol.* **2019**, *10*, 1145. [CrossRef]
159. Plotkin, S.A. Vaccines: Past, present and future. *Nat. Med.* **2005**, *11*, S5–S11. [CrossRef]
160. Choo, Q.L.; Kuo, G.; Ralston, R.; Weiner, A.; Chien, D.; Van Nest, G.; Han, J.; Berger, K.; Thudium, K.; Kuo, C.; et al. Vaccination of chimpanzees against infection by the hepatitis C virus. *Proc. Natl. Acad. Sci. USA* **1994**, *91*, 1294–1298. [CrossRef]

161. Houghton, M. Prospects for prophylactic and therapeutic vaccines against the hepatitis C viruses. *Immunol. Rev.* **2011**, *239*, 99–108. [CrossRef] [PubMed]
162. Frey, S.E.; Houghton, M.; Coates, S.; Abrignani, S.; Chien, D.; Rosa, D.; Pileri, P.; Ray, R.; Di Bisceglie, A.M.; Rinella, P.; et al. Safety and immunogenicity of HCV E1E2 vaccine adjuvanted with MF59 administered to healthy adults. *Vaccine* **2010**, *28*, 6367–6373. [CrossRef] [PubMed]
163. Ray, R.; Meyer, K.; Banerjee, A.; Basu, A.; Coates, S.; Abrignani, S.; Houghton, M.; Frey, S.E.; Belshe, R.B. Characterization of antibodies induced by vaccination with hepatitis C virus envelope glycoproteins. *J. Infect. Dis.* **2010**, *202*, 862–866. [CrossRef] [PubMed]
164. Law, J.L.; Chen, C.; Wong, J.; Hockman, D.; Santer, D.M.; Frey, S.E.; Belshe, R.B.; Wakita, T.; Bukh, J.; Jones, C.T.; et al. A hepatitis C virus (HCV) vaccine comprising envelope glycoproteins gpE1/gpE2 derived from a single isolate elicits broad cross-genotype neutralizing antibodies in humans. *PLoS ONE* **2013**, *8*, e59776. [CrossRef] [PubMed]
165. Wong, J.A.; Bhat, R.; Hockman, D.; Logan, M.; Chen, C.; Levin, A.; Frey, S.E.; Belshe, R.B.; Tyrrell, D.L.; Law, J.L.; et al. Recombinant hepatitis C virus envelope glycoprotein vaccine elicits antibodies targeting multiple epitopes on the envelope glycoproteins associated with broad cross-neutralization. *J. Virol.* **2014**, *88*, 14278–14288. [CrossRef] [PubMed]
166. Logan, M.; Law, J.; Wong, J.A.J.; Hockman, D.; Landi, A.; Chen, C.; Crawford, K.; Kundu, J.; Baldwin, L.; Johnson, J.; et al. Native Folding of a Recombinant gpE1/gpE2 Heterodimer Vaccine Antigen from a Precursor Protein Fused with Fc IgG. *J. Virol.* **2017**, *91*. [CrossRef]
167. Ruwona, T.B.; Giang, E.; Nieusma, T.; Law, M. Fine mapping of murine antibody responses to immunization with a novel soluble form of hepatitis C virus envelope glycoprotein complex. *J. Virol.* **2014**, *88*, 10459–10471. [CrossRef]
168. Krapchev, V.B.; Rychlowska, M.; Chmielewska, A.; Zimmer, K.; Patel, A.H.; Bienkowska-Szewczyk, K. Recombinant Flag-tagged E1E2 glycoproteins from three hepatitis C virus genotypes are biologically functional and elicit cross-reactive neutralizing antibodies in mice. *Virology* **2018**, *519*, 33–41. [CrossRef]
169. McCaffrey, K.; Boo, I.; Poumbourios, P.; Drummer, H.E. Expression and characterization of a minimal hepatitis C virus glycoprotein E2 core domain that retains CD81 binding. *J. Virol.* **2007**, *81*, 9584–9590. [CrossRef]
170. Vietheer, P.T.; Boo, I.; Gu, J.; McCaffrey, K.; Edwards, S.; Owczarek, C.; Hardy, M.P.; Fabri, L.; Center, R.J.; Poumbourios, P.; et al. The core domain of hepatitis C virus glycoprotein E2 generates potent cross-neutralizing antibodies in guinea pigs. *Hepatology* **2017**, *65*, 1117–1131. [CrossRef]
171. McCaffrey, K.; Boo, I.; Owczarek, C.M.; Hardy, M.P.; Perugini, M.A.; Fabri, L.; Scotney, P.; Poumbourios, P.; Drummer, H.E. An Optimized Hepatitis C Virus E2 Glycoprotein Core Adopts a Functional Homodimer That Efficiently Blocks Virus Entry. *J. Virol.* **2017**, *91*. [CrossRef] [PubMed]
172. Law, J.L.M.; Logan, M.; Wong, J.; Kundu, J.; Hockman, D.; Landi, A.; Chen, C.; Crawford, K.; Wininger, M.; Johnson, J.; et al. Role of the E2 Hypervariable Region (HVR1) in the Immunogenicity of a Recombinant Hepatitis C Virus Vaccine. *J. Virol.* **2018**, *92*. [CrossRef]
173. Torresi, J. The Rationale for a Preventative HCV Virus-Like Particle (VLP) Vaccine. *Front. Microbiol.* **2017**, *8*, 2163. [CrossRef] [PubMed]
174. Bachmann, M.F.; Jennings, G.T. Vaccine delivery: A matter of size, geometry, kinetics and molecular patterns. *Nat. Rev. Immunol.* **2010**, *10*, 787–796. [CrossRef] [PubMed]
175. Baumert, T.F.; Ito, S.; Wong, D.T.; Liang, T.J. Hepatitis C virus structural proteins assemble into viruslike particles in insect cells. *J. Virol.* **1998**, *72*, 3827–3836. [CrossRef] [PubMed]
176. Baumert, T.F.; Vergalla, J.; Satoi, J.; Thomson, M.; Lechmann, M.; Herion, D.; Greenberg, H.B.; Ito, S.; Liang, T.J. Hepatitis C virus-like particles synthesized in insect cells as a potential vaccine candidate. *Gastroenterology* **1999**, *117*, 1397–1407. [CrossRef]
177. Lechmann, M.; Murata, K.; Satoi, J.; Vergalla, J.; Baumert, T.F.; Liang, T.J. Hepatitis C virus-like particles induce virus-specific humoral and cellular immune responses in mice. *Hepatology* **2001**, *34*, 417–423. [CrossRef]
178. Jeong, S.H.; Qiao, M.; Nascimbeni, M.; Hu, Z.; Rehermann, B.; Murthy, K.; Liang, T.J. Immunization with hepatitis C virus-like particles induces humoral and cellular immune responses in nonhuman primates. *J. Virol.* **2004**, *78*, 6995–7003. [CrossRef]
179. Elmowalid, G.A.; Qiao, M.; Jeong, S.H.; Borg, B.B.; Baumert, T.F.; Sapp, R.K.; Hu, Z.; Murthy, K.; Liang, T.J. Immunization with hepatitis C virus-like particles results in control of hepatitis C virus infection in chimpanzees. *Proc. Natl. Acad. Sci. USA* **2007**, *104*, 8427–8432. [CrossRef]

180. Chua, B.Y.; Johnson, D.; Tan, A.; Earnest-Silveira, L.; Sekiya, T.; Chin, R.; Torresi, J.; Jackson, D.C. Hepatitis C VLPs delivered to dendritic cells by a TLR2 targeting lipopeptide results in enhanced antibody and cell-mediated responses. *PLoS ONE* **2012**, *7*, e47492. [CrossRef]
181. Christiansen, D.; Earnest-Silveira, L.; Chua, B.; Meuleman, P.; Boo, I.; Grubor-Bauk, B.; Jackson, D.C.; Keck, Z.Y.; Foung, S.K.H.; Drummer, H.E.; et al. Immunological responses following administration of a genotype 1a/1b/2/3a quadrivalent HCV VLP vaccine. *Sci. Rep.* **2018**, *8*, 6483. [CrossRef] [PubMed]
182. Earnest-Silveira, L.; Chua, B.; Chin, R.; Christiansen, D.; Johnson, D.; Herrmann, S.; Ralph, S.A.; Vercauteren, K.; Mesalam, A.; Meuleman, P.; et al. Characterization of a hepatitis C virus-like particle vaccine produced in a human hepatocyte-derived cell line. *J. Gen. Virol.* **2016**, *97*, 1865–1876. [CrossRef] [PubMed]
183. Collett, S.; Torresi, J.; Earnest-Silveira, L.; Christiansen, D.; Elbourne, A.; Ramsland, P.A. Probing and pressing surfaces of hepatitis C virus-like particles. *J. Colloid Interface Sci.* **2019**, *545*, 259–268. [CrossRef]
184. Christiansen, D.; Earnest-Silveira, L.; Grubor-Bauk, B.; Wijesundara, D.K.; Boo, I.; Ramsland, P.A.; Vincan, E.; Drummer, H.E.; Gowans, E.J.; Torresi, J. Pre-clinical evaluation of a quadrivalent HCV VLP vaccine in pigs following microneedle delivery. *Sci. Rep.* **2019**, *9*, 9251. [CrossRef]
185. Ura, T.; Okuda, K.; Shimada, M. Developments in Viral Vector-Based Vaccines. *Vaccines* **2014**, *2*, 624–641. [CrossRef] [PubMed]
186. Barnes, E.; Folgori, A.; Capone, S.; Swadling, L.; Aston, S.; Kurioka, A.; Meyer, J.; Huddart, R.; Smith, K.; Townsend, R.; et al. Novel adenovirus-based vaccines induce broad and sustained T cell responses to HCV in man. *Sci. Transl. Med.* **2012**, *4*, 115ra1. [CrossRef] [PubMed]
187. Capone, S.; Zampaglione, I.; Vitelli, A.; Pezzanera, M.; Kierstead, L.; Burns, J.; Ruggeri, L.; Arcuri, M.; Cappelletti, M.; Meola, A.; et al. Modulation of the immune response induced by gene electrotransfer of a hepatitis C virus DNA vaccine in nonhuman primates. *J. Immunol.* **2006**, *177*, 7462–7471. [CrossRef] [PubMed]
188. Swadling, L.; Capone, S.; Antrobus, R.D.; Brown, A.; Richardson, R.; Newell, E.W.; Halliday, J.; Kelly, C.; Bowen, D.; Fergusson, J.; et al. A human vaccine strategy based on chimpanzee adenoviral and MVA vectors that primes, boosts, and sustains functional HCV-specific T cell memory. *Sci. Transl. Med.* **2014**, *6*, 261ra153. [CrossRef]
189. Swadling, L.; Halliday, J.; Kelly, C.; Brown, A.; Capone, S.; Ansari, M.A.; Bonsall, D.; Richardson, R.; Hartnell, F.; Collier, J.; et al. Highly-Immunogenic Virally-Vectored T-cell Vaccines Cannot Overcome Subversion of the T-cell Response by HCV during Chronic Infection. *Vaccines* **2016**, *4*, 27. [CrossRef]
190. Trial Evaluating Experimental Hepatitis C Vaccine Concludes|NIH: National Institute of Allergy and Infectious Diseases. Available online: https://www.niaid.nih.gov/news-events/trial-evaluating-experimental-hepatitis-c-vaccine-concludes (accessed on 29 December 2019).
191. Beaumont, E.; Patient, R.; Hourioux, C.; Dimier-Poisson, I.; Roingeard, P. Chimeric hepatitis B virus/hepatitis C virus envelope proteins elicit broadly neutralizing antibodies and constitute a potential bivalent prophylactic vaccine. *Hepatology* **2013**, *57*, 1303–1313. [CrossRef]
192. Wei, S.; Lei, Y.; Yang, J.; Wang, X.; Shu, F.; Wei, X.; Lin, F.; Li, B.; Cui, Y.; Zhang, H. Neutralization effects of antibody elicited by chimeric HBV S antigen viral-like particles presenting HCV neutralization epitopes. *Vaccine* **2018**, *36*, 2273–2281. [CrossRef] [PubMed]
193. Garrone, P.; Fluckiger, A.C.; Mangeot, P.E.; Gauthier, E.; Dupeyrot-Lacas, P.; Mancip, J.; Cangialosi, A.; Du Chene, I.; LeGrand, R.; Mangeot, I.; et al. A prime-boost strategy using virus-like particles pseudotyped for HCV proteins triggers broadly neutralizing antibodies in macaques. *Sci. Transl. Med.* **2011**, *3*, 94ra71. [CrossRef] [PubMed]

vaccines

MDPI

Article

Broad Protection of Pigs against Heterologous PRRSV Strains by a GP5-Mosaic DNA Vaccine Prime/GP5-Mosaic rVaccinia (VACV) Vaccine Boost

Junru Cui, Caitlin M. O'Connell, Connor Hagen, Kim Sawicki, Joan A. Smyth, Paulo H. Verardi, Herbert J. Van Kruiningen and Antonio E. Garmendia *

Department of Pathobiology and Veterinary Science, College of Agriculture, Health and Natural Resources, University of Connecticut, Storrs, CT 06269, USA; junru.cui@uconn.edu (J.C.); caitlin.o'connell@uconn.edu (C.M.O.); connor.hagen@uconn.edu (C.H.); kimitt@gmail.com (K.S.); joan.smyth@uconn.edu (J.A.S.); paulo.verardi@uconn.edu (P.H.V.); herbert.vankruiningen@uconn.edu (H.J.V.K.)

* Correspondence: antonio.garmendia@uconn.edu; Tel.: +1-860-486-3945

Received: 22 January 2020; Accepted: 23 February 2020; Published: 28 February 2020

Abstract: Background: Porcine reproductive and respiratory syndrome (PRRS) viruses are a major cause of disease and economic loss in pigs worldwide. High genetic diversity among PRRSV strains is problematic for successful disease control by vaccination. Mosaic DNA and vaccinia (VACV) vaccines were developed in order to improve protection against heterologous PRRSV strains. Methods: Piglets were primed and boosted with GP5-Mosaic DNA vaccine and recombinant GP5-Mosaic VACV (rGP5-Mosaic VACV), respectively. Pigs vaccinated with rGP5-WT (VR2332) DNA and rGP5-WT VACV, or empty vector DNA and empty VACV respectively, served as controls. Virus challenge was given to separate groups of vaccinated pigs with VR2332 or MN184C. Necropsies were performed 14 days after challenge. Results: Vaccination with the GP5-Mosaic-based vaccines resulted in cellular reactivity and higher levels of neutralizing antibodies to both VR2332 and MN184C PRRSV strains. In contrast, vaccination of animals with the GP5-WT vaccines induced responses only to VR2332. Furthermore, vaccination with the GP5-Mosaic based vaccines resulted in protection against challenge with two heterologous virus strains, as demonstrated by the significantly lower viral loads in serum, tissues, porcine alveolar macrophages (PAMs), and bronchoalveolar lavage (BAL) fluids, and less severe lung lesions after challenge with either MN184C or VR2332, which have only 85% identity. In contrast, significant protection by the GP5-WT based vaccines was only achieved against the VR2332 strain. Conclusions: GP5-Mosaic vaccines, using a DNA-prime/VACV boost regimen, conferred protection in pigs against heterologous viruses.

Keywords: PRRSV Mosaic T-cell DNA vaccine VACV; PRRS; cross protection; heterologous virus challenge

1. Introduction

Porcine reproductive and respiratory syndrome (PRRS) is a major disease in pigs that causes significant economic losses to industry across the world. In the United States alone, PRRS causes over $600 million in losses a year [1]. PRRS causes reproductive failure in pregnant sows and respiratory disease in young pigs. The causal virus, PRRSV, is a positive-sense, single-stranded RNA virus with a lipid envelope, and belongs to the Family *Arteriviridae*, Order *Nidovirales* [2–4]. The genome is approximately 15 Kb long and encodes at least 22 different viral proteins including fourteen non-structural and eight structural proteins [5]. PRRSV induces both humoral and cellular immune responses in pigs and some of the viral proteins inducing such responses have been identified; however, protection against reinfection is incomplete [6–9]. Killed virus (KV) vaccines and modified live virus (MLV) vaccines for PRRS have been licensed for more than two decades. These vaccines generally reduce the severity of clinical signs and the transmission of virus; however, they do not induce sterilizing immunity. In general, the efficacy of MLV vaccines is superior to that of KV vaccines [10–13]. Importantly, however, highly variable and generally sub-optimal levels of protection against heterologous PRRSV strains have been reported [10,14–18]. The potential for reversion to the virulence of MLV vaccines and subsequent transmission to susceptible pigs is a concern [19–21].

The major challenge for the development of efficacious, broadly protective PRRS vaccines is the extraordinary genetic variation among disease producing PRRSV strains. Currently, two major PRRSV genotypes are recognized, Genotype 1 (European) and Genotype 2 (North American), which exhibit nearly 40% sequence dissimilarity [22,23]. Genotype 1 and Genotype 2 PRRSVs can be further divided into four subgroups and nine different lineages, respectively, based on phylogenetic analysis of ORF5 [24]. The co-existence of multiple variants within one farm, or even within individual pigs, possibly indicates the occurrence of quasispecies variation of PRRSV [25]. Thus, the development of vaccines that can induce protection against different subgroups and lineages is highly desirable. Multi-subunit vaccines [26], consensus vaccines [27], molecular breeding of different viral structural proteins [28], Mosaic T-cell vaccines [29,30], a polyvalent vaccine containing five different live-attenuated PRRSV strains [31] and DNA prime-MLV boost [32] are just some of the vaccines that are or have been under evaluation recently.

Studies on potential vaccines against human immune deficiency virus type 1 (HIV-1), have shown that Mosaic sequences designed from naturally occurring HIV sequences could effectively address genetic diversity when used as vaccines [33,34]. Mosaic vaccines have been shown to elicit broader immune responses successfully and to confer cross protection in non-human primates and these Mosaic HIV vaccines have been trialed in humans [34–38]. We previously reported that a PRRSV Mosaic vaccine based on 748 GP5 sequences of the Genotype 2 PRRSV strain was immunogenic [29] and induced reactivity to four divergent Genotype-2 PRRSV strains that had at least 10% or more difference in their GP5 sequence—as shown by the expression of interferon gamma (IFN-γ) by peripheral blood mononuclear cells—and, further, that vaccinated pigs were protected against challenge with VR2332 [30]. The present study demonstrates further that vaccination of pigs with the GP5-Mosaic by using a DNA prime and rVaccinia boost approach protects them against strains that are more than 10% divergent in their sequences (VR2332 and MN184C).

2. Materials and Methods

2.1. Viruses and Cells

The viruses used in the study included the VR2332 NA reference strain (ATCC VR-2332) and the MN184C strain provided kindly by Drs. Kelly Lager and Kay Faaberg at U.S. Department of Agriculture-Agriculture Research Service (USDA-ARS). The viruses were propagated in MARC-145 cells [39] grown in Dulbecco's modified Eagle's medium (DMEM) containing 2 mM L-glutamine, 100 U penicillin/mL, 100 μg streptomycin/mL and 10% fetal bovine serum (FBS). The Reed–Muench formula was used to calculate virus titers [40]. Viruses were purified over continuous cesium chloride gradients, quantified using a NanoDrop 1000 spectrophotometer (Thermo Scientific, Waltham, MA, USA) and stored at −80 °C for later use. Titrated viruses were used for ex vivo recall immune response assay and challenge experiments.

2.2. Transfer Vector Construction

A combination of gene synthesis (DNA 2.0, Menlo Park, CA, USA) and standard sub-cloning was utilized to generate three transfer vectors. Each transfer vector contained a cassette with the tetR gene (based on GenBank: X00694), and either a natural or Mosaic version of Genotype 2 PRRSV ORF 5 [29,30], followed by the EMCV IRES (based on GenBank: NC_001479.1) and the EGFP gene (based on plasmid pEGFP-1, GenBank: U55761). The tetR gene and the ORF 5–IRES-EGFP genetic segment were placed under back-to-back synthetic VACV early/late promoters [41]. The tetO2 operator sequence was inserted after the putative VACV D6R promoter, as described in [42]. The cassettes were flanked by 600 bp of the VACV D5R gene to the left and 600 bp of the VACV D6R gene to the right (based on GenBank: NC_006998.1). Restriction endonuclease analysis was used to confirm plasmid identity.

2.3. Generation of Recombinant VACVs and Preparation of High-Titer Stocks

Standard homologous recombination was used to generate Tetracycline-inducible recombinant VACVs after the transfection of transfer vectors with FuGene HD Transfection Reagent (Promega, Madison, WI, USA) into BS-C-1 cells, infected 1 h before with an IPTG-inducible VACV strain (based on the WR clone 9.2.4.8.) in the presence of 0.1 mM IPTG and 1 μg/mL doxycycline. Recombinant EGFP-positive tetracycline-inducible VACVs were plaque purified in the absence of Isopropyl β-d-1-thiogalactopyranoside (IPTG) and in the presence of 1 μg/mL doxycycline. The elimination of the parental virus was confirmed by PCR analysis of viral DNA that was purified using a Nucleospin® Blood kit (Macherey-Nagel, Düren, Germany). High-titer stocks were generated by infecting HeLa S3 cells with recombinant virus at a multiplicity of infection (MOI)of 0.1 in the presence of 1 μg/mL doxycycline. Infected cells were harvested and homogenized 4 days post-infection. Homogenates were clarified by centrifugation at 750× *g* for 10 min, purified over a sucrose cushion [43], and resuspended in 1X PBS pH 7.3 (with no doxycycline).

2.4. Protein Sequence Alignment and Phylogenetic Analysis

MEGA 7 (Molecular Evolutionary Genetics Analysis) (www.megasoftware.net) (NIH, Bethesda, MD, USA) was utilized to evaluate protein sequence alignments between GP5 sequences of VR2332, MN184C, Mosaic 1 and Mosaic 2 and to create a phylogenetic tree.

2.5. Vaccination and Collection of Samples

Cross-bred three- to four-week-old male and female piglets, which were free of PRRSV and porcine circovirus-2, were used in this study. The experimental design is summarized in Table 1. GP5-Mosaic, GP5-WT and vector-control vaccines were administered by both intradermal and intramuscular injection. Briefly, 1 mL vaccine containing 500 μg DNA and 100 μg Quil-A® as adjuvant was injected intradermally (0.1 mL) on the back of ear and intramuscularly (0.9 mL) in the neck region at day 0 and again on day 14. The animals were further boosted at day 28 with a 1 mL suspension containing 10^8 PFU VACV expressing GP5-Mosaic, GP5-WT or VACV and 100 μg Quil-A® as adjuvant. Pigs were challenged at day 35 with VR2332 and at day 37 with MN184C to their respective groups. A total of 10^6 $TCID_{50}$ of each virus was administered by intranasal and intramuscular challenge to each animal. Blood was collected at days 0, 7, 14, 21, 28, the challenge day, and 4, 7, 10, and 14 days after challenge.

Table 1. Experimental design.

Group	Vaccination [a]	Challenge [b]
A (*n* = 8)	DNA/Vector-control/VACV	VR2332 (*n* = 4) MN184C (*n* = 4)
B (*n* = 8)	DNA GP5-WT/VACV GP5 WT	VR2332 (*n* = 4) MN184C (*n* = 4)
C (*n* = 8)	DNA GP5-Mosaic/VACV GP5-Mosaic	VR2332 (*n* = 4) MN184C (*n* = 4)

[a] One mL vaccine containing 500 μg DNA and 100 μg Quil-A® as adjuvant was injected intradermally (0.1 mL) on the back of ear and intramuscularly (0.9 mL) in the neck region at day 0 and again at day 14. VACV 10^8 PFU and 100 μg Quil-A® as adjuvant was administered at day 28. [b] Pigs were challenged at day 35 with $10^6 TCID_{50}$ VR2332 (*n* = 4/group) and day 37 with $10^6 TCID_{50}$ MN184C (*n* = 4/group) both intranasally and intramuscularly.

The pigs were euthanized at 14 days post-challenge. The lungs were evaluated macroscopically, weighed, and bronchoalveolar lavage (BAL) was then performed. Tissue samples were collected from each lung lobe, tracheobronchial lymph nodes (TBLN), spleen, inguinal lymph nodes (ILN) and tonsils: portions of each were either fixed in 10% neutral buffered formalin or kept frozen. Fixed tissues were routinely processed to paraffin, and 4–5 μm sections were stained with hematoxylin and eosin and evaluated histologically. Lung lesion scores were calculated as reported before [44]. All animal work was performed under a protocol approved by the University of Connecticut Institutional Animal Care and Use Committee, the animal protocol number under which the study was conducted is IACUC A17-003.

2.6. *Measurement of IFN-γ Immune Response to PRRSV*

Peripheral blood mononuclear cells harvested from blood collected at days 0 and on the challenge day, were seeded in 24-well flat-bottom plates (5×10^5 cells/well). They were then stimulated, in duplicate, by adding 200 $TCID_{50}$ VR2332 or MN184C/well, or mock treated for 48 h at 37 °C in a 5% CO_2 atmosphere. The cells were then collected and total RNA was extracted for quantitative real-time PCR analysis.

2.7. *Serum Neutralization Test*

Virus neutralization testing was carried out as previously reported [30]. Briefly, each serum was mixed with equal volumes of DMEM containing 100 $TCID_{50}$ of VR2332 or MN184C and the mixtures were incubated at 37 °C for 1 h. The serum–virus mixtures were then added to 96-well plates containing 80–90% confluent MARC-145 cells and incubated for 48 h at 37 °C in a 5% CO_2 atmosphere (final serum dilution 1:4). The VR2332 or MN184C virus, negative serum, and uninfected cells served as the virus control, negative serum control and cell control, respectively. The neutralizing capacity of serum was quantified by measuring the viral copy numbers by RT-qPCR in supernatants 48 h after the addition of pre-incubated serum–virus mixtures to the cells.

2.8. *Quantitative Real-Time PCR*

TRIzol LS Reagent or TRIzol Reagent (Invitrogen, Grand Island, NY, USA) was used to extract total RNA from serum/ culture supernatants or tissues, respectively. The extracted RNA was quantified in a NanoDrop 1000 spectrophotometer (Thermo Scientific, Waltham, MA, USA). The cDNA was synthesized from each sample RNA using a 20 μL reaction mixture and random primers (Invitrogen, Grand Island, NY, USA) and the following reaction conditions: 26 °C for 10 min, 42 °C for 45 min and 75 °C for 10 min. The cDNA was then amplified by SYBR Green real-time PCR. To this effect, SYBR qPCR Master Mix (Bimake, Huston, TX, USA), the cDNA template and 5′-ATG ATG RCC TGG CAT TCT-3′and 5′-ACA CGG TCG CCC TAA TTG-3′ were utilized as the forward and reverse primers for ORF7, respectively. Real time PCR was then performed as follows: 2 min at 95 °C, followed by 40 cycles at 95 °C for 15 s and 61 °C for 1 min using Bio-Rad CFX96 Touch System (Bio-Rad, Hercules, CA, USA). For use in quantification, a standard curve was generated using serial dilutions of viral RNA which contained 10^2–10^7 copies/μL. Both positive and negative reference samples were run concurrently with the test samples. Viral loads were determined by plotting the Ct values against the standard curve. Melting curves were analyzed to verify the specificity of the PCR.

To test for IFN-γ expression, total RNA was extracted by TRIzol Reagent from virus-stimulated or mock-treated PBMCs; this was then used as template for cDNA synthesis and this, in turn, was used for real-time PCR following the protocol described above. Glyceraldehyde 3-phosphate dehydrogenase (GAPDH) (forward primer: 5′-CGT CCC TGA GAC ACG ATG GT-3′and reverse primer: 5′-CCC GAT GCG GCC AAA T-3′) was used as internal control to calculate the fold changes in the expression of IFN-γ (forward primer: 5′-TGG TAG CTC TGG GAA ACT GAA TG-3′and reverse primer: 5′-GGC TTT GCG CTG GAT CTG-3′) by the delta–delta method [44].

2.9. Lung Lesion Scoring

The scoring of lung lesions was done systematically, as previously described [45], by a board-certified veterinary pathologist, blinded to the treatment groups. Nine sections, representing all six lung lobes, were scored, with one section from each division of the left cranial lung lobe and two sections from each diaphragmatic lobe.

2.10. Statistical Analysis

Two-way ANOVA or Student's t-test was used to evaluate the differences in measurements between the samples within or between groups. The data were analyzed using GraphPad Prism (version 7.0) (GraphPad Software, San Diego, CA, USA).

3. Results

3.1. Sequence Alignment and Analysis of GP5

The GP5 amino acid (aa) sequences in Mosaic 1, Mosaic 2, MN184C and VR2332 (the prototype of Genotype 2 PRRSV) were all the same size, with no deletions or insertions. Sequence alignments showed aa identity from 85% to 93%. To further investigate the antigenic relationship of these strains, a phylogenetic tree was constructed using the neighbor-joining method b. The four sequences clustered into two subgroups (Figure 1), with the two most distant being Mosaic 1 and MN184C. Mosaic 1 and Mosaic 2 were, relatively, more closely related to VR2332 and MN184C, respectively.

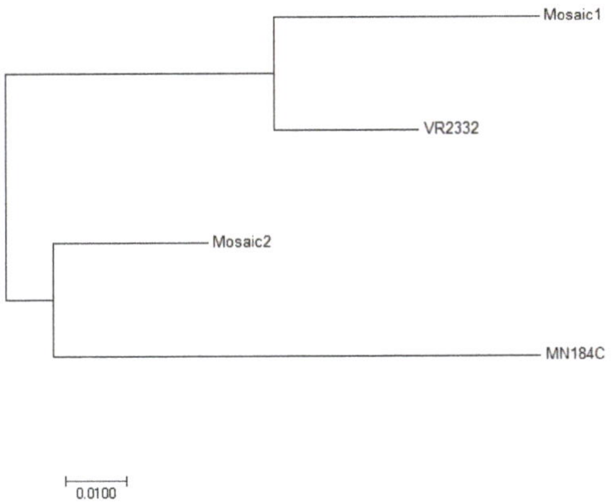

Figure 1. Phylogenetic analysis of the GP5 Amino acid sequence of the two Mosaic sequences, MN184C and VR2332. The analysis was done via the neighbor-joining method using MEGA7.0.

3.2. GP5-Mosaic Vaccines Induced Both Humoral and Cellular Response

GP5-Mosaic-vaccinated pigs had significantly higher levels of neutralizing antibodies in their serum compared to the vector-control animals, both to VR2332 ($p < 0.001$) and MN184C ($p < 0.05$) The virus neutralizing capability of serum from GP5-WT-vaccinated animals was greater against VR2332 ($p < 0.01$) and against MN184C ($p > 0.05$) when compared to serum from vector control animals (Figure 2A); vaccination with the GP5-Mosaic vaccine resulted in broader recall cellular responses than those induced with the GP5WT vaccine. Thus, a significantly higher ($p < 0.05$) relative fold-change in IFN-γ mRNA expression was detected upon stimulation of PBMCs derived from GP5-Mosaic-vaccinated pigs, with either VR2332 or MN184C strains, when compared to those in equally stimulated PMBCs from vector control pigs (Figure 2B). In contrast, the expression of IFN-γ mRNA in GP5-WT-vaccinated pigs was significantly higher only if their PBMCs were stimulated with

VR2332, when compared to those in the equally stimulated PBMCs of the control pigs at the same time points (Figure 2B). No changes were detected with the PBMCs of vector-control pigs with any type of stimulation.

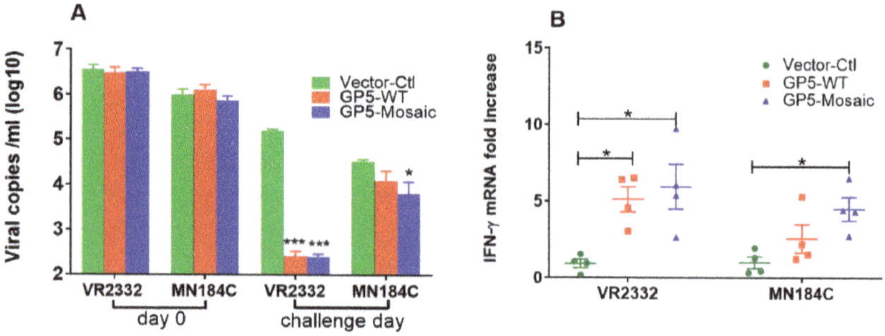

Figure 2. Vaccination-induced humoral and cellular responses. (**A**) The virus neutralization was expressed as viral copy numbers (log10 scale), as measured by RT-qPCR in cell supernatants after the infection of MARC-145 cells with pre-incubated serum–virus mixtures. (**B**) The expression of IFN-γ mRNA as fold changes, by either VR2332 or MN184C-stimulated PBMCs collected on the challenge day. Each dot represents the value of one animal. The variation is expressed as standard error of the means. There were three independent replications. Significant differences were calculated by a two-way ANOVA or Student's *t* test (* $p < 0.05$, *** $p < 0.0001$).

3.3. GP5-Mosaic Vaccination Induced Cross-Protection in Pigs

Viral loads in serum of both GP5-WT and GP5-Mosaic-vaccinated groups were significantly lower than those in the vector-control group at 7, 10 and 14 days after challenge with VR2332 (* $p < 0.05$, ** $p < 0.01$) (Figure 3A). Therefore, the capacity of reducing VR2332 virus loads in serum was relatively similar between the GP5-Mosaic and the GP5-WT vaccines. Furthermore, there was a steady decrease in viral loads from 4 days to 14 days after challenge in both GP5-WT and GP5-Mosaic vaccinated groups, while viral loads increased during the course of challenge and reached their peak at 10 days post-challenge (DPC), then declining slightly at 14 DPC in the vector-control group (Figure 3A). In contrast, the viral loads in serum of animals receiving the GP5-Mosaic-vaccine were significantly lower than those of animals receiving the GP5-WT vaccine or those of vector-control animals at 7 and 14 DPC with MN184C (* $p < 0.05$) (Figure 3B), which was different compared to VR2332-challenged groups. Viral load levels in GP5-WT vaccinated animals, increased during the infection with MN184C and reached their peak at 10DPC, which is comparable to the vector-control group. The viral loads in GP5-Mosaic vaccinated animals decreased steadily from 4 to 10 DPC and remained unchanged until 14 DPC (Figure 3B). Furthermore, the viral loads in lung, TBLN, spleen, ILN and tonsils were significantly lower in GP5-Mosaic-vaccinated animals than those in the vector-control group (* $p < 0.05$) after challenge with MN184C, while those of the GP5-WT group were similar or slightly lower compared to the vector-control group (Figure 3C). Viral loads in the lungs, TBLN, and tonsil were significantly lower in GP5-Mosaic-vaccinated animals than those in the vector-control group (* $p < 0.05$) after challenge with VR2332, while those of the GP5-WT group were significantly lower in the lungs, spleen and ILN compared to the vector-control group (* $p < 0.05$). There was no significant difference in VR2332 virus loads between the GP5-Mosaic and GP5-WT groups (Figure 3D).

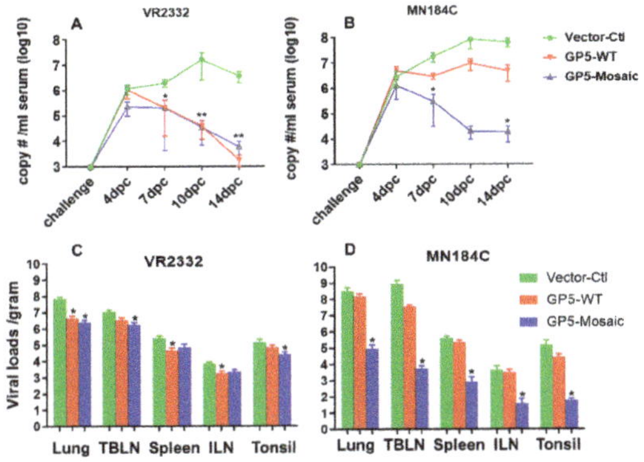

Figure 3. Virus clearance in sera and tissues. (**A**) Viral copy numbers in serum from 0 to 14 DPC upon VR2332 challenge. (**B**) The viral copy numbers in serum from 0 to 14 DPC upon MN184C challenge. Each dot represents the mean value of each group. The variation bars are expressed as the standard error of the mean. Three separate experiments were performed for each. A two-way ANOVA or Student's *t* test (* $p < 0.05$, ** $p < 0.01$, was used to calculate significant differences; days post-challenge (DPC). (**C**) The viral copy numbers in tissues at necropsy upon VR2332 challenge. (**D**) The viral copy numbers in tissues at necropsy upon MN184C challenge. Each bar represents the mean value of each group. The bars are the standard error of the mean. Three separate experiments were performed for each. Significant differences were calculated by Student's *t* test (* $p < 0.05$).

Tests in PAMs and BAL fluids showed a similar pattern in which the viral loads in both the GP5-Mosaic and GP5-WT groups were lower than those in the vector-control group after challenge with VR2332 (Figure 4A,C), meanwhile only the viral loads of GP5-Mosaic-vaccinated animals were significantly lower than those in the vector-control animals after challenge with MN184C (* $p < 0.05$ and ** $p < 0.01$, respectively), furthermore there was no apparent difference in MN184C viral loads between GP5-WT and vector-control animals (Figure 4B,D).

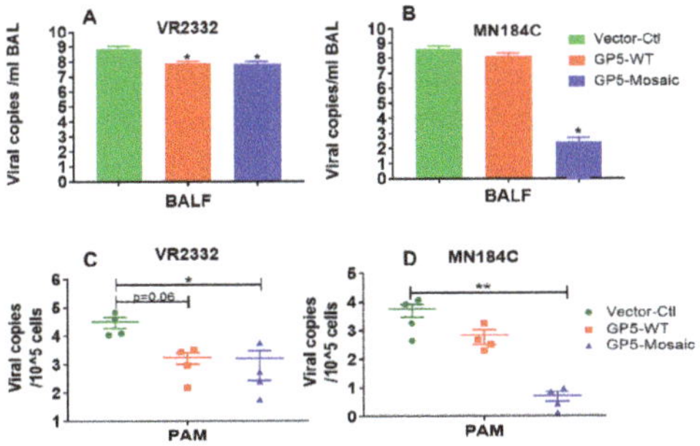

Figure 4. Virus clearance in bronchioalveolar lavage fluids (BAL) and PAMs. (**A**) The viral copy numbers in BAL fluids at necropsy upon challenge with VR2332. (**B**) The viral copy numbers in BAL fluids at necropsy upon challenge with MN184C. Each bar represents the mean value of each group. Bars represent the standard error of the mean. Three independent experiments were performed for each. Significant differences were calculated by Student's *t* test (* $p < 0.05$). (**C**) The viral copy numbers in PAMs at necropsy upon challenge with VR2332. (**D**) The viral copy numbers in PAMs at necropsy upon challenge with MN184C. Each dot represents the mean value of each animal. The bars represent the standard error of the mean. Three independent experiments were performed for each. Student's *t* test was used to calculate significant differences (* $p < 0.05$, ** $p < 0.01$).

3.4. Lower Lung Lesion Scores Detected in GP5-Mosaic-Vaccinated Animals

The lung lesion scores after challenge with MN184C were significantly lower in GP5-Mosaic-vaccinated animals than those in both GP5-WT and vector-control animals when evaluated using nine sections of lung (Figure 5 right panel, $p < 0.05$). In contrast, after VR2332 challenge, lung lesion scores were lower on average in both the GP5-Mosaic and GP5-WT groups than those in vector-control animals. There were no significant differences between the lung lesion scores of GP5-WT and GP5-Mosaic-vaccinated groups after challenge with VR2332 (Figure 5).

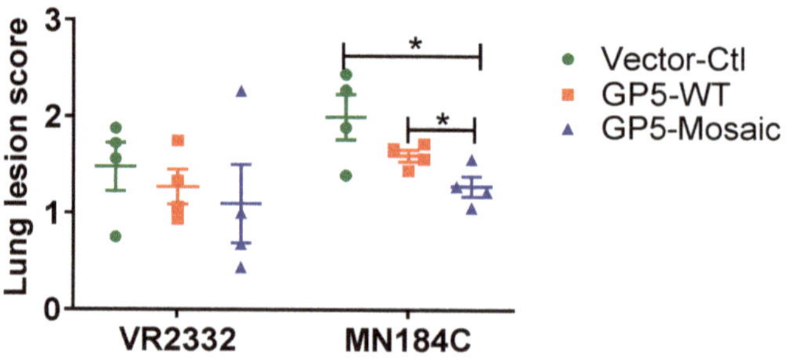

Figure 5. Lung lesion scores. The lung lesion scores of GP5-Mosaic-vaccinated animals were significantly lower ($p < 0.05$) than those of GP%-WT or vector-control animals after challenge with MN184C. Each figure represents the mean value of each individual. The bars represent the standard error of the mean. Three independent experiments were performed for each. Student's t test was utilized to calculate significant differences (days post-challenge (DPC)).

4. Discussion

There is extraordinary diversity among PRRSV strains. The diversity among PRRSV strains is as high as, or may even surpass that of, HIV. Recently, several vaccine candidates, including a synthetic consensus PRRSV strain [27], a chimeric PRRSV strain containing multiple ORFs DNA shuffled [46–48] and an intranasal live virus vaccine with adjuvant [49] induced various levels of heterologous protection in pigs. We have developed GP5-Mosaic vaccines that incorporate sequences derived from naturally circulating viruses. The data obtained from our GP5-Mosaic vaccinated pigs supports the Mosaic vaccine approach as an effective strategy to address PRRSV diversity. It has also been demonstrated that Mosaic T-cell vaccines have great potential for other viruses with extraordinary diversity, such as HIV [33–38]. In an earlier study, we demonstrated the immunogenicity of GP5-Mosaic vaccines in swine and their ability to induce cross-reactivity, as shown by their broad recall responses ex-vivo, and conferred the partial protection they provide in pigs [29,30]. The ability of the GP5-Mosaic vaccines to induce cross-protection in pigs against heterologous PRRSV strains was confirmed in the present study.

A sequence analysis of two GP5-Mosaic vaccines and the two Genotype 2 PRRSV strains utilized in the study, VR2332 and MN184C, that belong to lineage 5 and to lineage 1, respectively, revealed a 15% difference in the GP5 aa sequences. The aa sequences were used to generate a phylogenetic tree using the neighbor-joining method [24]. The GP5-Mosaic 1 was closer to VR2332 (93% aa identity), while GP5-Mosaic 2 was closer to MN184C (90% aa identity), which suggested that the two GP5-Mosaic sequences broaden the coverage to strains belonging to different lineages. Based on this analysis, a broader protection could be expected with GP5-Mosaic vaccines. The data of the present study supports clearly the capacity of the GP5-Mosaic vaccine to cross-protect pigs against VR2332 and MN184C that share only 85% aa identity.

VACV provides a very good platform for the development and testing of vaccines, including animal vaccines, human vaccines and cancer immunotherapy [50]. In our study, a GP5-Mosaic DNA vaccine prime/GP5-Mosaic rVaccinia (VACV) boost regime was used to immunize pigs. This type of prime-boost regime has previously been demonstrated to increase vaccination efficacy substantially [51,52]. In addition, Quil-A®, used as adjuvant for the priming of the GP5-Mosaic DNA vaccine, was previously shown to further increase the immune responses [53–55]. Therefore, the prime-boost vaccination regime used here for testing GP5-Mosaic vaccine efficacy, in terms of broad protection, proved appropriate for testing the hypothesis.

PBMCs collected on the challenge day from GP5-Mosaic-vaccinated pigs responded to a broader range of virus strains, as measured by IFN-γ mRNA expression, than those from GP5-WT vaccinates. Thus, PBMC from GP5-Mosaic-vaccinated pigs expressed higher levels of IFN-γ mRNA in response to stimulation with VR2332 or MN184C strains, respectively, compared to those of the vector-control pigs. In contrast, PBMC from GP5-WT vaccinated pigs expressed higher levels of IFN-γ mRNA only when stimulated with VR2332. These data were consistent with those of our previous study where the GP5-Mosaic vaccine induced broad recall cellular responses, as measured by significantly higher levels of IFN-γ mRNA expression in response to the four diverse Genotype 2 PRRSV strains tested, including VR2332, NADC9, NADC30 and SDSU73 [30]. The significant induction of IFN-γ is an important asset of a PRRSV vaccine, as IFN-γ reportedly plays a critical role in the control of and protection from PRRSV infection [56]. In addition, both the GP5-Mosaic and the GP5-WT vaccines induced relatively high levels of neutralizing antibodies in VR2332-challenged pigs. These data indicate that the GP5-Mosaic vaccine preserves virus-neutralizing epitopes that appear to contribute to the overall efficacy of this vaccine.

In terms of vaccine-induced protection, both GP5-Mosaic and GP5-WT-vaccinated pigs had significantly lower serum viral loads at 7, 10 and 14 DPC than the vector-control group after the VR2332 challenge. In contrast, only the GP5-Mosaic-vaccinated group showed significantly lower viral loads in sera at 7 and 14 DPC than the vector-control group after the MN184C challenge. These data demonstrate that the GP5-Mosaic vaccine is capable of cross-protecting pigs against two divergent PRRSV strains (15% difference) while the GP5-WT vaccine only provided protection in pigs against the homologous strain. Furthermore, a similar pattern was found with respect to viral loads in tissues, where the GP5-Mosaic-vaccinated pigs had significantly lower viral loads in their lungs, TBLN, spleen, ILN and tonsils compared to the vector-control group after challenge with MN184C, while the GP5-WT group only showed slightly lower (numerically, but not significant) viral loads. In the VR2332 challenge experiment, both the GP5-Mosaic and GP5-WT vaccinates had significantly lower viral loads in tissues generally—the viral loads in the GP5-Mosaic vaccinates were significantly lower in their lungs, TBLN and tonsils, while viral loads in the GP5-WT group were significantly lower in their lungs, ILN and spleen, compared to the vector-control group. Similar protective effects were also demonstrated in the GP5-Mosaic vaccine vaccinates, where lower viral loads were detected in the BAL fluids or PAMs after MN184C challenge, further confirming the cross-protective capability of the GP5-Mosaic vaccine. Indeed, this is finding may be particularly relevant since PAMs are the primary target of PRRSV infection. Lung lesion scoring is an essential and crucial method to evaluate vaccine efficacy, as infection by PRRSV tends to increase susceptibility to coinfection with other virus or bacterial pathogens [57–59] which may result in more severe lesions and mortality. Pigs vaccinated with the GP5-Mosaic vaccine had significantly lower lung lesion scores than both the GP5-WT and vector-control groups after challenge with MN184C, while both the GP5-Mosaic and GP5-WT groups had lower lung lesion scores compared to the vector-control group in the VR2332 challenge experiment.

5. Conclusions

Taken altogether, our results clearly demonstrate that the GP5-Mosaic vaccine provided cross-protection against two heterologous PRRSV strains, VR2332, the prototype Genotype 2 strain, and MN184C, a highly virulent strain, while the GP5-WT vaccine provided only homologous protection against VR2332. In summary, our results demonstrate that our GP5-Mosaic vaccine is able to induce broader protection against PRRS and warrants further research for field applications.

Author Contributions: Conceptualization, P.H.V. and A.E.G.; Methodology, J.C., C.M.O., J.A.S., P.H.V. and A.E.G.; Formal analysis, J.C. and A.E.G.; Investigation, J.C., C.M.O., C.H., K.S., J.A.S., P.H.V., H.J.V.K., and A.E.G.; Data curation, J.C. and A.E.G.; Writing—original draft preparation, J.C.; Writing—review and editing, J.C., C.M.O., J.A.S., P.H.V. and A.E.G.; Supervision, A.E.G.; Project administration, A.E.G.; Funding acquisition, J.A.S., P.H.V. and A.E.G. All authors have read and agreed to the published version of the manuscript.

Funding: This work was funded by USDA/NIFA Grant Number 2011 67015-30176 and NC229.

Acknowledgments: The authors thank Kay Faaberg and Kelly Lager kindly providing the PRRSV strains.

Conflicts of Interest: The authors declare no conflict of interest. The funders had no role in the design of the study; in the collection, analyses, or interpretation of data; in the writing of the manuscript, or in the decision to publish the results.

References

1. Holtkamp, D.J.; Kliebenstein, J.B.; Neumann, E.J.; Zimmerman, J.J.; Rotto, H.F.; Yoder, T.K.; Wang, C.; Yeske, P.E.; Mowrer, C.L.; Haley, C.A. Assessment of the economic impact of porcine reproductive and respiratory syndrome virus on United States pork producers. *J. Swine Health Prod.* **2013**, *21*, 72–84.
2. Collins, J.; Benfield, D.; Christianson, W.T.; Harris, L.; Hennings, J.C.; Shaw, D.P.; Goyal, S.M.; McCullough, S.; Morrison, R.B.; Joo, H.S.; et al. Isolation of Swine Infertility and Respiratory Syndrome Virus (Isolate ATCC VR-2332) in North America and Experimental Reproduction of the Disease in Gnotobiotic Pigs. *J. Veter Diagn. Investig.* **1992**, *4*, 117–126. [CrossRef] [PubMed]
3. Wensvoort, G.; Terpstra, C.; Pol, J.M.; Ter Laak, E.A.; Bloemraad, M.; de Kluyver, E.P.; Kragten, C.; van Buiten, L.; den Besten, A.; Wagenaar, F. Mystery swine disease in The Netherlands: The isolation of Lelystad virus. *Veter Q.* **1991**, *13*, 121–130. [CrossRef] [PubMed]
4. Cavanagh, D. Nidovirales: A new order comprising Coronaviridae and Arteriviridae. *Arch. Virol.* **1997**, *142*, 629–633. [PubMed]
5. Lunney, J.K.; Fang, Y.; Ladinig, A.; Chen, N.; Li, Y.; Rowland, B.; Renukaradhya, G. Porcine Reproductive and Respiratory Syndrome Virus (PRRSV): Pathogenesis and Interaction with the Immune System. *Annu. Rev. Anim. Biosci.* **2016**, *4*, 129–154. [CrossRef]
6. Mokhtar, H.; Eck, M.; Morgan, S.B.; Essler, S.E.; Frossard, J.-P.; Ruggli, N.; Graham, S. Proteome-wide screening of the European porcine reproductive and respiratory syndrome virus reveals a broad range of T cell antigen reactivity. *Vaccine* **2014**, *32*, 6828–6837. [CrossRef]
7. Parida, R.; Choi, I.-S.; Peterson, D.A.; Pattnaik, A.K.; Laegreid, W.; Zuckermann, F.A.; Osorio, F. Location of T-cell epitopes in nonstructural proteins 9 and 10 of type-II porcine reproductive and respiratory syndrome virus. *Virus Res.* **2012**, *169*, 13–21. [CrossRef]
8. Brown, E.; Lawson, S.; Welbon, C.; Gnanandarajah, J.; Li, J.; Murtaugh, M.P.; Nelson, E.; Molina, R.; Zimmerman, J.; Rowland, R.; et al. Antibody response to porcine reproductive and respiratory syndrome virus (PRRSV) nonstructural proteins and implications for diagnostic detection and differentiation of PRRSV types I and II. *Clin. Vaccine Immunol.* **2009**, *16*, 628–635. [CrossRef]
9. Vanhee, M.; Van Breedam, W.; Costers, S.; Geldhof, M.; Noppe, Y.; Nauwynck, H. Characterization of antigenic regions in the porcine reproductive and respiratory syndrome virus by the use of peptide-specific serum antibodies. *Vaccine* **2011**, *29*, 4794–4804. [CrossRef]
10. Zuckermann, F.A.; Garcia, E.A.; Luque, I.D.; Christopher-Hennings, J.; Doster, A.; Brito, M.; Osorio, F. Assessment of the efficacy of commercial porcine reproductive and respiratory syndrome virus (PRRSV) vaccines based on measurement of serologic response, frequency of gamma-IFN-producing cells and virological parameters of protection upon challenge. *Veter Microbiol.* **2007**, *123*, 69–85. [CrossRef]
11. Osorio, F.A.; Galeota, J.A.; Nelson, E.; Brodersen, B.; Doster, A.; Wills, R.; Zuckermann, F.; Laegreid, W.W. PRRSV: Comparison of commercial vaccines in their ability to induce protection against current PRRSV strains of high virulence. In Proceedings of the Allen D Leman Swine Conference, St. Paul, MN, USA, 14–17 September 2019; 1998; pp. 176–182.
12. Scortti, M.; Prieto, C.; Alvarez, E.; Simarro, I.; Castro, J.M. Failure of an inactivated vaccine against porcine reproductive and respiratory syndrome to protect gilts against a heterologous challenge with PRRSV. *Veter Rec.* **2007**, *161*, 809–813.

13. Geldhof, M.F.; Vanhee, M.; Van Breedam, W.; Van Doorsselaere, J.; Karniychuk, U.U.; Nauwynck, H.J. Comparison of the efficacy of autogenous inactivated Porcine Reproductive and Respiratory Syndrome Virus (PRRSV) vaccines with that of commercial vaccines against homologous and heterologous challenges. *BMC Veter Res.* **2012**, *8*, 182. [CrossRef] [PubMed]
14. Labarque, G.; Reeth KVan Nauwynck, H.; Drexler, C.; Gucht SVan Pensaert, M. Impact of genetic diversity of European-type porcine reproductive and respiratory syndrome virus strains on vaccine efficacy. *Vaccine* **2004**, *22*, 4183–4190. [CrossRef] [PubMed]
15. Okuda, Y.; Kuroda, M.; Ono, M.; Chikata, S.; Shibata, I. Efficacy of Vaccination with Porcine Reproductive and Respiratory Syndrome Virus Following Challenges with Field Isolates in Japan. *J. Veter Med. Sci.* **2008**, *70*, 1017–1025. [CrossRef]
16. Han, K.; Seo, H.W.; Park, C.; Chae, C. Vaccination of sows against type 2 Porcine Reproductive and Respiratory Syndrome Virus (PRRSV) before artificial insemination protects against type 2 PRRSV challenge but does not protect against type 1 PRRSV challenge in late gestation. *Veter Res.* **2014**, *45*, 12. [CrossRef]
17. Kim, T.; Park, C.; Choi, K.; Jeong, J.; Kang, I.; Park, S.-J.; Chae, C. Comparison of Two Commercial Type 1 Porcine Reproductive and Respiratory Syndrome Virus (PRRSV) Modified Live Vaccines against Heterologous Type 1 and Type 2 PRRSV Challenge in Growing Pigs. *Clin. Vaccine Immunol.* **2015**, *22*, 631–640. [CrossRef]
18. Trus, I.; Bonckaert, C.; van der Meulen, K.; Nauwynck, H.J. Efficacy of an attenuated European subtype 1 porcine reproductive and respiratory syndrome virus (PRRSV) vaccine in pigs upon challenge with the East European subtype 3 PRRSV strain Lena. *Vaccine* **2014**, *32*, 2995–3003. [CrossRef]
19. Bøtner, A.; Strandbygaard, B.; Sørensen, K.J.; Have, P.; Madsen, K.G.; Madsen, E.S.; Alexandersen, S. Appearance of acute PRRS-like symptoms in sow herds after vaccination with a modified live PRRS vaccine. *Veter Rec.* **1997**, *141*, 497–499. [CrossRef]
20. Madsen, K.G.; Hansen, C.M.; Madsen, E.S.; Strandbygaard, B.; Bøtner, A.; Sørensen, K.J. Sequence analysis of porcine reproductive and respiratory syndrome virus of the American type collected from Danish swine herds. *Arch. Virol.* **1998**, *143*, 1683–1700. [CrossRef]
21. Nielsen, H.S.; Stadejek, T.; Bøtner, A.; Oleksiewicz, M.B.; Forsberg, R. Reversion of a live porcine reproductive and respiratory syndrome virus vaccine investigated by parallel mutations. *J. Gen. Virol.* **2015**, *82*, 1263–1272. [CrossRef]
22. Nelsen, C.J.; Murtaugh, M.P.; Faaberg, K.S. Porcine reproductive and respiratory syndrome virus comparison: Divergent evolution on two continents. *J. Virol.* **1999**, *73*, 270–280. [CrossRef] [PubMed]
23. Kim, H.K.; Yang, J.S.; Moon, H.J.; Park, S.J.; Luo, Y.; Lee, C.S.; Song, D.; Kang, B.; Ann, S.; Jun, C.; et al. Genetic analysis of ORF5 of recent Korean porcine reproductive and respiratory syndrome viruses (PRRSVs) in viremic sera collected from MLV-vaccinating or non-vaccinating farms. *J. Veter Sci.* **2009**, *10*, 121–130. [CrossRef] [PubMed]
24. Shi, M.; Lam, T.T.-Y.; Hon, C.-C.; Murtaugh, M.P.; Davies, P.R.; Hui, R.K.-H.; Li, J.; Wong, L.; Yip, C.; Jiang, J.; et al. Phylogeny-Based Evolutionary, Demographical, and Geographical Dissection of North American Type 2 Porcine Reproductive and Respiratory Syndrome Viruses. *J. Virol.* **2010**, *84*, 8700–8711. [CrossRef] [PubMed]
25. Goldberg, T.L.; Lowe, J.F.; Milburn, S.M.; Firkins, L.D. Quasispecies variation of porcine reproductive and respiratory syndrome virus during natural infection. *Virology* **2003**, *317*, 197–207. [CrossRef]
26. Jiang, Y.; Xiao, S.; Fang, L.; Yu, X.; Song, Y.; Niu, C.; Chen, H. DNA vaccines co-expressing GP5 and M proteins of porcine reproductive and respiratory syndrome virus (PRRSV) display enhanced immunogenicity. *Vaccine* **2006**, *24*, 2869–2879. [CrossRef]
27. Vu, H.L.; Ma, F.; Laegreid, W.W.; Pattnaik, A.K.; Steffen, D.; Doster, A.R.; Osorio, F. A Synthetic Porcine Reproductive and Respiratory Syndrome Virus Strain Confers Unprecedented Levels of Heterologous Protection. *J. Virol.* **2015**, *89*, 12070–12083. [CrossRef]
28. Zhou, L.; Ni, Y.Y.; Pineyro, P.; Sanford, B.J.; Cossaboom, C.M.; Dryman, B.A.; Huang, Y.; Cao, D.; Meng, X. DNA shuffling of the GP3 genes of porcine reproductive and respiratory syndrome virus (PRRSV) produces a chimeric virus with an improved cross-neutralizing ability against a heterologous PRRSV strain. *Virology* **2012**, *434*, 96–109. [CrossRef]

29. Cui, J.; O'Connell, C.M.; Smith, J.D.; Pan, Y.; Smyth, J.A.; Verardi, P.H.; Garmendia, A.E. A GP5 Mosaic T-cell vaccine for porcine reproductive and respiratory syndrome virus is immunogenic and confers partial protection to pigs. *Vaccine Rep.* **2016**, *6*, 77–85. [CrossRef]
30. Cui, J.; O'Connell, C.M.; Costa, A.; Pan, Y.; Smyth, J.A.; Verardi, P.H.; Burgess, D.; Van Kruiningen, H.; Garmendia, A.E. A PRRSV GP5-Mosaic vaccine: Protection of pigs from challenge and ex vivo detection of IFNγ responses against several genotype 2 strains. *PLoS ONE* **2019**, *14*, e0208801. [CrossRef]
31. Mengeling, W.L.; Lager, K.M.; Vorwald, A.C.; Clouser, D.F. Comparative safety and efficacy of attenuated single-strain and multi-strain vaccines for porcine reproductive and respiratory syndrome. *Veter Microbiol.* **2003**, *93*, 25–38. [CrossRef]
32. Bernelin-Cottet, C.; Urien, C.; Fretaud, M.; Langevin, C.; Trus, I.; Jouneau, L.; Blanc, F.; Leplat, J.; Barc, C.; Boulesteix, O.; et al. A DNA Prime Immuno-Potentiates a Modified Live *Vaccine* against the Porcine Reproductive and Respiratory Syndrome Virus but Does Not Improve Heterologous Protection. *Viruses* **2019**, *11*, 576. [CrossRef] [PubMed]
33. Fischer, W.; Perkins, S.; Theiler, J.; Bhattacharya, T.; Yusim, K.; Funkhouser, R.; Kuiken, C.; Haynes, B.; Letvin, N.; Walker, B.; et al. Polyvalent vaccines for optimal coverage of potential T-cell epitopes in global HIV-1 variants. *Nat. Med.* **2007**, *13*, 100–106. [CrossRef] [PubMed]
34. Thurmond, J.; Yoon, H.; Kuiken, C.; Yusim, K.; Perkins, S.; Theiler, J.; Bhattacharya, T.; Korber, B.; Fisher, W. Web-based design and evaluation of T-cell vaccine candidates. *Bioinformatics* **2008**, *24*, 1639–1640. [CrossRef] [PubMed]
35. Kong, W.P.; Wu, L.; Wallstrom, T.C.; Fischer, W.; Yang, Z.Y.; Ko, S.Y.; Letvin, N.; Haynes, B.; Hahn, B.; Korber, B.; et al. Expanded breadth of the T-cell response to mosaic human immunodeficiency virus type 1 envelope DNA vaccination. *J. Virol.* **2009**, *83*, 2201–2215. [CrossRef]
36. Barouch, D.H.; O'Brien, K.L.; Simmons, N.L.; King, S.L.; Abbink, P.; Maxfield, L.F.; Sun, Y.; La Port, A.; Riggs, A.; Lynch, D.; et al. Mosaic HIV-1 vaccines expand the breadth and depth of cellular immune responses in rhesus monkeys. *Nat. Med.* **2010**, *16*, 319–323. [CrossRef]
37. Santra, S.; Liao, H.X.; Zhang, R.; Muldoon, M.; Watson, S.; Fischer, W.; Theiler, J.; Szinger, J.; Balachandran, H.; Buzby, A.; et al. Mosaic vaccines elicit CD8+ T lymphocyte responses that confer enhanced immune coverage of diverse HIV strains in monkeys. *Nat. Med.* **2010**, *16*, 324–328. [CrossRef]
38. Barouch, D.H.; Tomaka, F.L.; Wegmann, F.; Stieh, D.J.; Alter, G.; Robb, M.L.; Nelson, L.; Michael, N.L.; Peter, L.; Nkolola, J.P.; et al. Evaluation of a mosaic HIV-1 vaccine in a multicentre, randomised, double-blind, placebo-controlled, phase 1/2a clinical trial (APPROACH) and in rhesus monkeys (NHP 13–19). *Lancet* **2018**, *392*, 232–243. [CrossRef]
39. Kim, H.S.; Kwang, J.; Yoon, I.J.; Joo, H.S.; Frey, M.L. Enhanced replication of porcine reproductive and respiratory syndrome (PRRS) virus in a homogeneous subpopulation of MA-104 cell line. *Arch. Virol.* **1993**, *133*, 477–483. [CrossRef]
40. Reed, L.J.; Muench, H. A simple method of estimating fifty percent endpoints. *Am. J. Hyg.* **1938**, *27*, 493–497.
41. Chakrabarti, S.; Sisler, J.R.; Moss, B. Compact, synthetic, vaccinia virus early/late promoter for protein expression. *Biotechniques* **1997**, *23*, 1094–1097. [CrossRef]
42. Hagen, C.J.; Titong, A.; Sarnoski, E.A.; Verardi, P.H. Antibiotic-dependent expression of early transcription factor subunits leads to stringent control of vaccinia virus replication. *Virus Res.* **2014**, *181*, 43–52. [CrossRef] [PubMed]
43. Cotter, C.A.; Earl, P.L.; Wyatt, L.S.; Moss, B. Preparation of Cell Cultures and Vaccinia Virus Stocks. *Curr. Protoc. Protein Sci.* **2017**, *89*, 5121–5128. [CrossRef]
44. Livak, K.J.; Schmittgen, T.D. Analysis of Relative Gene Expression Data Using Real-Time Quantitative PCR and the $2-\Delta\Delta CT$ Method. *Methods* **2001**, *25*, 402–408. [CrossRef] [PubMed]
45. Halbur, P.G.; Paul, P.S.; Meng, X.J.; Lum, M.A.; Andrews, J.J.; Rathje, J.A. Comparative pathogenicity of nine US porcine reproductive and respiratory syndrome virus (PRRSV) isolates in a five-week-old cesarean-derived, colostrum-deprived pig model. *J. Veter Diagn. Investig.* **1996**, *8*, 11–20. [CrossRef]
46. Ni, Y.Y.; Opriessnig, T.; Zhou, L.; Cao, D.; Huang, Y.W.; Halbur, P.G.; Meng, X. Attenuation of porcine reproductive and respiratory syndrome virus by molecular breeding of virus envelope genes from genetically divergent strains. *J. Virol.* **2013**, *87*, 304–313. [CrossRef]

47. Zhou, L.; Ni, Y.-Y.; Piñeyro, P.; Cossaboom, C.M.; Subramaniam, S.; Sanford, B.J.; Dryman, B.; Huang, Y.; Meng, X. Broadening the heterologous cross-neutralizing antibody inducing ability of porcine reproductive and respiratory syndrome virus by breeding the GP4 or M genes. *PLoS ONE* **2013**, *8*, e66645. [CrossRef]
48. Tian, D.; Ni, Y.-Y.; Zhou, L.; Opriessnig, T.; Cao, D.; Piñeyro, P.; Yugo, D.; Overend, C.; Cao, Q.; Lynn Heffron, C.; et al. Chimeric porcine reproductive and respiratory syndrome virus containing shuffled multiple envelope genes confers cross-protection in pigs. *Virology* **2015**, *485*, 402–413. [CrossRef]
49. Dwivedi, V.; Manickam, C.; Patterson, R.; Dodson, K.; Murtaugh, M.; Torrelles, J.B.; Schlesinger, L.; Renukaradhya, G. Cross-protective immunity to porcine reproductive and respiratory syndrome virus by intranasal delivery of a live virus vaccine with a potent adjuvant. *Vaccine* **2011**, *29*, 4058–4066. [CrossRef]
50. Verardi, P.H.; Titong, A.; Hagen, C.J. A vaccinia virus renaissance. *Hum. Vaccines Immunother.* **2012**, *8*, 961–970. [CrossRef]
51. Chapman, R.; Jongwe, T.I.; Douglass, N.; Chege, G.; Williamson, A.L. Heterologous prime-boost vaccination with DNA and MVA vaccines, expressing HIV-1 subtype C mosaic Gag virus-like particles, is highly immunogenic in mice. *PLoS ONE* **2017**, *12*, e0173352. [CrossRef]
52. Deng, Y.; Chuai, X.; Chen, P.; Chen, H.; Wang, W.; Ruan, L.; Li, W.; Tan, W. Recombinant vaccinia vector-based vaccine (Tiantan) boosting a novel HBV subunit vaccine induced more robust and lasting immunity in rhesus macaques. *Vaccine* **2017**, *35*, 3347–3353. [CrossRef] [PubMed]
53. Lampe, K.; Gottstein, B.; Becker, T.; Stahl-Hennig, C.; Kaup, F.J.; Mätz-Rensing, K. Immunization of rhesus macaques with Echinococcus multilocularis recombinant 14-3-3 antigen leads to specific antibody response. *Parasitol. Res.* **2017**, *116*, 435–439. [CrossRef] [PubMed]
54. Tahoun, A.; Jensen, K.; Corripio-Miyar, Y.; McAteer, S.P.; Corbishley, A.; Mahajan, A.; Brown, H.; Frew, D.; Aumeunier, A.; Smith, D.G.; et al. Functional analysis of bovine TLR5 and association with IgA responses of cattle following systemic immunisation with H7 flagella. *Veter Res.* **2015**, *46*, 9. [CrossRef] [PubMed]
55. Gómez-Gascón, L.; Cardoso-Toset, F.; Tarradas, C.; Gómez-Laguna, J.; Maldonado, A.; Nielsen, J.; Olaya-Abril, A.; Rodriguez-Ortega, M.; Luque, I. Characterization of the immune response and evaluation of the protective capacity of rSsnA against Streptococcus suis infection in pigs. *Comp. Immunol. Microbiol. Infect. Dis.* **2016**, *47*, 52–59. [CrossRef] [PubMed]
56. Morgan, S.B.; Graham, S.P.; Salguero, F.J.; Sánchez Cordón, P.J.; Mokhtar, H.; Rebel, J.M.J.; Weesendorp, E.; Bodman-Smith, K.; Steinbach, F.; Frossard, J. Increased pathogenicity of European porcine reproductive and respiratory syndrome virus is associated with enhanced adaptive responses and viral clearance. *Veter Microbiol.* **2013**, *163*, 13–22. [CrossRef] [PubMed]
57. Thanawongnuwech, R.; Brown, G.B.; Halbur, P.G.; Roth, J.A.; Royer, R.L.; Thacker, B.J. Pathogenesis of Porcine Reproductive and Respiratory Syndrome Virus-induced Increase in Susceptibility to Streptococcus suis Infection. *Veter Pathol.* **2000**, *37*, 143–152. [CrossRef] [PubMed]
58. Van Reeth, K.; Nauwynck, H.; Pensaert, M. Dual infections of feeder pigs with porcine reproductive and respiratory syndrome virus followed by porcine respiratory coronavirus or swine influenza virus: A clinical and virological study. *Veter Microbiol.* **1996**, *48*, 325–335. [CrossRef]
59. Tsai, Y.C.; Chang, H.W.; Jeng, C.R.; Lin, T.L.; Lin, C.M.; Wan, C.H.; Pang, V. The effect of infection order of porcine circovirus type 2 and porcine reproductive and respiratory syndrome virus on dually infected swine alveolar macrophages. *BMC Veter Res.* **2012**, *8*, 174. [CrossRef]

vaccines

MDPI

Article

Significant Interference with Porcine Epidemic Diarrhea Virus Pandemic and Classical Strain Replication in Small-Intestine Epithelial Cells Using an shRNA Expression Vector

Da Shi †, Xiaobo Wang †, Hongyan Shi †, Jiyu Zhang, Yuru Han, Jianfei Chen, Xin Zhang, Jianbo Liu, Jialin Zhang, Zhaoyang Ji, Zhaoyang Jing and Li Feng *

State Key Laboratory of Veterinary Biotechnology, Harbin Veterinary Research Institute, Chinese Academy of Agricultural Sciences, Xiangfang District, Haping Road 678, Harbin 150069, China; dashi198566@163.com (D.S.); wxb1901@163.com (X.W.); shy2005y@163.com (H.S.); 18841618894@163.com (J.Z.); hyr1968274346@163.com (Y.H.); chenjianfei@126.com (J.C.); zhangxin2410@163.com (X.Z.); liujianbo@caas.cn (J.L.); zhangjialin0106@gmail.com (J.Z.); Zy_ji2010@163.com (Z.J.); 15204604415@163.com (Z.J.)

* Correspondence: fengli@caas.cn; Tel.: +86-0451-5105-1720

† These authors contributed equally to this work.

Received: 27 August 2019; Accepted: 16 October 2019; Published: 2 November 2019

Abstract: Porcine epidemic diarrhea (PED) re-emerged in China in 2010 and is now widespread. Evidence indicates that highly virulent porcine epidemic diarrhea virus (PEDV) strains belonging to genotype G2 caused a large-scale outbreak of diarrhea. Currently, vaccines derived from PEDV classical strains do not effectively prevent infection by virulent PEDV strains, and no specific drug is available to treat the disease. RNA interference (RNAi) is a novel and effective way to cure a wide range of viruses. We constructed three short hairpin RNA (shRNA)-expressing plasmids (shR-N307, shR-N463, and shR-N1071) directed against nucleocapsid (N) and determined their antiviral activities in intestine epithelial cells infected with a classical CV777 strain and LNCT2. We verified that shR-N307, shR-N463, and shR-N1071 effectively inhibited the expression of the transfected *N* gene in vitro, comparable to the control shRNA. We further demonstrated the shRNAs markedly reduced PEDV CV777 and LNCT2 replication upon downregulation of N production. Therefore, this study provides a new strategy for the design of antiviral methods against coronaviruses by targeting their processivity factors.

Keywords: porcine epidemic diarrhea virus; RNA interference; processivity factor; intestine epithelial cells; *N* gene

1. Introduction

Porcine epidemic diarrhea (PED), caused by porcine epidemic diarrhea virus (PEDV), is a highly contagious intestinal infectious disease. PED is an important disease in swine-producing countries. PED causes the death of newborn piglets and weight loss in pigs of all ages from PEDV-induced severe symptoms, such as serious diarrhea, vomiting, and dehydration, which seriously damage the swine industry [1]. Following reports in 1978 [1], PED had an outbreak in swine-farming countries in Asia, North America, South America, and Europe [2–5]. Starting from the end of 2010, highly virulent PEDV variants that differed from the classic European strain CV777 were widespread in China, resulting in high mortality of newborn piglets and huge economic losses [6–9]. PEDV can be divided into genotypes G1 and G2 based on phylogenetic analysis of full-length *S* gene sequences [10]. PEDV strains detected in China since 2010 mostly belonged to genotype G2, which differed genetically from the CV777 vaccine strain belonging to subtype G1 [11]. However, many studies demonstrated that commercially available PEDV vaccines derived from classical strains of PEDV do not provide effective protection against highly virulent PEDV variant infections in China [3]. Thus, PEDV infection remains a major veterinary problem. Understanding it is essential to developing novel antiviral drugs that will specifically inhibit PEDV propagation.

RNA interference (RNAi) is a short, double-strand RNA-induced process that targets and degrades the messenger RNA (mRNA) of specific sequences [12,13]. Post-transcriptional gene silencing can be mediated by exogenous small interfering RNAs (siRNAs), endogenous microRNAs (miRNAs), and short hairpin RNAs (shRNAs). Effective gene knockdown is achieved by shRNAs by inducing the endogenous RNAi process [14,15]. Transcribed shRNAs are exported from the nucleus by Exportin-5 and processed by the RNase III Dicer into small double-stranded RNA (dsRNA) molecules of 19 to 23 bp called siRNAs. The complementary guide strand of processed siRNA is incorporated into the RNA-induced silencing complex to mediate the cleavage of target mRNAs [16,17]. RNAi evolves in the host defense system directed at infectious viruses and transposable elements. Effective silencing of transgene expression and endogenous genes in vivo was shown by a number of groups [6,7,18]. These findings raised the possibility that RNAi could be another therapeutic approach for inhibiting virus infection. ShRNAs were employed for therapy against human viral diseases, as well as cancer and neurogenerative diseases [8]. PEDV primarily infects villous epithelial cells throughout the small intestine and causes serious injury of intestine epithelial cells (IECs), including superficial villous enterocyte swelling and severe diffuse atrophic enteritis [19]. Infection of PEDV variant strains in the field complicates the development of prophylactic and therapeutic strategies to protect suckling pigs from diarrhea. As an RNA virus, PEDV could be an ideal target for studying its biology and therapeutics using RNAi.

The PEDV nucleocapsid (N) protein, which is abundantly expressed in infected cells, has multiple functions. It is one of the structural proteins that forms complexes with genomic RNA, enhancing viral transcription and assembly. Therefore, the N protein may be a potential drug target for antiviral therapy against PEDV infection. In this study, we compared and analyzed *N* gene sequences from 25 different PEDV G1 and G2 isolates from different countries. Three novel shRNAs targeting conserved and unexploited regions in the *N* gene were tested for inhibition of PEDV CV777 and LNCT2 replication. Cell viability, viral titer, and protein expression were examined as indicators of the efficacy of targeted gene silencing by the shRNAs. All three shRNAs effectively inhibited PEDV replication and *N* expression of the G1 and G2 subtypes.

2. Materials and Methods

2.1. Viral Propagation and Titer Assays

Swine intestinal epithelial cells (IECs) were donated by Dr. Yanming Zhang (Northwest A&F University, China), and derived from the mid-jejunum of neonatal, unsuckled, one-day-old piglets. Primary intestinal epithelial cells were isolated by the tissue explant adherent method and purified by trypsin digestion with citric acid, forming an undifferentiated porcine intestinal epithelial cell line that was immortalized. Cells were maintained in a Dulbecco's minimum essential medium (DMEM; Gibco, Thermo Fisher Scientific, Waltham, MA, USA)/nutrient mixture F-12 (Ham) (1:1) containing 10% heat-inactivated fetal bovine serum (FBS; Gibco), 5 ng/mL epidermal growth factor (Life Technologies, Carlsbad, CA, USA), 5 mg/mL insulin-transferring selenium supplements (Life Technologies), and 1% penicillin–streptomycin (Life Technologies). Cell culture media were changed every two days, and cells were passaged every 3–4 days by trypsinization with 0.25% trypsin–ethylenediaminetetraacetic acid (EDTA) (Life Technologies). Vero E6 (African green monkey kidney cells, American Type Culture Collection (ATCC)) were grown and maintained in DMEM supplemented with 10% heat-inactivated FBS and penicillin–streptomycin, and incubated at 37 °C with 5% CO_2.

The PEDV G1 CV777 vaccine strain (GenBank accession: AF353511.1) was preserved at Harbin Veterinary Research Institute (Harbin, China). PEDV G2 strain LNCT2 (GenBank accession: KT323980.1) was isolated in Vero E6 cells in our laboratory. Vero E6 cells were cultured and used to amplify PEDV as previously described [9]. After 70% of virus-infected cells showed cytopathic effects (CPEs), cultures were collected for three freeze–thaw cycles. Viral titration used 96-well microplates with Vero E6 cells. Viral cultures were 10-fold serially diluted with virus replication medium containing trypsin (10 μg/mL). Confluent Vero E6 cells from microplates were washed three times with phosphate-buffered saline (PBS) and inoculated at 0.1 mL per well into eight wells. Following adsorption for 1 h at 37 °C, the inocula were removed, and cells were washed three times with PBS. Subsequently, 0.1 mL of fresh virus replication medium was transferred into each well, and cells were incubated 4–5 days at 37 °C. The 50% tissue culture infective dose ($TCID_{50}$) was expressed as the reciprocal of the highest dilution showing CPE by the Reed and Muench method. Assays were performed in triplicate in three independent experiments.

2.2. Plasmid Construction

Plasmids expressing GFP-tagged N and myc-Tagged N were described previously [20]. The design of shRNAs targeting the PEDV strain LNCT2 genome *N* gene (Figure 1A) used methods from the literature [21] and the web-based Block-iT^{TM} RNAi Designer program [22]. A Basic Local Alignment Search Tool (BLAST) search [23] was performed to exclude possible homologous sequences. Three individual targeting sites were selected and chemically synthesized (Sangon Biotech, Shanghai, China) (Table 1). Control shRNA was designed at the same time to have no homology with PEDV or the IEC cell genome. All sequences were arranged as *Bbs*I + sense + loop + antisense + termination signal + *BamHI* and cloned into the pGPU6-Hygro vector to make the shRNA-expressing plasmids shR-N307, shR-N463, shR-N1071, and shR-NC (Figure 1B,C). Expression of siRNAs was driven by the U6 promoter.

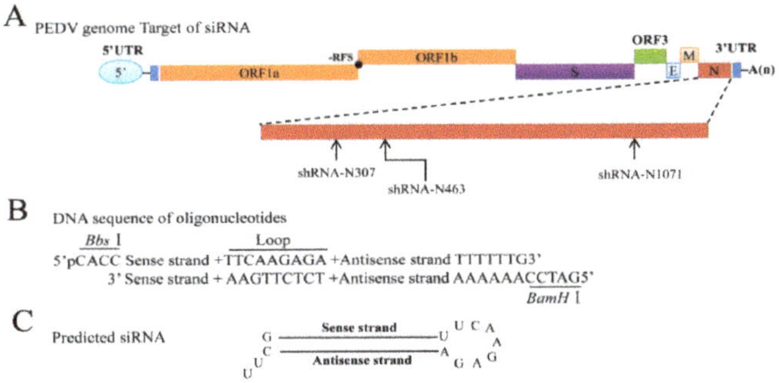

Figure 1. Schematic description of the target viral genome, and small interfering RNA (siRNA)-expressing cassette. (**A**) Genomic structure of porcine epidemic diarrhea virus (PEDV) and position of target short hairpin RNA (shRNA) at *N* gene. ShR-N307, shR-N463, and shR-N1071 indicate initial shRNA target sites; (**B**) sequences and design map for shRNA constructs; (**C**) structure of predicted shRNA.

Table 1. Gene sequence and position of RNA interference targets.

shRNA	Sequence	Position
shRNA-N307	GCAAAGACTGAACCCACTAAC	Position in *N* gene sequence: 307–327
shRNA-N463	GGCAACAACAGGTCCAGATCT	Position in *N* gene sequence: 463–483
shRNA-N1071	GCCAAAGTCTGATCCAAATGT	Position in *N* gene sequence: 1071–1091

2.3. Plasmid DNA Preparation

Plasmid DNA was transformed into electrocompetent DH5α *Escherichia coli* and purified with EndoFree Plasmid Maxi Kits (QIAGEN, Hilden, Germany).

2.4. Cell Transfection and Antiviral Activity In Vitro

We validated the inhibitory effects of the shRNAs against N by target gene expression in an in vitro transfection system. One day before transfection, IEC cells were seeded into 12-well plates at 5×10^4 cells per well without antibiotics and grown at 37 °C overnight with 5% CO_2. The 60–80% confluent cells were transiently transfected with the indicated plasmid using Lipofectamine 3000 (Invitrogen, Carlsbad, CA, USA), according to the manufacturer's instructions. At 48 h after transfection, *N* expression was analyzed by Western blot or inverted fluorescence microscope. To examine the inhibitory effects of shRNAs against N on target gene expression during PEDV replication, IEC cells were transfected with or without 1 µg, 2 µg, or 4 of µg shR-N307, shR-N463, and shR-N1071 or 4 µg of shR-NC for 24 h and infected with 100 $TCID_{50}$/mL PEDV strain CV777 or LNCT2. At 48 h post-infection (hpi), antigen slides were prepared to detect PEDV N protein expression by Western blot. In parallel experiments, cells from individual wells were collected and frozen and thawed twice, followed by centrifugation at low speed (1000× *g*), and supernatants were serially diluted, inoculated with Vero E6 cells, and titrated by the Reed and Muench method.

2.5. Sodium Dodecyl Sulfate Polyacrylamide Gel Electrophoresis and Western Blots

IEC cells grown in 12-well plates were transfected and infected as described. Cells were harvested at the indicated time points after transfection or virus infection, washed once with cold PBS, and lysed in radioimmunoprecipitation assay (RIPA) buffer (Sigma-Aldrich, St. Louis, MO, USA) to determine protein concentrations. Equal amounts of protein were subjected to sodium dodecyl sulfate polyacrylamide gel electrophoresis (SDS-PAGE) followed by blotting onto nitrocellulose membranes. Membranes were washed twice in Tris-buffered saline (TBS) and incubated 2 h in Superblock blocking buffer (ThermoFisher, Waltham, MA, USA). Membranes were incubated with anti-N monoclonal antibody (mAb) 3G2 (prepared by our laboratory, diluted 1:1000), anti-myc monoclonal (Sigma, diluted 1:1000) or anti-glyceraldehyde 3-phosphate dehydrogenase (GAPDH) monoclonal antibody (Sigma, diluted 1:10,000). Proteins were revealed by IRDye 800CW goat anti-mouse immunoglobulin G (IgG) (H + L) (1:10,000) (LiCor BioSciences, Lincoln, NE, USA), and blots were visualized using an Odyssey infrared imaging system (LiCor BioSciences).

2.6. Cell Viability Assays

Cell viability assays were performed using cell counting kit-8 (CCK-8) (CK04; Dojindo, Shanghai, China), according to the manufacturer's protocol. In brief, IEC cells were seeded in 96-well plates at 10,000 per well and incubated at 37 °C for 24 h. Cells were transfected or not with shRNAs, and plates were incubated for 48 h before 10 µL of CCK-8 was added to wells for incubation for 2 h. Optical density at 450 nm was measured. Viability of treated cells was expressed as a percentage relative to untreated cells.

2.7. Immunofluorescence Assays

IEC cells were seeded in 12-well plates, and confluent cell monolayers were transfected with shR-N307, shR-N463 and shR-N1071, or shR-NC (4 µg) with Lipofectamine 3000 (Invitrogen) before PEDV infection. Cells were infected with PEDV strain CV777 or LNCT2 at 100 $TCID_{50}$/mL. PEDV infection was analyzed using immunofluorescence assays (IFAs) at 48 hpi. Cells were fixed with 4% paraformaldehyde at 4 °C for 30 min and washed with PBS. Fixed cells were permeabilized with 0.2% Triton X-100 for 15 min at room temperature and blocked with blocking buffer (PBS with 5% bovine serum albumin (BSA)) for 2 h. Preparations were labeled with the mouse anti-PEDV N mAb (1:100 dilution) at 37 °C for 2 h followed by labeling with Alexa Fluor 488 goat anti-mouse IgG antibody (1:200 dilution) (ThermoFisher) for 1 h at 37 °C. Cell nuclei were stained with 4′,6-diamidino-2-phenylindole (DAPI) (0.05 µg/mL) (D9542; Sigma) for 15 min and analyzed using an AMG EVOS F1 florescence microscope.

2.8. *Statistical Analysis*

All statistical data are expressed as means ± standard deviation (SD) of three independent experiments and analyzed using the Student's *t*-test. A *p*-value <0.05 was considered statistically significant.

3. Results

3.1. *IEC Cells and PEDV Infection*

Phylogenetic analysis of CV777 and LNCT2 was based on complete genomic sequences (Figure 2A). CV777 clustered with PEDV G1 genotype (classic strains), whereas LNCT2 clustered with PEDV G2 genotype (epidemic strains), with >98% nucleotide identity to these strains. To determine PEDV propagation in IEC cells, CPEs and IFAs were used to monitor after infection (Figure 2B). At 48 hpi, CV777 and LNCT2 caused similar CPEs in IEC cells, characterized by rounding, aggregation, and rupturing. The morphology of negative control cells remained unchanged and did not exhibit any signs of CPEs. Inoculation of CV777 and LNCT2 with IEC cells resulted in positive immunofluorescent staining with mAb that recognized the virus N protein. Controls were negative for immunostaining.

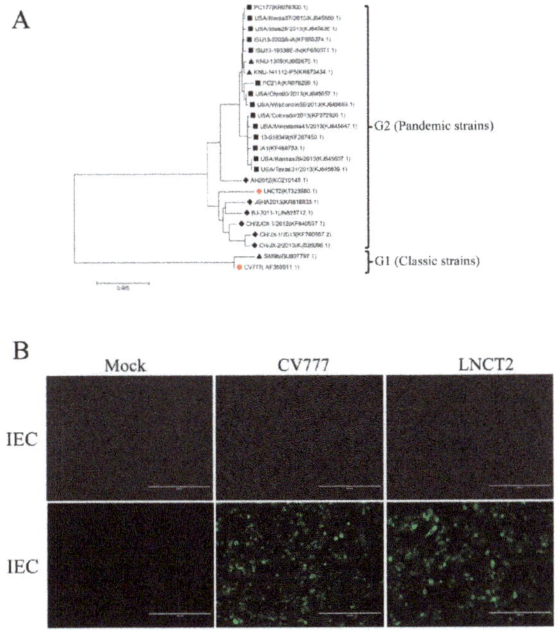

Figure 2. Phylogenetic analysis and virus-induced cytopathic effect (CPE) in intestine epithelial cells (IECs). (**A**) Phylogenetic trees of PEDV based on complete genomic DNA. Black squares, strains in United States of America (USA); black triangles, strains in South Korea; black rhombuses, strains in China; red circle, G1 CV777 strain from this study; red rhombus, G2 LNCT2 strain from this study. (**B**) Production and growth properties of PEDV CV777 and LNCT2 in IEC cells. CPE 48 h post-infection (hpi) (upper panels, bar: 400 μm) and immunofluorescence assay (IFA) 48 hpi (lower panels, bar: 200 μm) of CV777 and LNCT2 in IEC cells. IEC cells were infected with PEDV CV777 or LNCT2 at 100 50% tissue culture infective dose ($TCID_{50}$)/mL. CPE and IFA were examined at 48 hpi, and cell images were captured.

3.2. *Selection of Targeted Sites for N Gene-Specific shRNAs*

The prevalent strains that caused the outbreak of PEDV in China in 2010 and in North America in recent years belonged to the G2 genotype. PEDV is a positive-stranded RNA virus with higher mutation rates than DNA viruses [24]. Specific shRNAs were designed to target the conserved gene. We used the *N* gene of LNCT2 as the target sequence. Using nucleotide substitutions in the *N* gene and previous reports [25], we chose three unused regions that were well conserved in *N* genes among 25 isolates of PEDV G1 and G2 genogroups. The sites were at +307 to +327 nt, +463 to +483 nt, and +1071 to +1091 nt relative to the 5′ ATG initiation codon (Table 1).

3.3. *Cell Viability Is Not Affected by Plasmids with shRNAs*

ShRNAs induce large amounts of cell death when transfected at large volume, resulting in interference with experimental results. To detect if the three shRNAs we used led to cytotoxicity at 4 μg, IEC cells were seeded in 96-well microplates and transfected with shR-N307, shR-N463, shR-N1071, or shR-NC (4 μg) using Lipofectamine 3000 (Invitrogen), or transfected with transfection reagent alone as mock. After transfecting for 48 h, CCK-8 solution (10 μL) was added to wells, and plates were incubated at 37 °C for 2 h. Absorbance was measured at 450 nm using a microtiter plate reader (Bio-Rad, Hercules, CA, USA). Viable cells that were mock transfected with transfection reagent alone were the reference of 100% cell viability. ShR-N307, shR-N463, and shR-N1071 exhibited no obvious cytotoxicity in transfected Vero E6 and IEC cells at 4 μg (Figure 3).

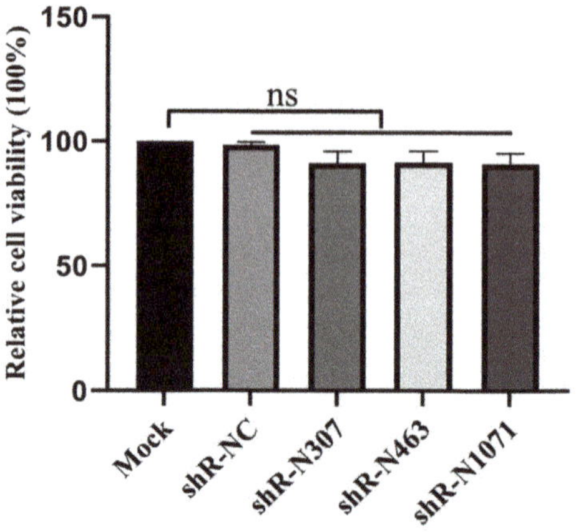

Figure 3. ShRNA treatment did not affect cell viability. Cell viability was detected by cell counting kit-8 (CCK-8) assays after transfection of IEC cells with shRNAs for 48 h. Absorption at 450 nm was recorded and expressed as a percentage of relative cell viability. Values are means ± SD (n = 3). Significant differences were assessed by Student's t-test; ns, no significant difference compared to control; $p > 0.05$.

3.4. *Efficient Inhibition of PEDV Myc-N or AcGFP-N Expression by shRNA Expression Cassettes*

We designed three shRNAs specifically targeting regions shown in Figure 1, named shR-N307, shR-N463, and shR-N1071. Western blots determined the inhibitory effects of the shRNAs on *N* gene expression. PMyc-N was co-transfected into IEC cells with increasing doses of shR-N307, shR-N463, or shR-N1071 using Lipofectamine 3000. At 48 h after transfection, N protein expression was analyzed by Western blots using mouse anti-Myc mAb. Western blots demonstrated that shR-N307, shR-N463, and shR-N1071 inhibited Myc-tagged N protein expression in a dose-dependent manner (Figure 4A).

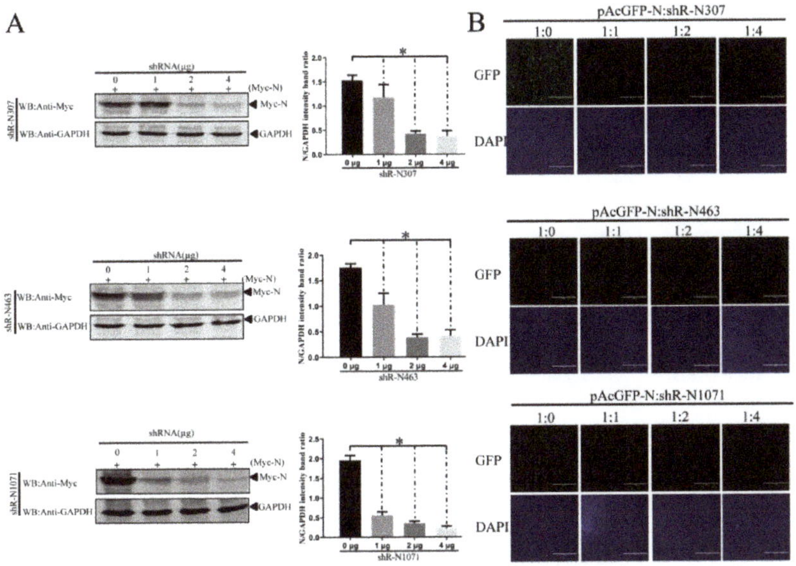

Figure 4. Inhibitory effects of shR-N307, shR-N463, and shR-N1071 on the PEDV N protein. (**A**) Western blots for effect of shR-N307, shR-N463, and shR-N1071 on *N* gene expression. PMyc-N was co-transfected with increasing doses of shR-N307, shR-N463, or shR-N1071 into IEC cells. After 48 h, transfected cells were lysed. Equal amounts of cell lysates were resolved by 12.5% SDS-PAGE. Reaction products were probed with anti-Myc or anti-glyceraldehyde 3-phosphate dehydrogenase (GAPDH). Densitometric data for N/GAPDH from three independent experiments are shown as means ± SD. * $p < 0.05$. The p value was calculated using Student's t-test; (**B**) shR-N307, shR-N463, and shR-N1071 influence on pAcGFP-N expression in cultured IEC cells. PAcGFP-N was co-transfected with increasing doses of shR-N307, shR-N463, or shR-N1071 into IEC cells. PAcGFP-N expression plasmid was the unrelated control. Images show enhanced GFP (EGFP) expression at 48 h post-transfection.

The *N* gene was fused with the *AcGFP* gene to make pAcGFP-N. The effect of shRNAs on *N* gene expression was monitored by *AcGFP* expression. Plasmid pAcGFP-N was transfected into IEC cells alone or with the indicated concentrations of shR-N307, shR-N463, or shR-N1071 expression cassettes. At 48 h post-transfection, the effects of shRNA on enhanced GFP (EGFP) expression were monitored by fluorescence microscopy. The shR-N307, shR-N463, and shR-N1071 expression cassettes targeting *N* gene inhibited the expression of *AcGFP* to some extent compared with cells transfected with plasmid pAcGFP-N alone. The shR-N307, shR-N463, and shR-N1071 expression cassettes targeting the *N* sequence were similar, with weak fluorescence observed from cells transfected with 4 µg of shRNAs (Figure 4B).

3.5. ShRNA-Mediated Inhibition of N Expression and PEDV Production in Infected IEC Cells

To examine the inhibitory effects of shRNAs against N on target gene expression during CV777 and LNCT2 replication, IEC cells were transfected with indicated plasmids for 24 h and then infected with PEDV CV777 orLNCT2 strain (100 $TCID_{50}$/mL). At 48 hpi, PEDV-infected cells were lysed with RIPA buffer containing 1 mM phenylmethylsulfonyl fluoride (PMSF), and Western blots were used to analyze *N* expression using mAb 3G2. Treatment with shR-N307, shR-N463, and shR-N1071 significantly reduced *N* expression compared to shR-NC- or mock-transfected IEC cells. The inhibitory effects of the three shRNAs on *N* expression were elevated with increased shRNA concentration (Figures 5A and 6A). These results show that *N*-targeted shRNA efficiently inhibited target gene expression during PEDV replication.

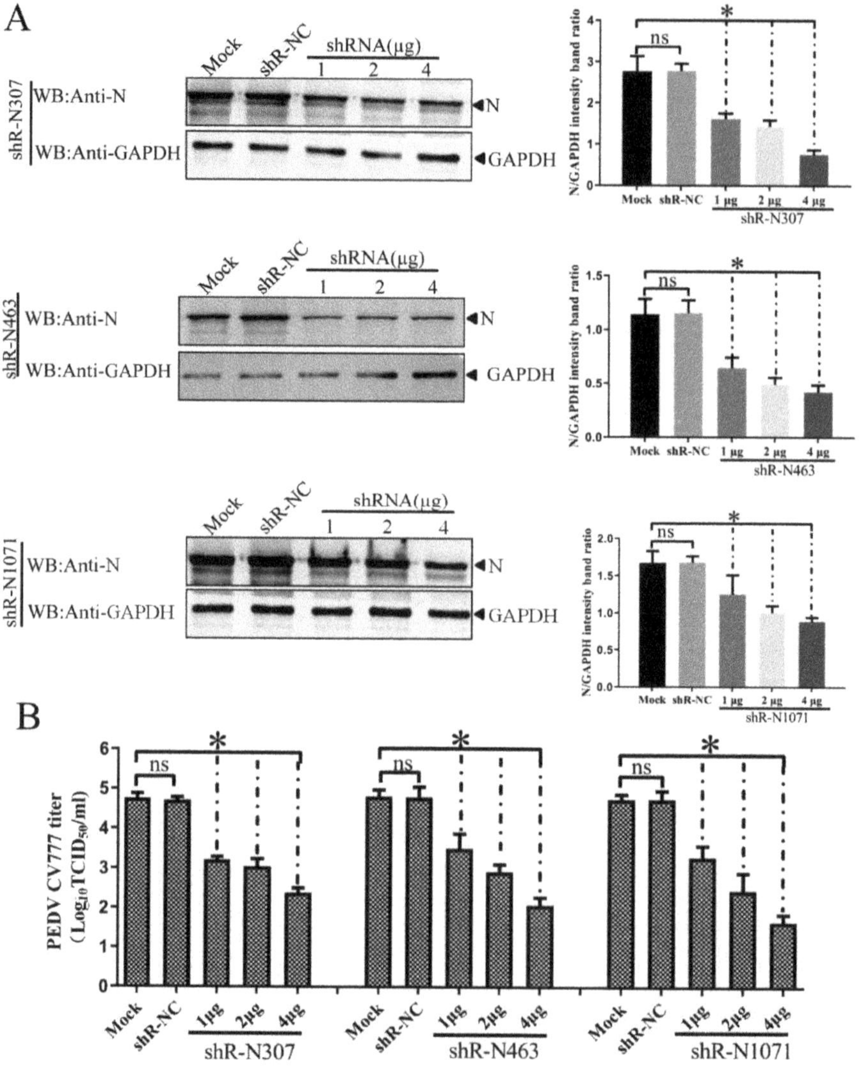

Figure 5. Dose-dependent inhibitory effects of shR-N307, shR-N463, and shR-N1071 against N on target gene expression and PEDV CV777 replication in infected IEC cells. IEC cells with shRNA (1, 2, 4 μg) for 24 h before infection with PEDV CV777 for 48 h. (**A**) PEDV N protein by Western blot with anti-N protein monoclonal antibody (mAb). Densitometric data for N/GAPDH from three independent experiments, shown as means ± SD. * $p < 0.05$. The p value was calculated using Student's t-test; (**B**) PEDV CV777 titers in shRNA-transfected IEC cells. ShRNA transfection and viral infection were as in panel A. Viral titers in supernatants collected at 48 hpi were determined using the Reed–Muench method. Error bars represent standard errors of the mean from three independent experiments. * $p < 0.05$. The p value was calculated using Student's t-test.

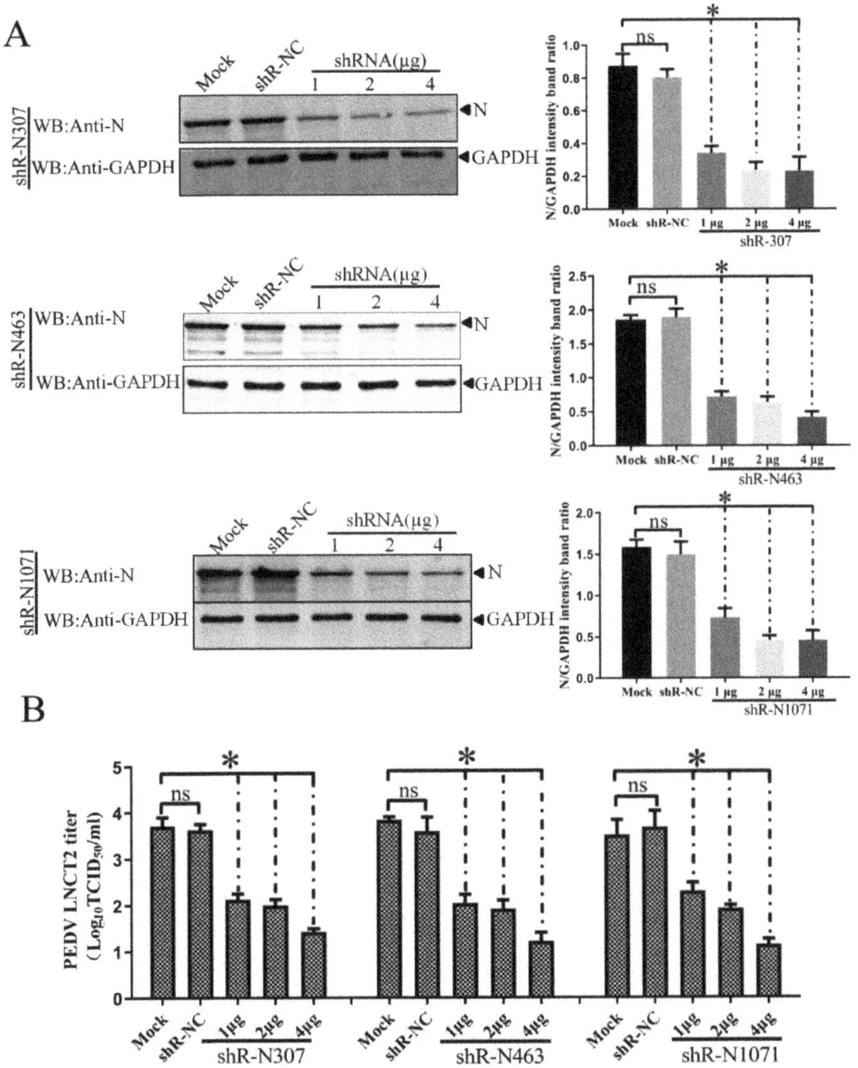

Figure 6. Dose-dependent inhibitory effects of shR-N307, shR-N463, and shR-N1071 directed against N on target gene expression and PEDV LNCT2 replication in infected IEC cells. IEC cells with shRNA (1, 2, 4 μg) for 24 h were infected with PEDV LNCT2 for 48 h. (**A**) PEDV N protein was detected by Western blot with anti-N protein mAb. Densitometric data for N/GAPDH from three independent experiments are shown as means ± SD. * $p < 0.05$. The p value was calculated using Student's t-test; (**B**) PEDV LNCT2 titers in shRNA-transfected IEC cells. ShRNA transfection and viral infection were as in panel A. Viral titers in supernatants collected at 48 hpi were determined using the Reed–Muench method. Error bars represent standard errors of the mean from three independent experiments. * $p < 0.05$. The p value was calculated using Student's t-test.

To determine if downregulation of *N* expression by shRNAs decreased PEDV CV777 and LNCT2 strain replication, IEC cells were transfected with indicated plasmids for 24 h and infected with CV777 or LNCT2 (100 $TCID_{50}$/mL). Cell cultures were collected at 48 hpi, and viral titers were determined.

Transfection with shR-N307, shR-N463, or shR-N1071 significantly reduced PEDV CV777 and LNCT2 replication compared to shR-NC- or mock-transfected IEC cells ($p < 0.05$) (Figures 5B and 6B). Although differences in inhibition of PEDV CV777 and LNCT2 strain replication induced by 1 µg, 2 µg, or 4 µg of shR-N307, shR-N463, and shR-N1071 were seen, PEDV replication gradually reduced with increased shRNA concentrations.

4. Discussion

In this study, we demonstrated that shRNAs against PEDV N protein broadly inhibited PEDV G1 and G2 strains. This report found that shRNAs inhibit swine coronavirus replication in epithelia. Most coronaviruses such as severe acute respiratory syndrome coronavirus (SARS-CoV), Middle East respiratory syndrome coronavirus (MERS-CoV), and PEDV infect epithelial cells in the respiratory and/or enteric tracts. The control of coronavirus diseases is important for human public health security. Further developing RNAi as a potential therapeutic agent against coronavirus infection is worthwhile.

The PEDV N protein is predominantly produced in susceptible cells, which makes it a major target for early and accurate diagnosis [26]. The N protein forms complexes with coronavirus genomic RNA and enhances the viral transcription and assembly. Because of the importance of N protein in viral replication and the coronavirus *N* gene long used as a major target for shRNA design, we focused on the inhibition of PEDV infection using RNAi targeting the *N* gene of PEDV and systematically evaluated suppression efficiency. Alterations of viral genomes such as nucleotide substitution, insertion, and deletion have the potential to decrease the inhibitory effect of shRNA. We analyzed 25 *N* gene sequences derived from PEDV genotypes G1 and G2 and only found single-nucleotide substitutions. Considering the nucleotide substitutions in the *N* gene, we chose three conserved and unexploited regions for the design of shRNAs. PEDV is primarily transmitted through the fecal–oral route and infects intestinal villous epithelial cells in vivo [27]. Current in vitro cell cultures of PEDV include Vero E6 cells, MARC-145 cells (another monkey kidney cell line), and HEK293 cells [28]. Most are non-porcine intestinal epithelial cells and, thus, not ideal in vitro cellular models for studying the interaction between PEDV infection and the host response due to interspecific variation. The IEC cell line represented a better model of normal porcine intestinal epithelium than transformed cell lines, and provided a unique opportunity to explore host–pathogen interactions in an in vitro system [29]. Using this cell model, we showed that shRNA expression did not affect the viability of IEC cells. Co-transfection of recombinant plasmid pMyc-N and different concentrations of shRNAs highlighted the success of the gene knockdown at the protein level. GFP was an important reporter for *N* gene expression. For example, if the *N* gene was silenced by the shRNAs, the translation of GFP protein in frame with the *N* gene in the recombinant plasmid would also be inhibited. This hypothesis was consistent with our findings. Our shRNAs shR-N307, shR-N463, and shR-N1071 strongly reduced GFP expression, and the inhibition was dose-dependent. In addition, the model system was exploited to further study the pathological functions of PEDV genes. We assessed the capacity of shR-N307, shR-N463, and shR-N1071 for inhibiting the gene and protein expressions of PEDV CV777 and LNCT2 strains in vitro. We observed that shR-N307, shR-N463, and shR-N1071 were able to knock down target gene expression of PEDV CV777 and LNCT2 strains at 48 hpi. We also showed that shR-N307, shR-N463, and shR-N1071 against the *N* gene suppressed PEDV CV777 and LNCT2 strain replication.

Currently, siRNA import into cells requires vectors such as plasmids and recombinant lentiviruses that express shRNAs efficiently and stably. As recombinant lentiviruses have a higher adaptability and replication ability in host cells, and as their genes can be integrated into cellular genomes, the silencing effect of lentiviruses is more efficient than plasmids [30]. However, this kind of gene integration may induce host genome mutations and cause cellular injury. In addition, excessive expression of shRNAs competitively inhibits cell endogenous miRNAs and causes cytotoxicity [31]. Therefore, RNAi mediated by a plasmid is currently safer for high gene silencing efficiency. However, off-target effects from using plasmid-based siRNA are still a shortfall [32]. To solve this problem, designing improved siRNA sequences, as well as developing novel and progressive vectors, is necessary.

In conclusion, plasmids expressing three shRNAs targeting different sites of the *N* gene of PEDV were constructed and transfected into IEC cells. Infection of PEDV CV777 (G1) or LNCT2 (G2) occurred post transfection. Detection by Western blot and viral titer assays was used to measure levels of viral replication in cells. The results demonstrated that PEDV G1 and G2 strains were susceptible to RNAi pathways targeting the *N* gene. All shRNA tests led to the silencing of *N* gene expression and suppressed proliferation of PEDV G1 and G2 strains in IEC cells. In sum, our data showed the potential for the shRNA expression vectors to precisely and effectively interfere with the replication of PEDV G1 and G2 strains in vitro. To our knowledge, this is the first report of the inhibition of PEDV G1 and G2 strain infection with shRNAs in IEC cells. Therefore, this report enriches the antiviral spectrum of RNAi treatment. Although IEC cells are a non-transformed porcine intestinal epithelial cell line, these cells lack the complexity of the cell types found in the architecture of the intestinal epithelium and, thus, do not satisfactorily mimic the natural infection process. This method merits further investigation in animal studies to define its therapeutic potential. Determining if the technology could be used in vivo for anti-PEDV therapy is still under investigation.

Author Contributions: Conceptualization, L.F.; data curation, D.S., X.W., and H.S.; funding acquisition, L.F.; METHODOLOGY, D.S., X.W., and H.S.; project administration, L.F.; resources, J.C.; software, X.Z., J.L., J.Z. (Jialin Zhang), Z.J. (Zhaoyang Ji), and Z.J. (Zhaoyang Jing); supervision, L.F.; writing—original draft, D.S., X.W., H.S., and L.F.; writing—review and editing, J.Z. (Jiyu Zhang) and Y.H.

Funding: This work was supported by grants from the National Natural Science Foundation of China (31602072 and 31572541), the China Postdoctoral Science Foundation (2017M610136), and the Natural Science Foundation of Heilongjiang Province of China (C2017079 and C2018066).

Conflicts of Interest: The authors declare no conflicts of interest.

References

1. Shi, D.; Lv, M.; Chen, J.; Shi, H.; Zhang, S.; Zhang, X.; Feng, L. Molecular characterizations of subcellular localization signals in the nucleocapsid protein of porcine epidemic diarrhea virus. *Viruses* **2014**, *6*, 1253–1273. [CrossRef] [PubMed]
2. Fouchier, R.A.; Hartwig, N.G.; Bestebroer, T.M.; Niemeyer, B.; de Jong, J.C.; Simon, J.H.; Osterhaus, A.D. A previously undescribed coronavirus associated with respiratory disease in humans. *Proc. Natl. Acad. Sci. USA* **2004**, *101*, 6212–6216. [CrossRef] [PubMed]
3. Li, W.; Li, H.; Liu, Y.; Pan, Y.; Deng, F.; Song, Y.; Tang, X.; He, Q. New variants of porcine epidemic diarrhea virus, China, 2011. *Emerg. Infect. Dis.* **2012**, *18*, 1350–1353. [CrossRef] [PubMed]
4. Zhou, P.; Fan, H.; Lan, T.; Yang, X.L.; Shi, W.F.; Zhang, W.; Zhu, Y.; Zhang, Y.W.; Xie, Q.M.; Mani, S.; et al. Fatal swine acute diarrhoea syndrome caused by an HKU2-related coronavirus of bat origin. *Nature* **2018**, *556*, 255–258. [CrossRef]
5. Lai, M.M.; Cavanagh, D. The molecular biology of coronaviruses. *Adv. Virus Res.* **1997**, *48*, 1–100.
6. Duenas-Carrera, S.; Alvarez-Lajonchere, L.; Alvarez, J.C.; Ramos, T.; Pichardo, D.; Morales, J. Repeated administration of hepatitis C virus core-encoding plasmid to mice does not necessarily increase the immune response generated against this antigen. *Biotechnol. Appl. Biochem.* **2001**, *33*, 47–51. [CrossRef]
7. Madden, C.R.; Finegold, M.J.; Slagle, B.L. Expression of hepatitis B virus X protein does not alter the accumulation of spontaneous mutations in transgenic mice. *J. Virol.* **2000**, *74*, 5266–5272. [CrossRef]
8. Reifenberg, K.; Deutschle, T.; Wild, J.; Hanano, R.; Gastrock-Balitsch, I.; Schirmbeck, R.; Schlicht, H.J. The hepatitis B virus e antigen cannot pass the murine placenta efficiently and does not induce CTL immune tolerance in H-2(b) mice in utero. *Virology* **1998**, *243*, 45–53. [CrossRef]
9. Reifenberg, K.; Lohler, J.; Pudollek, H.P.; Schmitteckert, E.; Spindler, G.; Kock, J.; Schlicht, H.J. Long-term expression of the hepatitis B virus core-e- and X-proteins does not cause pathologic changes in transgenic mice. *J. Hepatol.* **1997**, *26*, 119–130. [CrossRef]
10. Chen, J.; Liu, X.; Shi, D.; Shi, H.; Zhang, X.; Li, C.; Chi, Y.; Feng, L. Detection and molecular diversity of spike gene of porcine epidemic diarrhea virus in China. *Viruses* **2013**, *5*, 2601–2613. [CrossRef]

11. Wang, X.; Chen, J.; Shi, D.; Shi, H.; Zhang, X.; Yuan, J.; Jiang, S.; Feng, L. Immunogenicity and antigenic relationships among spike proteins of porcine epidemic diarrhea virus subtypes G1 and G2. *Arch. Virol.* **2016**, *161*, 537–547. [CrossRef] [PubMed]
12. Aagaard, L.; Rossi, J.J. RNAi therapeutics: Principles, prospects and challenges. *Adv. Drug Deliv. Rev.* **2007**, *59*, 75–86. [CrossRef] [PubMed]
13. Battistella, M.; Marsden, P.A. Advances, Nuances, and Potential Pitfalls When Exploiting the Therapeutic Potential of RNA Interference. *Clin Pharm. Ther.* **2015**, *97*, 79–87. [CrossRef] [PubMed]
14. Brummelkamp, T.R.; Bernards, R.; Agami, R. A system for stable expression of short interfering RNAs in mammalian cells. *Science* **2002**, *296*, 550–553. [CrossRef] [PubMed]
15. Fire, A.; Xu, S.; Montgomery, M.K.; Kostas, S.A.; Driver, S.E.; Mello, C.C. Potent and specific genetic interference by double-stranded RNA in Caenorhabditis elegans. *Nature* **1998**, *391*, 806–811. [CrossRef] [PubMed]
16. Grimm, D.; Wang, L.; Lee, J.S.; Schurmann, N.; Gu, S.; Borner, K.; Storm, T.A.; Kay, M.A. Argonaute proteins are key determinants of RNAi efficacy, toxicity, and persistence in the adult mouse liver. *J. Clin. Investig.* **2010**, *120*, 3106–3119. [CrossRef] [PubMed]
17. Hammond, S.M. Dicing and slicing: The core machinery of the RNA interference pathway. *FEBS Lett.* **2005**, *579*, 5822–5829. [CrossRef]
18. Ontiveros, E.; Kuo, L.L.; Masters, P.S.; Perlman, S. Inactivation of expression of gene 4 of mouse hepatitis virus strain JHM does not affect virulence in the murine CNS. *Virology* **2001**, *289*, 230–238. [CrossRef]
19. Wang, D.; Fang, L.; Xiao, S. Porcine epidemic diarrhea in China. *Virus Res.* **2016**, *226*, 7–13. [CrossRef]
20. Shi, D.; Shi, H.; Sun, D.; Chen, J.; Zhang, X.; Wang, X.; Zhang, J.; Ji, Z.; Liu, J.; Cao, L.; et al. Nucleocapsid Interacts with NPM1 and Protects it from Proteolytic Cleavage, Enhancing Cell Survival, and is Involved in PEDV Growth. *Sci. Rep.* **2017**, *7*, 39700. [CrossRef]
21. Fingerote, R.J.; Cruz, B.M.; Gorczynski, R.M.; Fung, L.S.; Hubbell, H.R.; Suhadolnik, R.J.; Levy, G.A. A 2′,5′-Oligoadenylate Analog Inhibits Murine Hepatitis-Virus Strain-3 (Mhv-3) Replication in-Vitro but Does Not Reduce Mhv-3-Related Mortality or Induction of Procoagulant Activity in Susceptible Mice. *J. Gen. Virol.* **1995**, *76*, 373–380. [CrossRef] [PubMed]
22. BLOCK-iT™ RNAi Designer. Available online: http://rnaidesigner.thermofisher.com/rnaiexpress/ (accessed on 19 October 2019).
23. Basic Local Alignment Search Tool. Available online: http://www.ncbi.nlm.nih.gov/BLAST (accessed on 19 October 2019).
24. Tokuriki, N.; Oldfield, C.J.; Uversky, V.N.; Berezovsky, I.N.; Tawfik, D.S. Do viral proteins possess unique biophysical features? *Trends Biochem. Sci.* **2009**, *34*, 53–59. [CrossRef] [PubMed]
25. Shen, H.; Zhang, C.; Guo, P.; Liu, Z.; Zhang, J. Effective inhibition of porcine epidemic diarrhea virus by RNA interference in vitro. *Virus Genes* **2015**, *51*, 252–259. [CrossRef] [PubMed]
26. Kuo, L.; Hurst-Hess, K.R.; Koetzner, C.A.; Masters, P.S. Analyses of Coronavirus Assembly Interactions with Interspecies Membrane and Nucleocapsid Protein Chimeras. *J. Virol.* **2016**, *90*, 4357–4368. [CrossRef]
27. Lin, C.M.; Saif, L.J.; Marthaler, D.; Wang, Q. Evolution, antigenicity and pathogenicity of global porcine epidemic diarrhea virus strains. *Virus Res.* **2016**, *226*, 20–39. [CrossRef]
28. Zhang, J.; Guo, L.; Xu, Y.; Yang, L.; Shi, H.; Feng, L.; Wang, Y. Characterization of porcine epidemic diarrhea virus infectivity in human embryonic kidney cells. *Arch. Virol.* **2017**, *162*, 2415–2419. [CrossRef]
29. Liu, F.; Li, G.; Wen, K.; Bui, T.; Cao, D.; Zhang, Y.; Yuan, L. Porcine small intestinal epithelial cell line (IPEC-J2) of rotavirus infection as a new model for the study of innate immune responses to rotaviruses and probiotics. *Viral Immunol.* **2010**, *23*, 135–149. [CrossRef]
30. Pfeiffenberger, E.; Sigl, R.; Geley, S. Conditional RNAi Using the Lentiviral GLTR System. *Methods Mol. Biol.* **2016**, *1448*, 121–138.
31. Khan, A.A.; Betel, D.; Miller, M.L.; Sander, C.; Leslie, C.S.; Marks, D.S. Transfection of small RNAs globally perturbs gene regulation by endogenous microRNAs. *Nat. Biotechnol.* **2009**, *27*, 549–555. [CrossRef]
32. Olejniczak, M.; Polak, K.; Galka-Marciniak, P.; Krzyzosiak, W.J. Recent advances in understanding of the immunological off-target effects of siRNA. *Curr. Gene Ther.* **2011**, *11*, 532–543. [CrossRef]

vaccines

MDPI

Article

A Single Dose of Dendrimer B_2T Peptide Vaccine Partially Protects Pigs against Foot-and-Mouth Disease Virus Infection

Rodrigo Cañas-Arranz [1], Mar Forner [2], Sira Defaus [2], Patricia de León [1], María J. Bustos [1], Elisa Torres [1], Francisco Sobrino [1,*], David Andreu [2,*] and Esther Blanco [3,*]

1 Centro de Biología Molecular "Severo Ochoa" (CSIC-UAM), 28049 Madrid, Spain; rcannas@cbm.csic.es (R.C.-A.); pdeleon@cbm.csic.es (P.d.L.); mjbustos@cbm.csic.es (M.J.B.); elisa.torres@cbm.csic.es (E.T.)

2 Departament de Ciències Experimentals i de la Salut, Universitat Pompeu Fabra, 08003 Barcelona, Spain; mar.forner@upf.edu (M.F.); sira.defaus@upf.edu (S.D.)

3 Centro de Investigación en Sanidad Animal (CISA-INIA), Valdeolmos, 28130 Madrid, Spain

* Correspondence: fsobrino@cbm.csic.es (F.S.); david.andreu@upf.edu (D.A.); blanco@inia.es (E.B.)

Received: 16 December 2019; Accepted: 8 January 2020; Published: 10 January 2020

Abstract: Foot-and-mouth disease virus (FMDV) causes a highly contagious disease of cloven-hoofed animals whose control relies on efficient vaccination. We have reported that dendrimer peptide B_2T, with two copies of FMDV B-cell epitope VP1 (136–154) linked through maleimide units to T-cell epitope 3A (21–35)], elicits potent B- and T-cell specific responses and confers solid protection in pigs to type-O FMDV challenge after two doses of peptide. Herein we now show that B_2T evokes specific protective immune responses after administration of a single dose of either 2 or 0.5 mg of peptide. High titers of ELISA and neutralizing antibodies against FMDV were detectable at day 15 post-immunization. Likewise, activated T cells and induced IFN-γ response to in vitro recall with FMDV peptides were also detected by the same day. Further, in 70% of B_2T-vaccinated pigs, full protection—no clinical signs of disease—was observed upon virus challenge at day 25 post-immunization. These results strengthen the potential of B_2T as a safe, cost-effective candidate vaccine conferring adequate protection against FMDV with a single dose. The finding is particularly relevant to emergency scenarios permitting only a single shot immunization.

Keywords: FMDV; peptide vaccine; single dose; amount; pig

1. Introduction

Vaccination remains the most effective approach to prevent human and animal diseases [1]. In animal health, development of safe, cost-effective and marker vaccines, capable of telling infected from vaccinated animals (DIVA), remains a challenge for many diseases, particularly viral ones [2,3]. Conventional vaccines based on inactivated or attenuated viruses entail risks such as accidental escape or incomplete inactivation of infectious viruses, as well as possible reversion of attenuated into virulent forms. Subunit or epitopic vaccines represent an alternative that solves most such problems by excluding the infectious agent and allowing targeting to well characterized viral epitopes relevant for protection [4–6].

Foot-and-mouth disease virus (FMDV) is the prototype member of the *Aphthovirus* genus within the *Picornaviridae* family [7] and the etiological agent of FMD, a highly transmissible infection of pigs and other cloven-hoofed animals, with huge economic impact worldwide [8,9]. FMD underscores paradigmatically the challenge of finding alternative strategies to the classic vaccines still used to prevent this highly contagious disease [10]. The massive amplification and shedding of FMDV in infected pigs turns this species to a key epidemiological factor for the spread of the virus over the course of outbreaks in many regions of the world [11]. In addition, the growing numbers of domestic pigs worldwide, particularly in Asian countries, make the development of pig-suited FMD vaccines a strategic task.

Conventional FMDV vaccines based on chemically inactivated virus have allowed FMD control and eradication in some countries, although their manufacturing process—not upgraded over recent decades—poses significant biosafety concerns that have been related to occasional escape episodes of diverse consequence [12–14]. This risk plus other limitations, such as the need for a strict cold chain to preserve stability, and the use of updated vaccine strains, because of the high potential antigenic diversity of the virus, underlie the adoption of non-vaccination policies in FMDV-free countries, a controversial and by no means risk-free practice, as borne out by not infrequent outbreaks in those locations. In crisis scenarios of this kind [15], vaccines incorporating outbreak-relevant epitopes, eliciting protective responses and generated as a quick response to the epidemic, can become an invaluable emergency resource for FMD containment [16]. Among such emergency vaccines, those based on synthetic peptides [6] are particularly appealing because of their (i) total lack of biological hazard; (ii) possibility of displaying various epitopes on a single platform; (iii) DIVA compliance; (iv) efficient synthetic production and characterization as pharmaceuticals, and (v) no cold-chain required; easy transport and storage [17].

The main B-cell antigenic site in FMDV, located at the GH loop of capsid protein VP1 (residues ca. 140–160), is structurally continuous [18,19]. Linear peptides reproducing this loop, either alone or in combination with T-cell FMDV epitopes, have been shown to confer limited protection in natural hosts [20–23].

A substantial enhancement in immunogenicity can be achieved by multiple display of B- and/or T-cell epitopes on a single molecular scaffold [17] inspired on the multiple antigenic peptide (MAP) platform of Tam [24]. In an initial realization in this regard, a peptide spanning residues 21–35 of FMDV protein 3A [thereafter T3A], which delimit an immunodominant T-cell epitope in domestic pigs [25], was N-terminally elongated into a Lys tree to which four copies of a B-cell epitope (residues 140–158 of VP1; containing the RGD motif that mediates binding to integrins, the cell receptors) were covalently linked in a dendrimeric (branched) fashion. The sequence of the B-cell epitope corresponded to that of the epidemiologically relevant O/UKG/11/01 isolate, belonging to serotype O the most prevalent worldwide [26]. This multivalent construct (named B_4T) elicited high titers of FMDV-neutralizing antibodies, activated specific T cells, and fully protected pigs against FMDV challenge [27]. Interestingly, a simpler version (i.e., two B-cell epitope branches) of the peptide vaccine candidate, termed B_2T, also elicited potent specific responses and conferred solid protection in pigs to challenge [28] (Table 1). In both B_4T and B_2T trials, animals were immunized with two 2-mg doses of peptide (3 weeks apart from each other) before challenge.

Table 1. Synthetic peptides used in this study.

Peptide	FMDV Protein (Residues)	Sequence
B	VP1 (136–154)	PVTNVRGDLQVLAQKAART-amide
T	3A (21–35)	AAIEFFEGMVHDSIK-amide
B_2T	VP1 (136–154), 3A (21–35)	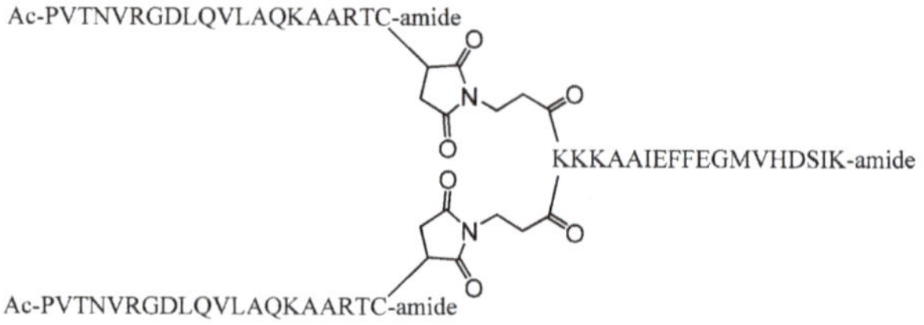

As mentioned above, emergency FMD vaccines, eliciting protective responses upon a single shot, are particularly valuable in containing uncontrolled FMDV outbreaks [14]. The modular nature of B_2T affords considerable versatility in the sequences that can be integrated into the constructions, either as part of a single molecule or as mixtures of different molecules. Thus, incorporation of VP1 GH-loop sequences from different FMDV isolates can modulate/enhance the protective spectrum of the candidates. This is particularly relevant because of the high FMDV antigenic diversity reflected in seven serotypes and many variants within each of them, which makes matching of vaccine strains with circulating virus a critical issue for vaccine efficacy [11,15]. On the other hand, the T3A sequence mentioned above is highly conserved among FMDV serotypes and therefore can evoke heterologous responses, again contributing to broaden the protective response conferred by B_2T. In addition to versatile, readily adaptable responses to new virus threats, emergency vaccines require fast and cost-effective manufacturing programs, which are ideally met by the expediency and flexibility inherent to chemical synthesis production.

Herein we have explored the possibility of: (i) Eliciting protective responses in pigs upon administration of a single B_2T dose, and (ii) reducing the amount of antigen required to elicit protective responses. Thus, we report results with both the 2 mg dose of previous experiments [28] and with a reduced 0.5 mg inoculum. Remarkably, the latter dose elicits a rapid immune response involving high titers of FMDV neutralizing antibodies and specific IFN-γ secreting T cells at 15 days post-immunization (dpi). In addition, solid protection is observed in 80% of pigs vaccinated with 0.5 mg B_2T, with no clinical signs upon viral challenge at day 25 dpi. Taken together, our results highlight the value of B_2T as candidate FMD vaccine for pigs in emergency scenarios.

2. Results

2.1. A Single B_2T Dose Elicits Rapid Humoral Specific Responses Including FMDV Neutralizing Antibodies

Domestic pigs, in two different groups of five animals each, were immunized once with 2 or 0.5 mg of B_2T (pigs 1 to 5 and 6 to 10, respectively), and two additional non-immunized animals were kept as controls (pigs 11 and 12 inoculated with PBS). Total FMDV-specific IgG antibodies were determined by ELISA at 0, 15, and 21 dpi. Both 2 and 0.5 mg doses elicited consistent and comparable IgG titers ($\log_{10}$) at 15 (4.3 ± 0.4 vs. 3.7 ± 0.3) and 21 (4.2 ± 0.2 vs. 4.3 ± 0.3) dpi (Figure 1A). Upon FMDV challenge (day 25) these titers were not boosted up, remaining similar in both B_2T-immunized groups (4.3 ± 0.1 vs. 4.6 ± 0.5). Non-immunized control pig 11 that survived 10 days post-challenge (dpc) showed anti-FMDV titers >2$\log_{10}$ units lower than those of the immunized and challenged groups (Figure 1A).

Regarding induction of FMDV neutralizing antibodies, as observed with the ELISA results, no major differences were noticed between virus neutralization titers (VNT) in the groups immunized with either 2 or 0.5 mg B_2T at day 15 (1.5 ± 0.2 vs. 1.4 ± 0.4) or day 21 pi (1.9 ± 0.4 vs. 2 ± 0.5) (Figure 1B). On the other hand, and in contrast to ELISA antibody titers, post-challenge VNT increased at 10 dpc (35 dpi) in both groups (3.1 ± 0.3 vs. 3.2 ± 0.4). As expected, no neutralizing antibodies were detected in the two control animals before challenge. The non-vaccinated animal that survived the challenge (pig 11), showed VNT (3.1) similar to those in immunized groups (Figure 1B), showing that neutralizing antibody levels in B_2T-immunized/challenged pigs—including those found to be protected—were as high as those in infected and recovered animals.

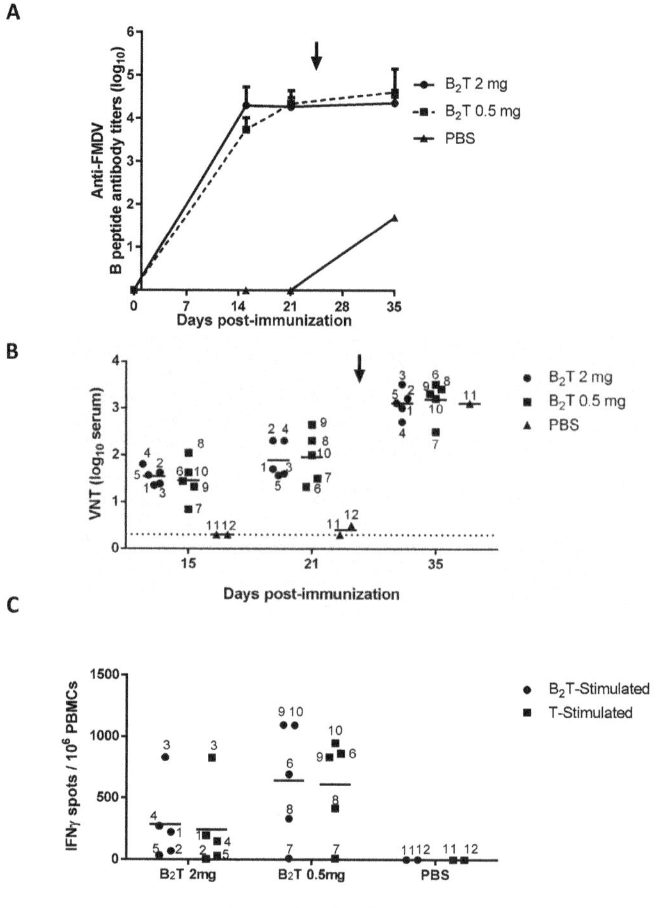

Figure 1. B- and T-cell responses in pigs immunized with a single dose and different amounts of B_2T. Time course of the specific antibody responses in sera collected on the indicated days pi. (**A**) Total anti peptide B IgG titers analyzed by ELISA. Each point depicts mean antibody titers (calculated as described in Methods) ± SD for each group of pigs ($n = 5$). (**B**) Virus neutralization titers, VNT, expressed as the reciprocal log10 of the last serum dilution that neutralized 100 TCID50 of FMDV isolate O/UKG 11/01. Each symbol represents the value for an individual pig (numbering is included). Horizontal lines indicate the geometric mean for each animal group. In no case individual spontaneous reactivity was observed in the titers determined at day 0. Dotted lines denotes the assay detection limit. In (**A**,**B**) arrows point FMDV challenge (day 25 pi). (**C**) Specific T-cell responses measured by an ex vivo IFN-γ ELISPOT at days 15 pi. The frequency of FMDV-specific IFN-γ secreting cells was determined as detailed in Methods. Horizontal bars represent the mean frequencies of IFN-γ release spots of triplicates of peripheral blood mononuclear cells (PBMCs) from pigs stimulated in vitro with B_2T (circles) or T (T3A) (squares) peptides (pig numbering is included).

2.2. *B_2T Elicits Early FMDV-Specific IFN-γ Responses*

Specific T cell responses elicited by B_2T at 15 dpi were determined by ELISPOT analysis of IFNγ-expressing PBMCs. High frequencies of spot-forming cells were found at day 15 in pigs immunized with either dose of B_2T in response to in vitro recall with homologous peptide (284.8 ± 321.1 vs. 645.6 ± 467.9). On average, pigs in the 0.5 mg group showed higher frequencies of IFNγ-expressing

PBMCs than those in the 2 mg group (Figure 1C). All responses were specific, as no peptide-driven IFN-γ-producing cells were detected in the two non-immunized pigs. PBMC stimulation with T3A peptide paralleled those observed with B_2T (241.3 ± 365.8 vs. 614.4 ± 403.1) (Figure 1C), supporting the recognition of T3A as a T-cell epitope.

2.3. A Single Dose of B_2T Peptide Confers Clinical Protection against FMDV Challenge

At 25 dpi, pigs in all three groups were challenged with FMDV. Animals were examined daily for clinical signs (see Methods) and considered protected when lesions were not observed or appeared only at the inoculation site [29]. As expected, PBS-inoculated control pigs 11 and 12 showed full FMD signs upon challenge, developing vesicular lesions on all four feet at 4 dpc and on the snout at 7 and 5 dpc, respectively (Table 2). The acute FMDV infection caused myocarditis, leading to heart failure and sudden death, of pig 12 at 5 dpc. In contrast, only 3 out of 10 peptide-immunized animals developed lesions outside the inoculation site: two pigs (3 and 5) in the 2 mg group and one (pig 10) in the 0.5 mg group. The remaining immunized animals did not develop any clinical signs, the cumulative lesion score of immunized groups being significantly lower than that of the non-immunized one (Table 2). In general, a correlation between lower body temperature and protection was observed, being the protected animals immunized with 0.5 mg B_2T those that did not develop fever.

Table 2. Evidences for protection in immunized pigs.

Inoculum	Pig	VNT/IFNγ [a]	Fever [b]	Lesion Score [c]	Protected [d]	RNA [e]
B_2T (2 mg)	1	1.7/221	39.8 (6)	0	++	ND
	2	2.3/68	39.7 (6)	0	++	ND
	3	1.6/830	41.7 (7)	3 (7)	−	1.8×10^4 (5)
	4	2.3/270	39.6 (7)	0	++	ND
	5	1.6/33	39.9 (10)	2 (10)	+	ND
B_2T (0.5 mg)	6	1.3/696	No fever	0	++	ND
	7	1.5/10	No fever	0	++	ND
	8	2.3/332	No fever	0	++	ND
	9	2.6/1096	No fever	0	++	ND
	10	2/1093	39.6 (8)	5 (7)	−	10^8 (3); 2×10^6 (5)
Non-immunized	11		40.7 (5)	7 (5)	−	1.4×10^8 (3); 4.5×10^6 (5)
	12		No fever	7 (5)	− [f]	1.1×10^8 (3)

[a] VNT and IFNγ spots/10^6 PBMCs determined at day 21 and 15 post-immunization, respectively. [b] Temperature (°C) and (in parenthesis) day pi when maximum temperature registered. No fever: ≤39.0–39.5 °C. [c] Animals were monitored up to 10 days pc for lesions. Lesion score (maximum value of 7): 1 point/vesicle in foot (up to 4 points); 1 point/mouth, tongue or snout lesion; 1 point/>2 lesions of diameter ≥10 mm. In parenthesis, day pc when lesion(s) was first observed. [d] Animals were considered fully protected (++) if lesion score ≤ 1; partially protected (mild/delayed disease) (+) if lesion score ≤ 2, or non-protected (−) if lesion score > 2. [e] Detection of FMDV RNA in serum samples. ND: RNA not detected. The amount of RNA in positive animals are expressed as viral RNA copies (VRC)/mL serum. Detection limit: 5×10^3 VRC/mL serum. The values from RNA positive animals are presented as VRC/mL serum. The day(s) post-challenge when RNA was detected is shown in brackets. [f] Animal died on day 5 pc.

Detection of FMDV RNA in serum samples from challenged pigs by RT-qPCR showed the presence of viral RNA in non-immunized control pigs 11 (days 3 and 5 pc) and 12 (day 3 pc), as well as in the two immunized but non-protected pigs 10 (days 3 and 5 pc) and 3 (only at day 5 pc), which showed the higher lesion score at day 7 pc (Table 2). Hence, virus detection in sera associated with the severity of the lesions of challenged pigs. Further work is necessary to assess the potential contribution of viruses circulating in non-protected animals, and to a lesser extent in protected animals, to the spread of the disease under field conditions.

In conclusion, immunization with a single 2 mg dose and, remarkably, even more with a 0.5 mg dose of B_2T dendrimer afforded substantial protection against conventional FMDV challenge.

3. Discussion

Protection after a single inoculation is a must for effective FMD vaccines, as it reduces both the cost of the vaccine as well as the logistics and labor expenses associated with the double immunization schedules. The application of a single dose vaccination program to the pig population can favor disease eradication, considering that pigs serve as amplifiers of FMDV and therefore a rapid control of the infection in swine is essential for disease control [11]. This is particularly relevant in settings such as diseases outbreaks occurring in areas where FMD is not enzootic and livestock remains unvaccinated [30]. To our knowledge, with the exception of adenovirus-vectored vaccines expressing FMDV empty capsids [31], few studies exist on the capability of FMD subunit vaccines alternative to classical ones to confer protection in relevant hosts after a single administration [32]. In this context, our optimization of the minimal amount of B_2T dendrimer still conferring protection is pertinent, both for understanding the response mechanisms to B_2T and for scaling down production costs, a relevant issue for FMD vaccine development.

We had previously shown that two 2 mg doses of B_2T conferred solid protection to FMDV challenge in swine, and that protection correlated with the induction of strong B- and T-cell specific responses [28]. Here, we explore the feasibility of B_2T as a protective, single dose subunit vaccine alternative to conventional FMD formulations. To this end, the original 2 mg dose and a four-fold lower one (0.5 mg) have been compared.

The challenge protocol followed in our experiment was as recommended by the OIE manual, for evaluation of protection against podal generalization (PPG) test, except that virus was inoculated 3 days earlier than indicated [33]. Under such conditions, full protection, considered as the absence of lesions at points other than the inoculation site, was observed in 70% of pigs vaccinated with B_2T; 3 out of 5 in the 2 mg dose group, and 4 out of 5 in the 0.5 mg group. This level of protection correlated with an average increase in virus neutralizing (VN) antibodies that was not observed for B-specific IgG antibodies detected by ELISA (Figure 1), suggesting the recall upon viral infection of a subset of FMDV-specific memory B cells, as well as of memory T cells capable to promote B-cell maturation. This increment of VN antibodies in protected animals, matching that of a non-immunized pig, might reflect virus multiplication to a limited extent not resulting in detectable viremia (Table 2). Similar levels of VN antibodies boost upon virus challenge have been reported in pigs and cattle immunized with live-vectored vaccines or FMDV-like particles [34,35].

Non-protected (pigs 3 and 10) and partially protected (pig 5) animals showed lower levels of VN antibodies at the day of challenge, albeit animals with lower VNT yet protected were also observed (Figure 1B); the lack of correlation in a fraction of protected animals immunized with different FMDV vaccines has been described [21,36]. Experiments aimed at assessing the amount of antibodies that may target the FMDV receptor [37] as well as at examining cross-neutralization among other type O FMDVs will be foreseen to further characterize the antibody response evoked by the dendrimer peptide vaccines.

In addition, and supporting T3A recognition as a T-cell epitope, specific IFN-γ releasing activated T cells were detected rather early, at 15 dpi, in 7 of the 10 immunized pigs. The average frequencies of IFN-γ releasing cells in PBMCs from pigs in the 0.5 mg dose group were higher than those in the 2 mg group (Figure 1C and Table 2), possibly reflecting differences in the in vitro dose-effect of peptide stimulation and/or on the MHC allele composition of the animals analyzed. High doses of antigen might also facilitate its capture by APC/DC subsets with suboptimal costimulatory capacity that favor the development of regulatory T cells, which could limit the activation of B cells and subsequent antibody production as well as the development of IFN-γ producing cells [38]. In any case, additional studies of the effector mechanisms triggered by the dendrimers will be necessary to understand the effect on the protective responses of different peptide vaccine doses. One animal that was low responder at 15 dpi (pig 7), turned out to be protected upon challenge and pig 5, also low responder, was partially protected. Among responder animals, no clear correlation between IFN-γ releasing cell frequency at 15 dpi and protection to FMDV challenge was observed, i.e., non-protected pigs 3 and 10 showed high responses. Thus, as previously observed [21], VNT and T-cell stimulation do not fully correlate with the protection conferred by FMD peptide vaccines.

A potential problem of epitopic vaccines such us the dendrimeric peptides used in this study is the selection in non-protected animals of escape viruses capable to avoid antibody neutralization [21] and/or T cell recognition. In our experiment, we could not rule out that possibility since the limited number and size of the vesicles developed by non-protected animals did not allow virus recovery for sequencing analyses.

Our evidence of the level of full protection conferred by a single B_2T dose upon challenge at 25 dpi is particularly remarkable with regard to the 0.5 mg dose group (80% of the pigs), as it opens the way to significant savings in manufacturing costs. Incidentally, on a related note, we have found that long-lasting (up to 19/20 weeks post-boost) reduced susceptibility to FMDV infection can be attained with two B_2T doses and, remarkably, a similarly lasting protective response with a single dose of B_2T (Cañas-Arranz et al., submitted).

Attempts to use B_2T and B_4T dendrimer peptides as vaccines in cattle showed a trend toward a reduced capacity to confer protection relative to swine, including the need for a third immunization to elicit protective levels on neutralizing antibodies [39,40]. Failure in conferring protection in cattle has been described for linear FMDV peptide vaccines containing a heterologous T cell epitope [41]. Further work on the requirements of the interactions between neutralizing epitopes and B cells, as well as the identification of new, effective T helper epitopes frequently recognized by individuals will contribute to the improvement of the effectiveness of this kind of vaccines for cattle and, eventually, other host species.

In summary, our findings portray the B_2T peptide as a safe, potentially cost-effective candidate to be included in FMD vaccine formulations conferring single-shot protection in pigs. Formulation of dendrimers with alternative adjuvants as well as the incorporation of peptides corresponding to other T cell epitopes previously identified in pigs [42,43] can contribute to improve their immunogenicity in swine.

4. Methods

4.1. Peptides

Peptides identified as B- and T-cell epitopes of FMDV O/UKG/11/01 (Table 1) were assembled by Fmoc-solid phase synthesis, purified by reverse-phase liquid chromatography, and characterized by mass spectrometry. Dendrimeric B_2T construct was conjugated in solution using two previously synthesized precursors: (i) B epitope (VP1, residues 136–154) plus a C-terminal Cys residue (free thiol form) and (ii) T epitope (3A, residues 21–35) elongated at the N-terminal with two Lys residues followed by an additional Lys branching derivatized as two maleimide groups. The B_2T peptide was efficiently obtained after the thiol-maleimide ligation at pH = 6, RP-HPLC purification and MS characterization [27,28,44].

4.2. Virus

A virus stock derived from FMDV isolate O/UKG/11/01 [45] by two amplifications in swine kidney cells (IB-RS-2 cells) was used. The resulting virus maintained the consensus sequences at the capsid region [46].

4.3. Animals and Experimental Design

The immune response to B_2T dendrimer peptide was assessed in ten 9-weeks-old white cross-bred Landrace female pigs (Agropardal SA breed), free of antibodies to FMDV. The study was approved (CBS2014/015 and CEEA2014/018) by the INIA Committees on Ethics of Animal Experiments and Biosafety, and by the National Committee on Ethics and Animal Welfare (PROEX 218/14). Pigs were randomly assigned to two groups of five animals each and immunized once (days 0) by intramuscular injection with 2 mL of Montanide ISA 50V2 emulsion (Seppic, Paris, France) containing 2 or 0.5 mg of B_2T peptide. Two additional non-vaccinated pigs were kept as infection controls (#11 and 12). Animals were housed in separate units of the high-containment facility and challenged at day 25 with 1.6×10^4 plaque forming units (pfu) of FMDV O/UKG/11/01, by inoculation at two sites of both main claws of the left-hindfoot pad (0.1 mL/site). Animals were monitored for clinical signs of disease during the 10 days (Table 2), and then euthanized at day 35.

4.4. *Viral RNA Detection after Challenge*

Serum samples were examined for the presence of viral RNA by real time RT-qPCR. Briefly, the cDNA obtained in a RT reaction using primer A (5′-CACACGGCGTTCACCCA(A/T)CGC-3′) [47] was amplified by qPCR using the "Light Cycler RNA Master SYBR Green I" kit (Roche, Basel, Switzerland) and LightCycler equipment following the instructions of the manufacturer. The amplicon synthesized spanned a conserved region of 290 pb length in the 3D protein coding sequence, and was amplified using primers A (5′-CACACGGCGTTCACCCA(A/T)CGC-3′) and B (5′-GACAAAGGTTTTGTTCTTGGTC-3′). The values for the quantification of the samples were obtained from a standard curve from a RNA transcript derived from the infectious clone pMT-28 codifying the genomic RNA from FMDV C-S8c1 [48].

4.5. *Virus Neutralization Test (VNT)*

Serial two-fold dilutions of sera were incubated with 100 infection units—50% tissue culture infective doses (TCID50) of FMDV O/UKG 11/01, for 1 h at 37 °C. End-point titers were calculated as the reciprocal of the serum dilution that neutralized FMDV infection in 50% of the wells [28].

4.6. *Detection of Specific Anti-FMDV Antibodies by ELISA*

Total anti-FMDV antibodies were determined by ELISA. Briefly, 96-well plates (Nunc, Rochester, NY, USA) were coated with peptide B (1 µg) overnight at 4 °C. Duplicate three-fold dilution series of each serum sample were prepared in 50 µL, starting at 1/100. Pre-immune sera from peptide-immunized pigs and sera from non-immunized animals were used as negative controls. Specific antibodies were detected with HRP-conjugated protein A (Thermo Fisher, Rochester, NY, USA), diluted 1/4000. Color development was obtained after addition of 100 µL/well of TMB (Sigma Aldrich, St. Louis, MO, USA) and stopped by an equal volume of 1M H_2SO_4. Plates were read at 450 nm, titers expressed as the reciprocal of the last dilution giving the absorbance recorded in the control wells (serum at day 0) plus 2 SD.

4.7. *PBMC Isolation and IFN-γ Detection by ELISPOT*

Porcine peripheral blood mononuclear cells (PBMCs) were isolated by density gradient centrifugation using Histopaque-1077 (Sigma, St. Louis, MO, USA) and cryopreserved prior to assay. Vials were defrosted and resuspended in complete RPMI 1640 and incubated overnight at 37 °C, 5% CO_2. Cell counting and viability were tested by Trypan blue staining. For the IFN-γ ELISPOT assay 2.5×10^5 PBMCs were shed in triplicate wells of Immobilon-P plates (Merck Millipore, Burlington, MA, USA) coated with 5 µg/mL of anti-pig IFN-γ antibody (clone P2G10, Becton Dickinson, Franklin Lakes, NJ, USA). For in vitro antigen recall, PBMCs were stimulated with 25 µg/mL of the peptide used for pig immunization [49]. As positive control, PBMCs were incubated with 5 µg/mL of phytohaemagglutinin (Sigma) using cells incubated without antigen as negative control. After 48 h at 37 °C, 5% CO_2, plates were washed and incubated with 2 µg/mL of biotinylated anti-mouse IFN-γ antibody (clone P2C11, BD) and HRP-streptavidin (BD). Antibody was visualized with 3-amino-9-ethyl carbazole (BD). The frequency of peptide-specific T cells in was expressed as the mean number of spot-forming cells/10^6 PBMCs, with background values (number of spots in negative control wells) subtracted from the respective counts of stimulated cells.

4.8. Statistical Analyses

Differences among the peptide-immunized groups in FMDV-antibody titers and number of IFN-γ producing cells were analyzed by two-way ANOVA, followed by Tukey's post-hoc comparisons tests. Values are cited in the text as means ± SD. All p values are two sided, and p values < 0.05 were considered significant. Statistical analyses were conducted using GraphPad Prism Software 5.0 (Graphpad Software, San Diego, CA, USA).

Author Contributions: Conception, design and funding of the work (D.A., E.B. and F.S.). Data Acquisition and analysis (R.C.-A., M.F., S.D., P.d.L., M.J.B. and E.T.). Interpretation of data for the work (R.C.-A., M.F., S.D., P.d.L., D.A., F.S. and E.B.). Drafting the work (R.C.-A., M.F., S.D., P.d.L., F.S. and E.B.). Revising the data critically for important intellectual content (D.A., E.B. and F.S.). All authors have read and agreed to the published version of the manuscript.

Funding: This work was supported by the Spanish Ministry of Science, Innovation and Universities (grant AGL2017-89097-C2 to FS and DA; AGL2016-76445-R to EB), Comunidad de Madrid co-financed with ECFEDER funds (S2013/ABI-2906-PLATESA and P2018/BAA-4370 to FS and EB) and Generalitat de Catalunya (2009SGR492 to DA). Work at Centro de Biología Molecular "Severo Ochoa" and at UPF was supported by Fundación Ramón Areces and by the Maria de Maeztu Program of the Spanish Ministry of Science, Innovation and Universities, respectively. R.C.-A. and M.F. were holders of a PhD fellowship from the Spanish Ministry of Science, Innovation and University (FPI programme). Article processing free of charge.

Acknowledgments: We thank P. Pallarés for her advice and support.

Conflicts of Interest: The authors declare no conflicts of interest.

References

1. Sallusto, F.; Lanzavecchia, A.; Araki, K.; Ahmed, R. From vaccines to memory and back. *Immunity* **2010**, *33*, 451–463. [CrossRef] [PubMed]
2. van Oirschot, J.T. Present and future of veterinary viral vaccinology: A review. *Vet. Q.* **2001**, *23*, 100–108. [CrossRef] [PubMed]
3. Brun, A.; Barcena, J.; Blanco, E.; Borrego, B.; Dory, D.; Escribano, J.M.; Le Gall-Recule, G.; Ortego, J.; Dixon, L.K. Current strategies for subunit and genetic viral veterinary vaccine development. *Virus Res.* **2011**, *157*, 1–12. [CrossRef] [PubMed]
4. Correia, B.E.; Bates, J.T.; Loomis, R.J.; Baneyx, G.; Carrico, C.; Jardine, J.G.; Rupert, P.; Correnti, C.; Kalyuzhniy, O.; Vittal, V.; et al. Proof of principle for epitope-focused vaccine design. *Nature* **2014**, *507*, 201–206. [CrossRef] [PubMed]
5. Sette, A.; Fikes, J. Epitope-based vaccines: An update on epitope identification, vaccine design and delivery. *Curr. Opin. Immunol.* **2003**, *15*, 461–470. [CrossRef]
6. Purcell, A.W.; McCluskey, J.; Rossjohn, J. More than one reason to rethink the use of peptides in vaccine design. *Nat. Rev. Drug Discov.* **2007**, *6*, 404–414. [CrossRef]
7. Saiz, M.; Nunez, J.I.; Jimenez-Clavero, M.A.; Baranowski, E.; Sobrino, F. Foot-and-mouth disease virus: Biology and prospects for disease control. *Microbes Infect.* **2002**, *4*, 1183–1192. [CrossRef]
8. Rweyemamu, M.; Roeder, P.; MacKay, D.; Sumption, K.; Brownlie, J.; Leforban, Y. Planning for the progressive control of foot-and-mouth disease worldwide. *Transbound. Emerg. Dis.* **2008**, *55*, 73–87. [CrossRef]
9. Knight-Jones, T.J.; Rushton, J. The economic impacts of foot and mouth disease—What are they, how big are they and where do they occur? *Prev. Vet. Med.* **2013**, *112*, 161–173. [CrossRef]
10. Grubman, M.J.; Baxt, B. Foot-and-mouth disease. *Clin. Microbiol. Rev.* **2004**, *17*, 465–493. [CrossRef]
11. Perez, A.M.; Willeberg, P.W. Editorial: Foot-and-Mouth Disease in Swine. *Front. Vet. Sci.* **2017**, *4*, 133. [CrossRef] [PubMed]
12. Rodriguez, L.L.; Gay, C.G. Development of vaccines toward the global control and eradication of foot-and-mouth disease. *Expert Rev. Vaccines* **2011**, *10*, 377–387. [CrossRef] [PubMed]
13. Doel, T.R. Natural and vaccine induced immunity to FMD. *Curr. Top. Microbiol. Immunol.* **2005**, *288*, 103–131. [PubMed]
14. Robinson, L.; Knight-Jones, T.J.; Charleston, B.; Rodriguez, L.L.; Gay, C.G.; Sumption, K.J.; Vosloo, W. Global Foot-and-Mouth Disease Research Update and Gap Analysis: 3—Vaccines. *Transbound. Emerg. Dis.* **2016**, *63* (Suppl. 1), 30–41. [CrossRef]

15. Kitching, R.P. Diagnosis and Control of Foot-and-Mouth Disease. In *Foot and Mouth Disease: Current Perspectives*; Sobrino, F., Domingo, E., Eds.; Horizon Press: Norfolk, UK, 2004.
16. Lyons, N.A.; Lyoo, Y.S.; King, D.P.; Paton, D.J. Challenges of Generating and Maintaining Protective Vaccine-Induced Immune Responses for Foot-and-Mouth Disease Virus in Pigs. *Front. Vet. Sci.* **2016**, 3, 102. [CrossRef]
17. Blanco, E.; Andreu, D.; Sobrino, F. Peptide vaccines against foot-and-mouth disease. In *Foot-and-Mouth Disease Virus. Current Research and Emerging Trends*; Sobrino, F., Domingo, E., Eds.; Caister Academis Press: Norfolk, UK, 2017; pp. 231–317.
18. Acharya, R.; Fry, E.; Stuart, D.; Fox, G.; Rowlands, D.; Brown, F. The three-dimensional structure of foot-and-mouth disease virus at 2.9 A resolution. *Nature* **1989**, *337*, 709–716. [CrossRef] [PubMed]
19. Mateu, M.G.; Verdaguer, N.; Sobrino, F.; Domingo, E. Functional and structural aspects of the interaction of foo-and-outh disease virus with antibodies. In *Foot-and-Mouth Disease: Current Perspectives*; Mateu, M.G., Verdaguer, N., Eds.; Horizon Bioscience: Norfolk, UK, 2004; p. 37.
20. Bittle, J.L.; Houghten, R.A.; Alexander, H.; Shinnick, T.M.; Sutcliffe, J.G.; Lerner, R.A.; Rowlands, D.J.; Brown, F. Protection against foot-and-mouth disease by immunization with a chemically synthesized peptide predicted from the viral nucleotide sequence. *Nature* **1982**, *298*, 30–33. [CrossRef] [PubMed]
21. Taboga, O.; Tami, C.; Carrillo, E.; Nunez, J.I.; Rodriguez, A.; Saiz, J.C.; Blanco, E.; Valero, M.L.; Roig, X.; Camarero, J.A.; et al. A large-scale evaluation of peptide vaccines against foot-and-mouth disease: Lack of solid protection in cattle and isolation of escape mutants. *J. Virol.* **1997**, *71*, 2606–2614. [CrossRef]
22. Cubillos, C.; de la Torre, B.G.; Barcena, J.; Andreu, D.; Sobrino, F.; Blanco, E. Inclusion of a specific T cell epitope increases the protection conferred against foot-and-mouth disease virus in pigs by a linear peptide containing an immunodominant B cell site. *Virol. J.* **2012**, *9*, 66. [CrossRef]
23. Collen, T.; Dimarchi, R.; Doel, T.R. A T cell epitope in VP1 of foot-and-mouth disease virus is immunodominant for vaccinated cattle. *J. Immunol.* **1991**, *146*, 749–755.
24. Tam, J.P. Synthetic peptide vaccine design: Synthesis and properties of a high-density multiple antigenic peptide system. *Proc. Natl. Acad. Sci. USA* **1988**, *85*, 5409–5413. [CrossRef] [PubMed]
25. Blanco, E.; Garcia-Briones, M.; Sanz-Parra, A.; Gomes, P.; De Oliveira, E.; Valero, M.L.; Andreu, D.; Ley, V.; Sobrino, F. Identification of T-cell epitopes in nonstructural proteins of foot-and-mouth disease virus. *J. Virol.* **2001**, *75*, 3164–3174. [CrossRef]
26. Mahapatra, M.; Parida, S. Foot and mouth disease vaccine strain selection: Current approaches and future perspectives. *Expert Rev. Vaccines* **2018**, *17*, 577–591. [CrossRef] [PubMed]
27. Cubillos, C.; de la Torre, B.G.; Jakab, A.; Clementi, G.; Borras, E.; Barcena, J.; Andreu, D.; Sobrino, F.; Blanco, E. Enhanced mucosal immunoglobulin A response and solid protection against foot-and-mouth disease virus challenge induced by a novel dendrimeric peptide. *J. Virol.* **2008**, *82*, 7223–7230. [CrossRef] [PubMed]
28. Blanco, E.; Guerra, B.; de la Torre, B.G.; Defaus, S.; Dekker, A.; Andreu, D.; Sobrino, F. Full protection of swine against foot-and-mouth disease by a bivalent B-cell epitope dendrimer peptide. *Antivir. Res.* **2016**, *129*, 74–80. [CrossRef] [PubMed]
29. Francis, M.J.; Black, L. Response of young pigs to foot-and-mouth disease oil emulsion vaccination in the presence and absence of maternally derived neutralising antibodies. *Res. Vet. Sci.* **1986**, *41*, 33–39. [CrossRef]
30. Smitsaart, E.; Bergmann, I. Quality and attributes of current inactivated foot-and-mouth disease vaccines and their effects on the success of vaccination programmes. In *Foot-and-Mouth Disease Virus. Current Research and Emerging Trends*; Sobrino, F., Domingo, E., Eds.; Caister Academic Press: Norfolk, UK, 2017; pp. 287–316.
31. Pacheco, J.M.; Brum, M.C.; Moraes, M.P.; Golde, W.T.; Grubman, M.J. Rapid protection of cattle from direct challenge with foot-and-mouth disease virus (FMDV) by a single inoculation with an adenovirus-vectored FMDV subunit vaccine. *Virology* **2005**, *337*, 205–209. [CrossRef]
32. Lyons, N.A.; Knight-Jones, T.J.D.; Bartels, C.; Paton, D.J.; Ferrari, G.; Vermillion, M.S.; Brooks, A.W.; Motroni, R.; Parker, E.; Hefferin Berquist, M.L.; et al. Considerations for design and implementation of vaccine field trials for novel foot-and-mouth disease vaccines. *Vaccine* **2019**, *37*, 1007–1015. [CrossRef]
33. OIE. *Manual of Diagnositic Tests and Vaccines for Terrestrial Animals (Terrestrial Manual)*; OIE: Paris, France, 2017.
34. Sitt, T.; Kenney, M.; Barrera, J.; Pandya, M.; Eckstrom, K.; Warner, M.; Pacheco, J.M.; LaRocco, M.; Palarea-Albaladejo, J.; Brake, D.; et al. Duration of protection and humoral immunity induced by an adenovirus-vectored subunit vaccine for foot-and-mouth disease (FMD) in Holstein steers. *Vaccine* **2019**, *37*, 6221–6231. [CrossRef]

35. Guo, H.C.; Sun, S.Q.; Jin, Y.; Yang, S.L.; Wei, Y.Q.; Sun, D.H.; Yin, S.H.; Ma, J.W.; Liu, Z.X.; Guo, J.H.; et al. Foot-and-mouth disease virus-like particles produced by a SUMO fusion protein system in Escherichia coli induce potent protective immune responses in guinea pigs, swine and cattle. *Vet. Res.* **2013**, *44*, 48. [CrossRef]
36. McCullough, K.C.; Bruckner, L.; Schaffner, R.; Fraefel, W.; Muller, H.K.; Kihm, U. Relationship between the anti-FMD virus antibody reaction as measured by different assays, and protection in vivo against challenge infection. *Vet. Microbiol.* **1992**, *30*, 99–112. [CrossRef]
37. Polacek, C.; Gullberg, M.; Li, J.; Belsham, G.J. Low levels of foot-and-mouth disease virus 3C protease expression are required to achieve optimal capsid protein expression and processing in mammalian cells. *J. Gen. Virol.* **2013**, *94*, 1249–1258. [CrossRef]
38. Bilate, A.M.; Lafaille, J.J. Induced CD4+Foxp3+ regulatory T cells in immune tolerance. *Annu. Rev. Immunol.* **2012**, *30*, 733–758. [CrossRef]
39. Soria, I.; Quattrocchi, V.; Langellotti, C.; Gammella, M.; Digiacomo, S.; Garcia de la Torre, B.; Andreu, D.; Montoya, M.; Sobrino, F.; Blanco, E.; et al. Dendrimeric peptides can confer protection against foot-and-mouth disease virus in cattle. *PLoS ONE* **2017**, *12*, e0185184. [CrossRef] [PubMed]
40. Soria, I.; Quattrocchi, V.; Langellotti, C.; Perez-Filgueira, M.; Pega, J.; Gnazzo, V.; Romera, S.; Schammas, J.; Bucafusco, D.; Di Giacomo, S.; et al. Immune Response and Partial Protection against Heterologous Foot-and-Mouth Disease Virus Induced by Dendrimer Peptides in Cattle. *J. Immunol. Res.* **2018**, *2018*, 3497401. [CrossRef] [PubMed]
41. Rodriguez, L.L.; Barrera, J.; Kramer, E.; Lubroth, J.; Brown, F.; Golde, W.T. A synthetic peptide containing the consensus sequence of the G-H loop region of foot-and-mouth disease virus type-O VP1 and a promiscuous T-helper epitope induces peptide-specific antibodies but fails to protect cattle against viral challenge. *Vaccine* **2003**, *21*, 3751–3756. [CrossRef]
42. Blanco, E.; McCullough, K.; Summerfield, A.; Fiorini, J.; Andreu, D.; Chiva, C.; Borras, E.; Barnett, P.; Sobrino, F. Interspecies major histocompatibility complex-restricted Th cell epitope on foot-and-mouth disease virus capsid protein VP4. *J. Virol.* **2000**, *74*, 4902–4907. [CrossRef]
43. Garcia-Briones, M.M.; Blanco, E.; Chiva, C.; Andreu, D.; Ley, V.; Sobrino, F. Immunogenicity and T cell recognition in swine of foot-and-mouth disease virus polymerase 3D. *Virology* **2004**, *322*, 264–275. [CrossRef]
44. Monso, M.; de la Torre, B.G.; Blanco, E.; Moreno, N.; Andreu, D. Influence of conjugation chemistry and B epitope orientation on the immune response of branched peptide antigens. *Bioconjug. Chem.* **2013**, *24*, 578–585. [CrossRef]
45. Sumption, K.; Rweyemamu, M.; Wint, W. Incidence and distribution of foot-and-mouth disease in Asia, Africa and South America; combining expert opinion, official disease information and livestock populations to assist risk assessment. *Transbound. Emerg. Dis.* **2008**, *55*, 5–13. [CrossRef]
46. Nunez, J.I.; Molina, N.; Baranowski, E.; Domingo, E.; Clark, S.; Burman, A.; Berryman, S.; Jackson, T.; Sobrino, F. Guinea pig-adapted foot-and-mouth disease virus with altered receptor recognition can productively infect a natural host. *J. Virol.* **2007**, *81*, 8497–8506. [CrossRef] [PubMed]
47. Saiz, M.; De La Morena, D.B.; Blanco, E.; Nunez, J.I.; Fernandez, R.; Sanchez-Vizcaino, J.M. Detection of foot-and-mouth disease virus from culture and clinical samples by reverse transcription-PCR coupled to restriction enzyme and sequence analysis. *Vet. Res.* **2003**, *34*, 105–117. [CrossRef] [PubMed]
48. García-Arriaza, J.; Manrubia, S.C.; Toja, M.; Domingo, E.; Escarmís, C. Evolutionary transition toward defective RNAs that are infectious by complementation. *J. Virol.* **2004**, *78*, 11678–11685. [CrossRef] [PubMed]
49. Saiz, J.C.; Rodriguez, A.; Gonzalez, M.; Alonso, F.; Sobrino, F. Heterotypic lymphoproliferative response in pigs vaccinated with foot-and-mouth disease virus. Involvement of isolated capsid proteins. *J. Gen. Virol.* **1992**, *73*, 2601–2607. [CrossRef] [PubMed]

vaccines

MDPI

Article

MVA Vectored Vaccines Encoding Rift Valley Fever Virus Glycoproteins Protect Mice against Lethal Challenge in the Absence of Neutralizing Antibody Responses

Elena López-Gil †, Sandra Moreno, Javier Ortego, Belén Borrego, Gema Lorenzo and Alejandro Brun *

Animal Health Research Centre (CISA), National Institute for Agriculture and Food Research and Technology (INIA), Valdeolmos, 28130 Madrid, Spain; melenalopezgil@gmail.com (E.L.-G.); sandramorenofdez@gmail.com (S.M.); ortego@inia.es (J.O.); borrego@inia.es (B.B.); lorenzo.gema@inia.es (G.L.)

* Correspondence: brun@inia.es; Tel.: +34-916-202-300

† Present address: Diagnostic and Therapeutic Applications Laboratory (Diater S. A). Avda. Gregorio Peces Barba, 2. Leganés Technology Park, Leganés, 28918 Madrid, Spain.

Received: 10 January 2020; Accepted: 10 February 2020; Published: 12 February 2020

Abstract: In vitro neutralizing antibodies have been often correlated with protection against Rift Valley fever virus (RVFV) infection. We have reported previously that a single inoculation of sucrose-purified modified vaccinia Ankara (MVA) encoding RVFV glycoproteins (rMVAGnGc) was sufficient to induce a protective immune response in mice after a lethal RVFV challenge. Protection was related to the presence of glycoprotein specific CD8+ cells, with a low-level detection of in vitro neutralizing antibodies. In this work we extended those observations aimed to explore the role of humoral responses after MVA vaccination and to study the contribution of each glycoprotein antigen to the protective efficacy. Thus, we tested the efficacy and immune responses in BALB/c mice of recombinant MVA viruses expressing either glycoprotein Gn (rMVAGn) or Gc (rMVAGc). In the absence of serum neutralizing antibodies, our data strongly suggest that protection of vaccinated mice upon the RVFV challenge can be achieved by the activation of cellular responses mainly directed against Gc epitopes. The involvement of cellular immunity was stressed by the fact that protection of mice was strain dependent. Furthermore, our data suggest that the rMVA based single dose vaccination elicits suboptimal humoral immune responses against Gn antigen since disease in mice was exacerbated upon virus challenge in the presence of rMVAGnGc or rMVAGn immune serum. Thus, Gc-specific cellular immunity could be an important component in the protection after the challenge observed in BALB/c mice, contributing to the elimination of infected cells reducing morbidity and mortality and counteracting the deleterious effect of a subneutralizing antibody immune response.

Keywords: Rift Valley fever virus (RVFV); modified vaccinia Ankara (MVA); cellular response; neutralizing antibodies; Gn Gc glycoproteins; passive serum:virus transfer

1. Introduction

Rift Valley fever virus (RVFV), a mosquito-borne bunyavirus, is widely distributed in Sub-Saharan countries, Egypt and the Arabian Peninsula, causing disease in both humans and livestock [1]. RVFV is considered an emerging threat for non-endemic countries due to the movement of infected animals and/or translocation of infected mosquitoes [2,3]. The ample range of RVFV competent mosquito vectors present in many areas of the Mediterranean basin suggests that RVF outbreaks in non-endemic areas could potentially end-up in the establishment of enzootic infection cycles [4]. Should this happen it would cause serious concern for both public and animal health. It is therefore desirable to develop control tools as well as enhance our knowledge about the immune mechanisms that correlate with the protection elicited by RVFV vaccines. The modified vaccinia Ankara (MVA) virus has been widely used as a carrier of vaccine antigens due to its safety and immunogenicity profile [5]. The MVA vector is a highly attenuated version of a vaccinia virus strain that has lost around 30 kb of sequence upon passage in primary avian cells (CEF) so that many host range and immune-modulatory genes are absent or nonfunctional [6]. This restricts the replication of the virus in most mammalian cells. Besides, it has been demonstrated that MVA itself is very immunogenic (induces humoral responses and is an excellent inducer of T-cell responses). It has been used in human preclinical and clinical trials [7] and more recently it has also been evaluated for different animal diseases, including zoonotic diseases [8]. In the case of zoonotic diseases the data obtained in animal field trials may also help to accelerate the development of corresponding human vaccines.

In order to control RVF it is generally accepted that the induction of neutralizing antibodies is an important correlate of protection [9]. Therefore, the Gn and Gc glycoproteins are the main vaccine antigen targets since both glycoproteins are membrane proteins forming spikes on the surface of the virions that can be accessible to neutralizing antibodies [10–12], precluding either internalization and/or nucleocapsid uncoating. Both glycoproteins are synthesized as a polyprotein precursor that becomes localized in Golgi membranes where they are glycosylated and cotranslationally processed by a yet unidentified cellular protease that releases one end of the membrane attachment sites, allowing both ectodomains to interact and the glycoproteins to acquire their final conformation on the surface of the virion [13,14]. The structure of GnGc architecture has been recently elucidated indicating that Gn shields Gc in the viral particles avoiding to expose the Gc fusion loop to antibodies [15] and offers an hypothesis for the neutralizing mechanisms of protective antibodies [16]. Our previous works using recombinant MVA (rMVA) as vector vaccines expressing both glycoprotein antigens (rMVAGnGc) showed an intriguingly low level of in vitro neutralizing antibody induction upon single dose administration, particularly when compared to other similar rMVA vaccines encoding RNA virus glycoprotein antigens [17]. In our system, the lack of a humoral protective antiglycoprotein response was observed in both mouse models and disease natural hosts [18]. Particularly, for sheep no neutralizing antibody induction was demonstrated either after one or two serial rMVAGnGc vaccine doses, questioning the efficacy of this vaccine in this species [18]. The lack of neutralizing antibody induction could be related to the vector platform used in those experiments (MVA) since the same coding glycoproteins expressed by means of an adenovirus vector induced a potent set of neutralizing antibodies [19,20].

In this work we show that rMVA vaccines expressing independently versions of the glycoprotein Gc or Gn were able to confer substantial protection in mice, albeit inducing no detectable in vitro neutralizing antibody responses. Rather, the protection observed upon challenge was related to a strong T-cell response, which appeared more prominent against Gc epitopes. Intriguingly, the immune response elicited by the rMVA vaccine encoding both glycoproteins or glycoprotein Gn endowed the serum with the capacity to exacerbate disease when a serum:virus mixture was passively transferred to naive mice, as shown in experiments using either mouse or sheep immune sera obtained from rMVA vaccinated animals. It therefore appears that evoking a strong cellular response counteracts the failure in inducing protective humoral responses when an MVA vaccine is used. Conversely, the absence of an effective cell-mediated immune response may lead to disease exacerbation when subneutralizing antibody responses are elicited. These results warrant the optimization of our rMVA vaccines towards the induction of optimal humoral responses.

2. Materials and Methods

2.1. Generation of Recombinant rMVA Encoding RVFV Gn and Gc Glycoproteins

The rMVA-GnGc recombinant virus generated by homologous recombination of wild type MVA DNA and a plasmid construct encoding RVFV-MP12 glycoproteins (GB accession: DQ380208.1) into the TK locus of MVA was described previously [17]. For the generation of rMVA-Gn and rMVA-Gc, the recombination (shuttle) plasmid encoding an RVFV-MP12 GnGc tagged sequence (plasmid #1389 produced at the Viral Vector Core Facility (VVCF), Jenner Institute, Oxford) was used as a template of an inverse PCR reaction using specific 5′ phosphorylated primers (Supplementary file, Table S1). After religation of the PCR fragments, two new shuttle vectors were generated, in which the Gn ectodomain (encoding amino acids Met131 to His580 of the translated polyprotein precursor) and a Gc including the C-terminal transmembrane-cytosolic tail (amino acids Cys690 to Ser1197) were placed under the control of the vaccinia p7.5 early/late promoter. The N-terminus of each recombinant polypeptide contained an in-frame fusion of the human tissue plasminogen activator leader sequence (tPA), known to enhance transgene expression and immunogenicity [21]. The C-terminus of each protein contained an H-$2K^d$ restricted CD8+ T cell epitope from *Plasmodium berghei* circumsporozoite protein (pb9) and an antiV5 monoclonal antibody recognition sequence. The plasmid for MVA construction also includes GFP as a reporter gene under the control of the vaccinia p11 late promoter. Both shuttle vectors were transfected into DF-1 cells (ATCC-CRL-12203) using lipofectamine 2000 (Thermo Fisher Scientific, Waltham, MA, USA), then infected with parental MVA and homologous recombination allowed the insertion of either Gn ectodomain (eGn) or Gc ORFs and the GFP marker gene at the TK locus of the MVA. Three consecutive rounds of green plaque purification were performed in order to obtain a pure preparation of each recombinant virus. The recombinant viruses (named rMVAGn and rMVAGc) were then further expanded in DF-1 cells. Semipurified, concentrated, virus preparations were obtained upon ultracentrifugation of infected cell extracts in a 36% sucrose cushion. The sucrose-purified virus fractions were titrated into DF-1 cells and stored at −80 °C until use.

2.2. Western Blot Analysis

Expression of recombinant RVFV glycoproteins was analyzed by western blots of infected cell lysates using either specific antiGn or Gc antibodies [22] or a monoclonal antibody against V5 peptide tag (Bio-Rad, Hercules, CA, USA)). BHK-21 cells (ATCC CCL-10) were infected with the different recombinant MVA viruses described above, at 5 pfu/cell or were mock infected. At 24 h post infection the cells were harvested, pelleted, washed in PBS-containing protease inhibitor cocktail (Sigma-Aldrich, San Luis, MO, USA), and lysed with cytoplasmic extraction buffer (10 mM HEPES pH 7.9, 10 mM KCl, 0.1 mM EDTA, and 0.3% NP−40). After a centrifugation step to release intact nuclei, extracts were mixed with an equal amount of 2X Laemmli buffer, including DTT as a reducing agent and proteins were resolved in 12% SDS-PAGE and blotted onto nitrocellulose membranes. After a blocking step with 5% low fat dry milk in PBS (blocking buffer), antiRVFV Gn monoclonal antibody 84a (1:3000 dilution), monoclonal antiV5 tag (1:5000), or a rabbit antiGc polyclonal antibody (1:5000) were applied to membranes in blocking buffer with 0.01% Tween-20 and incubated for 1 h at room temperature. Horseradish peroxidase conjugated antimouse or antirabbit antibodies (1:5000) were incubated to the membranes after three washing steps with PBS Tween-20 (PBST). The resulting immunocomplexes were detected by enhanced chemiluminescence (GE Healthcare, Little Chalfont, Buckinghamshire, UK) and X-ray film exposure.

2.3. Indirect Immunofluorescence and Laser Confocal Microscopy

Cells were grown in either multi-well 96 (MW96) plates or in glass coverslips (CS) and infected with the recombinant MVA viruses at a multiplicity of infection (MOI) of 1. 24 h after infection the cells were fixed and permeabilized with 100% ice-cold methanol (MW96) or fixed with 4% paraformaldehyde and permeabilized with 0.5% Triton-X100 (CS). Fixed cells were blocked with 10% FBS in PBS (10% blocking solution) for 30 min at room temperature (rt). AntiV5tag mAb, glycoprotein specific antibodies or antibodies specific to ER and Golgi proteins calreticulin and human mannosidase II (Bio-Rad's AHP516 and AHP674 antibodies) were incubated for 1 h at rt in 2% blocking solution with 0.01 Tween-20. After three serial washing steps with PBST Alexa 488 conjugated antimouse, or Alexa-Fluor 594-conjugated antirabbit or antigoat mabs (Thermo) were incubated for 30 min at rt. Stained cells in MW96 were visualized using a Zeiss AX10 inverted fluorescence microscope (Zeiss Gmbh, Oberkochen, Germany). Stained CS preparations were mounted onto glass microscopy slides with or without DAPI staining (Thermo Fisher) and were visualized analyzed in a Zeiss LSM880 confocal laser microscope. Images were further processed using the Zen Zeiss software.

2.4. Immunoprecipitation Analysis

For immunoprecipitation, monolayers of Vero cells were infected with RVFV-MP12 virus in the presence of 300 µCi/mL of [S35]-Methionine-Cysteine solution (Grupo Taper S.L, Alcobendas, Madrid, Spain). After 24 h the cells were lysed in radioimmunoprecipitation assay buffer (150 mM NaCl, 1% NP-40, 0.1% SDS, and 50 mM Tris, pH 7.5) and 20 µl of pooled sera from mice vaccinated with different rMVA viruses were incubated for 1 h at room temperature in a rotary shaker. Paramagnetic protein-G beads (Thermo Fisher) were added and incubated for an additional hour. The immunocomplexes were washed three times with the RIPA buffer and then separated by 12% SDS-PAGE. Fixed gels were subjected to fluorographic enhancement using Amplify solution (GE). After drying the gels were exposed to X-ray film.

2.5. Immunization, Sampling for Immunological Assays and RVFV Challenge

Groups of 5–10 BALB/c mice eight to ten weeks-old (Envigo RMS, Barcelona, Spain) were immunized intraperitoneally with 10^7 pfu of sucrose-cushion purified rMVA in phosphate-buffered saline (PBS). One or two weeks postvaccination, blood samples were taken either for neutralization assays (serum) or IFN-γ ELISpot (PBLs), and splenocytes for ex-vivo IFNγ ELISPOT at 7 or 14 dpi (n = 4). The remaining mice (n = 5), together with additional groups of unvaccinated BALB/c mice and immunized with nonrecombinant MVA (MVA control, expressing only GFP), were all challenged intraperitoneally with 10^3 plaque-forming units (pfu) of the South African RVF virus strain 56/74 [23]. The immunization and challenge studies were also performed in a similar manner using 129SvEv mice (B&K Universal Group Ltd, Hull, UK). To monitor viremia, blood samples were taken at 72 h after RVFV infection, and tested for virus isolation on cell culture as described [24]. Briefly, blood dilutions were incubated with Vero cells cultures and examined for the viral cytophatic effect (cpe). After 96 h the extent of cytophatic effect was recorded and cells were fixed and stained with 2% Crystal Violet in 10% formaldehyde solution. The extent of cpe was quantified to estimate a tissue culture infective titer ($TCID_{50}$). Serum samples collected at later times postinfection in surviving mice were analyzed for the presence of neutralizing antibodies as described below. Vaccine efficacy estimation was evaluated in terms of morbidity and mortality monitoring daily over three weeks. All surviving mice were culled after 21 days of follow-up. Procedures involving animals received institutional approval (INIA's ethics and biosafety Committee) as well as granted permits from regional veterinary authorities (Comunidad de Madrid PROEX 108/15).

2.6. Assessment of RVFV Serum Neutralizing Antibodies

Serum neutralizing antibody titers were measured in Vero cell monolayers by serial dilutions of serum mixed with an equal volume of medium containing MP-12 RVF virus strain and incubated for 1 h at 37 °C. After 72–96 h the cells were fixed and stained in a solution containing 10% formaldehyde and 2% crystal violet in PBS. The neutralization titer defined as the highest serum dilution at which cell lysis was reduced by 50% relative to cells incubated with RVF virus only. The assays were performed in triplicate and scored by an operator blinded to the vaccination regimen.

2.7. Analysis of T-Cell Responses Against RVFV Glycoproteins

Viral glycoprotein-specific T cells were measured by ex vivo IFNγ ELISPOT assay on splenocytes and pooled PBLs as described [17]. Gn, Gc-specific and nonspecific class-I restricted peptides were used for restimulation at a final concentration of 5 µg/mL in all assays for 18 h. IL-2, IL-6, IL-4, and IL-5 cytokine capture ELISAs (BD Pharmingen) were also performed using supernatants from peptide restimulated spleen cell cultures. Known concentrations of mouse IL-2, IL-6, IL-4, or IL-5 were used to generate a standard curve to correlate optical densities with cytokine concentration. The sensitivity limit of the assay was estimated in (61.25 pg/mL for IL-6, 250 pg/mL for IL-2, 3.75pg/mL for IL-4, and 37.5 pg/mL for IL-5).

2.8. Passive Transfer of Antibodies

The sera for passive transfer protection studies were generated by pooling sera from mice immunized with the different rMVA constructs expressing the same antigens. Serum pools were prepared from day 14 post immunization and analyzed by virus neutralization and immunoprecipitation assays. As a positive control, antiRVFV immune mouse serum was used while antihuman adenovirus 5 (AdHu5) pooled mouse serum (collected also at 14 days post immunization) was used as a negative control serum. For passive protection experiments each serum pool was ten-fold diluted in the virus inoculum used to challenge each group of 5 animals. 100 μL of each virus/serum mixture was injected intraperitoneally into adult female BALB/c mice. The virus challenge dose per mouse corresponded to 5×10^3 pfu. Animals were monitored for clinical signs and mortality during three weeks and were weighed daily to quantify the extent of morbidity after challenge. Additionally, serum from sheep immunized with the rMVAGnGc vaccine, rMVA or from mock vaccinated was also pooled and passively transferred to mice.

2.9. Statistical Analysis

The log rank (Mantel–Cox) test was used to check for differences in survival analysis following RVFV challenge. Individual ELISPOT values were determined by subtracting background values obtained after stimulation with media only. Statistical significance was calculated by one-way analysis of variance (ANOVA) transforming ELISPOT counts to $\log_{10}$ to limit the range of variation found among individual mice. All analyses were done using the GraphPad 6.0 software (San Diego, CA). Differences were considered significant when p value <0.05

3. Results

3.1. Expression of Recombinant Gn and Gc Glycoproteins in rMVA Infected Cells

Expression was assessed by western blot analysis (Figure 1A). Both glycoprotein sequences were tagged with the V5 epitope sequence to compare their relative expression levels. It was observed that the infection of cells with both recombinant MVAGn and rMVAGc rendered detectable expression levels for both glycoproteins. This ruled out the possibility of low level expression conditioning the immunity conferred by each vaccine. Expression of glycoproteins was also confirmed using antiGn or Gc specific antibodies [22]. The detecting signal was similar to that of RVFV MP12 infected BHK-21 cells. The size of Gn expressed by rMVAGn was in accordance with its theoretical mass (50.6 kDa) but slightly lower when expressed by rMVAGnGc. Gc expression was also in good agreement with the expected size and similar in size to the one expressed by RVFV infection, although a smaller truncated polypeptide was also evident using the antiGc or the antiV5 tag antibodies. Detection of the expressed antigens was performed also by immunofluorescence assay (IFA)of rMVA infected Vero cell monolayers with an antiV5 tag monoclonal antibody. The subcellular staining pattern of each glycoprotein was in good agreement with intracellular membrane trafficking as it has been described for both glycoproteins (Figure 1B). Gn expression was predominantly cytoplasmatic with no evident association with endoplasmic reticulum (ER). In contrast Gc interaction with ER structures was more obvious as shown by the colocalization with the ER marker calreticulin. No clear association of Gn or Gc was found with Golgi structures at least at the time point assayed (24 hpi), as evidenced by the lack of costaining with an antihuman mannosidase-II mAb.

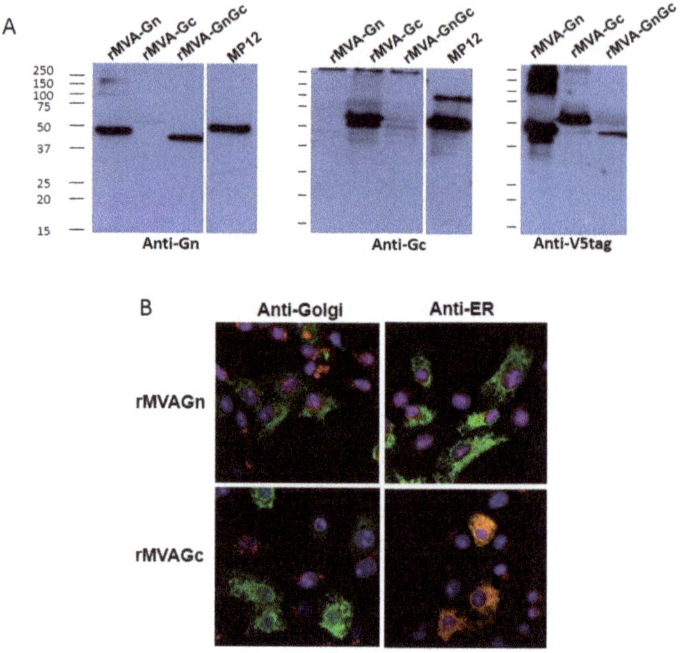

Figure 1. Expression and subcellular localization of recombinant Gn and Gc upon modified vaccinia Ankara (MVA) infection. (**A**). Western blot of different MVA infected BHK-21 cell extracts probed with mAb 84a antiGn or a rabbit polyclonal serum antiGc. The antiV5 tag mAb was used to compare the Gn and Gc expression levels and to confirm the expression of the full-length antigen. As a positive control a RVFV-MP12 infected cell extract was used. Numbers indicate relative molecular mass in kilodaltons. (**B**). Confocal immunofluorescence images of MVA infected Vero cells. Expression of Gn or Gc was detected with anti V5 tag mAb (green). Intracellular membranes were labeled with either antihuman mannosidase-II (Golgi) or anticalreticulin (ER) mAbs (red fluorescence) as indicated. Nuclei were labeled with DAPI stain (blue). All panels correspond to merged fluorescence images. Colocalization of Gc and ER membranes is evidenced by yellow-orange fluorescence.

3.2. Efficacy Assessment of MVA Vaccines in Mice

The protective ability of a single dose of our rMVA vaccines was tested in BALB/c mice (Figure 2A). Mice immunized with rMVAGc virus showed an 80% survival after challenge. In this group at 11 dpi one mouse showed signs compatible to a delayed-onset neurological disease, dying at day 14 pi. In contrast, two of the mice vaccinated with rMVAGn showed earlier clinical disease dying at day 4 and 6 post challenge respectively. As expected, in the group of mice vaccinated with the rMVAGnGc construct the survival after challenge was 100%, with only one animal showing mild clinical signs between 3 and 4 dpi. In the mice from both control groups (either nonrecombinant MVA and unvaccinated) the mortality was 80% and 100% respectively with an earlier onset of disease in both groups. Differences in the survival rates observed for each group were statistically significant ($\chi^2 = 09.503$; df = 3; $p = 0.023$) when compared to the control MVA vaccine (Mantel–Cox log-rank test).

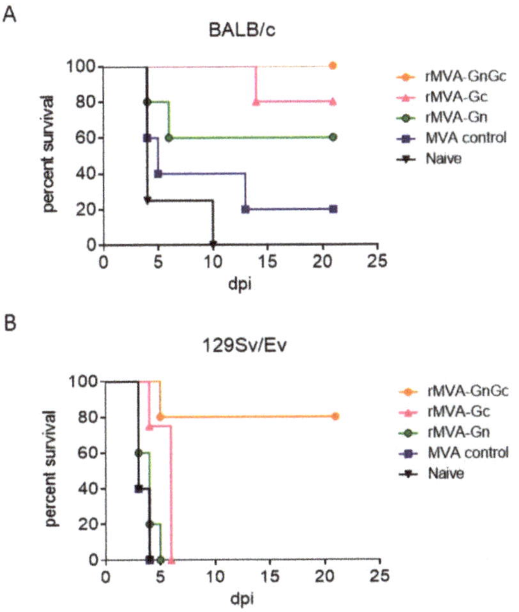

Figure 2. Survival of MVA vaccinated mice ($n = 5$) upon challenge with virulent Rift Valley fever virus (RVFV). Kaplan–Meier plots of BALB/c mice (haplotype $H2^d$ (**A**) or 129EvSv mice (haplotype $H2^b$) (**B**). The mice were vaccinated with a single intraperitoneal dose of 10^7 pfu of each recombinant virus or were mock-vaccinated (naive). Two weeks after immunization the mice were challenged with 10^3 pfu of RVFV 56/74. The mice were monitored for 3 weeks for the presence of signs of disease.

Since the protective effect of our rMVAGnGc single dose vaccine relies mainly in the induction of specific CD8+T-cell responses [17] we questioned whether its efficacy in a different inbred mouse strain would be compromised. Thus we tested the protective ability of our rMVA vaccines in the context of a different genetic background by using the 129SvEv mouse model (H-2^b-haplotype). The sensitivity of this mouse strain to the RVFV challenge is higher than that of the H-2^d BALB/c strain (our unpublished data). Survival rates upon the RVFV challenge in the 129SvEv mice immunized with rMVAGnGc reached 80% with only one animal dying at 5 dpi. Contrarily, to what was observed in the BALB/c experiments, all of the 129SvEv mice that were vaccinated with rMVAGc or rMVAGn died upon challenge, with a slight delay in mortality in the rMVAGc group with respect to the MVA control group (Figure 2B). Differences in survival times of rMVAGnGc were highly significant ($\chi^2 = 17.48$; df = 3; $p = 0.0006$).

3.3. *Analysis of Humoral Responses in rMVA Vaccinated Mice*

We had previously reported the low level of in vitro neutralizing antibody induction induced by a rMVAGnGc vaccine in BALB/c mice and sheep [17,18]. As expected, levels of neutralizing antibodies in the serum from immunized BALB/c mice remained below the established detection threshold (1.3 log10, 1:20 serum dilution; Figure 3A).

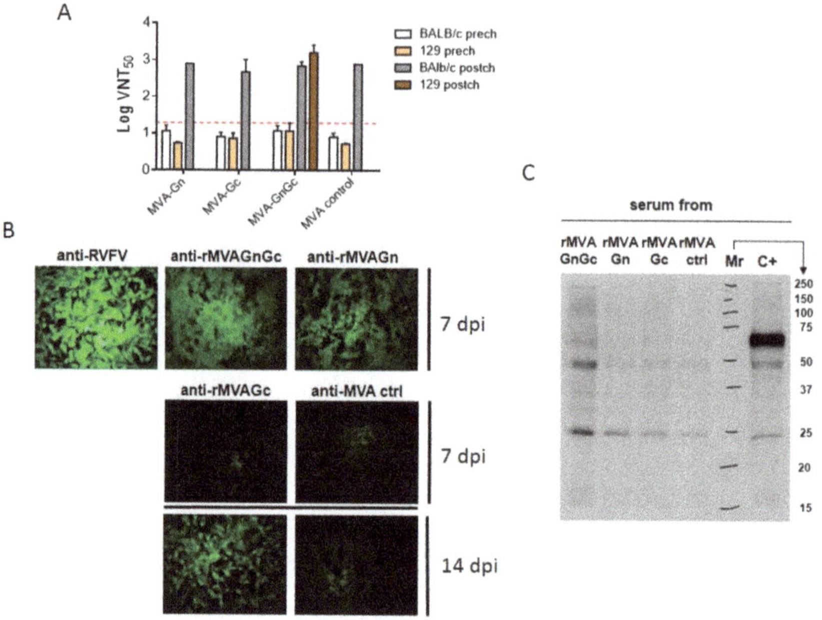

Figure 3. Humoral responses upon MVA vaccination in mice. (**A**). Virus neutralization titers (VNT) in serum samples taken 14 days after immunization (prech.) of either BALB/c or 129SvEv mice. Neutralization titers were also estimated in mice that survived the challenge (postch.). Bars represent mean plus SD. (**B**). Detection of RVFV-infected cells by IFA with serum from MVA vaccinated mice at 7 or 14 days post immunization (dpi). The figure shows representative images of viral plaques detected on cells. (**C**). Immunoprecipitation of RVFV-infected BHK21 cell extracts with serum from MVA vaccinated BALB/c mice. C+: positive control serum from mice immunized with an adenovirus vector encoding GnGc. Mr: relative mass in kDa.

Only two 129SvEv mice from the rMVAGnGc group showed titers slightly above the threshold limit (1.6 log10, serum dilution 1:40). The rest of mice, either vaccinated with rMVAGn or rMVAGc did not show titers above the detection limit in any of the mouse models used. Moreover, one animal from the MVA control group showed a VNT_{50} titer of 1:20 indicating that the observed neutralization at this dilution could be unspecific. When a more stringent neutralization determination was applied (i.e., VNT_{100}), no single prechallenge serum showed neutralization in all microtiter wells (not shown). Upon RVFV 56/74 challenge, all surviving animals showed elevated neutralization titers reaching around 3 logs. Although these data could indicate a successful priming of the vaccines, a similar titer observed in a surviving mouse from the control group ruled out this possibility. Interestingly, the mean postchallenge neutralization titer of the rMVAGnGc vaccinated 129EvSv mice was slightly higher, in agreement with the two mice showing prechallenge neutralization titers over the sensitivity limit. In spite of the lack of a clear in vitro neutralization activity, both vaccines induced antibodies able to label RVFV-MP12 infected cells as shown by indirect immunofluorescence (Figure 3B). In the case of the rMVAGc serum, antiGc antibodies developed later, since a clearly positive fluorescent signal on infected cells was only detected in serum collected 14 days post immunization (Figure 3B). However, none of these prechallenge sera was able to inmunoprecipitate metabolically labeled RVFV glycoproteins in infected cell extracts (Figure 3C).

3.4. Analysis of Cellular Immune Responses to Vaccination

ELISPOT assay using 14 dpi pooled peripheral blood leukocytes (PBLs) from BALB/c mice immunized with rMVAGc showed the highest numbers of IFN-γ secreting cells upon restimulation with two different Gc-specific, MHC-I-restricted, peptides #13 (SYKPMIDQL) and #14 (GGPLKTILL; Figure 4A).

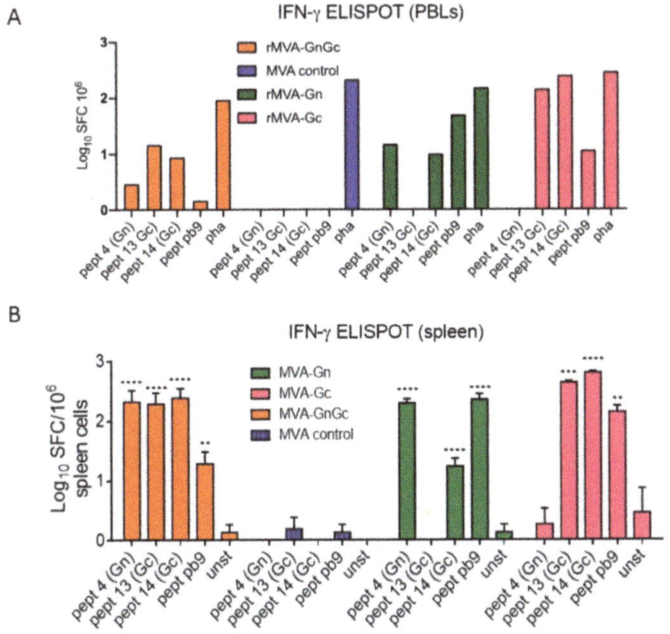

Figure 4. Cellular responses upon MVA immunization. (**A**). Interferon gamma ELISPOT assay of pooled ($n = 5$) BALB/c peripheral blood leukocytes (PBLs) taken at day 14 postimmunization with the different MVA vaccines. Each pool was restimulated with either Gn (#4), or Gc (#13 or #14) specific peptides or with peptide pb9. Nonspecific stimulation was induced with phytohemaglutinin (pha). (**B**). Mean ± SD log spot forming cells (SFC) values obtained in spleen cells from BALB/c mice ($n = 2$) at day 7 post MVA immunization. As above, the peptides 4, 13, and 14 were selected on the basis of their ability to stimulate Gn and Gc specific T-cell responses. Cell culture medium with no added peptide (unst) was used to measure the background of the assay. The pb9 peptide was used as a specific positive control for each recombinant MVA (rMVA) vaccinated mice. In all groups asterisks indicate significance levels for each peptide when compared to the unstimulated control (unst) using Dunnett's multiple comparisons test (** $p < 0.01$; *** $p < 0.001$; **** $p < 0.0001$).

Accordingly, lower numbers of cells were found upon stimulation with the Gn specific peptide (SYAHHRTLL). The rest of the groups showed lower numbers of IFN-γ secreting cells, with the only exception of the rMVAGn group restimulated with the pb9 control peptide. The highest number of IFNγ secreting cells was also found in the MVAGc group in an ELISPOT assay using splenocytes collected at 7 dpi (Figure 4B) or 14 dpi (data not shown). In contrast to the PBL assay, the number of spots was higher for the rMVAGnGc and rMVAGn upon restimulation with a Gn specific peptide. Higher responses were observed upon stimulation with pb9 control peptide in the rMVAGn group in comparison with rMVAGc or rMVAGnGc groups. Of note, the rMVAGn PBLs and spleen cells were also stimulated with Gc peptide 14, although at lower levels. The peptides used for restimulation of BALB/c spleen cells were not able to stimulate IFNγ secretion in 129SvEv spleen cells (not shown), indicative of the restriction imposed by the specific haplotypes. The ELISPOT data correlated with the higher secretion of IL-2 and IL-6 cytokines, involved in T-cell survival that were detected by ELISA in the supernatants of restimulated cultures (Figure 5), indicative of the induction of a lymphoproliferative environment. Again, the group vaccinated with the rMVAGc vaccine displayed the highest amounts of both cytokines. On the other hand, IL-4 or IL-5, two of the main cytokines involved into B-cell proliferation, class switching, and differentiation to effectors were not detected in the same supernatants (not shown).

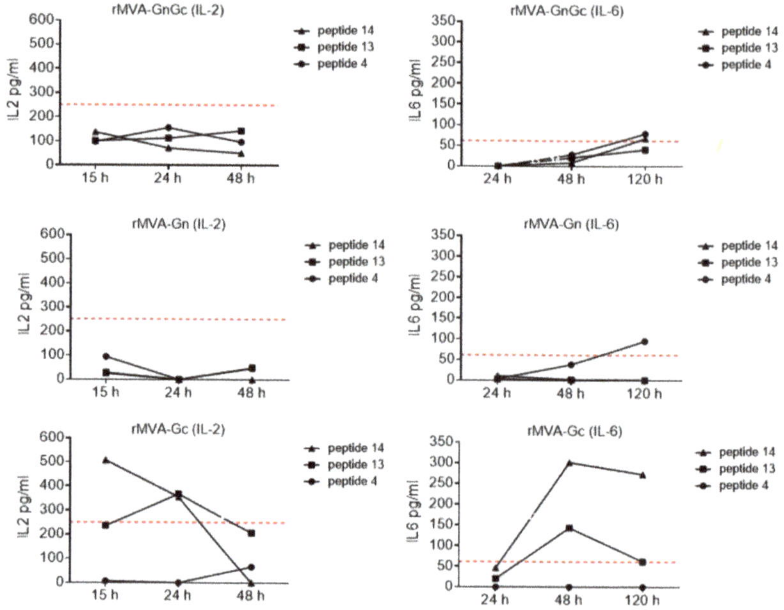

Figure 5. Detection of IL-6 and IL-2 secretion in ex-vivo restimulated spleen cells with peptides. The levels of each cytokine were estimated, using a capture ELISA, in supernatants collected at different times after stimulation. A standard curve was generated to correlate ELISA absorbance values with cytokine concentrations. The graph represents values after background subtraction from nonstimulated cells. The red dotted line determines the lower range of the standard curve.

3.5. Assessment of Efficacy of Humoral Responses by Passive Serum Transfer Experiments

In order to gain insights in the role of the humoral response induced by the rMVA vaccines, a passive serum transfer experiment was designed. In this experiment individual sera from BALB/c mice collected 14 days after immunization with the different rMVA vaccines were pooled. The challenge virus dose (5×10^3 pfu/mouse) was preincubated in the presence of each serum pool (final serum dilution 1/14) for 30 min, prior to the inoculation of mice. All mice that received the challenge dose in the presence of RVFV convalescent serum survived with no clinical display nor significant weigh loss (Figure 6A and Supplementary file, Figure S1). In contrast, all mice from the rMVAGn group and most of the mice inoculated with serum pooled from the rMVAGnGc or Ad5 control vaccinated groups died shortly after inoculation (Figure 6A). Interestingly, four out of five mice transferred with virus plus donor serum from rMVAGc or MVA control survived longer than mice from the rMVAGnGc group ($\chi^2 = 12.11$; df = 3; $p = 0.0070$) and eventually recovered from infection (Supplementary file, Figure S1). Accordingly with the survival data, mean viremia titers were more elevated in rMVAGn and rMVAGnGc groups when compared to rMVAGc or MVA control (Figure 6B), and the differences between means were statistically significant ($p < 0.01$, ANOVA test). Of note, the surviving mouse from the rMVAGnGc group had no conclusive viremia determination but it did not seroconverted (not shown), suggesting that this mouse was not efficiently infected.

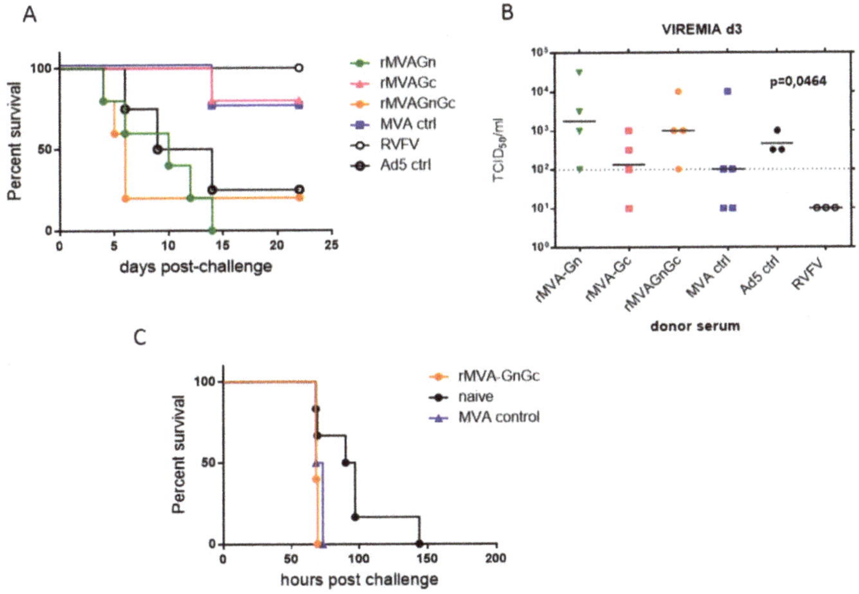

Figure 6. Effect of rMVA immune serum in BALB/c survival. Mice ($n = 5$) were passively transferred with a mixture of immune serum from MVA vaccinated mice and 5×10^3 pfu of virulent 56/74 RVFV. For positive and negative control groups $n = 4$ was used. (**A**). Kaplan–Meier plots of survival proportions. The mice were monitored for 3 weeks for the presence of signs of disease. (**B**). Viremia at day three post inoculation tested by tissue culture infection doses in Vero cells. The infectious titer of each sample is defined as the reciprocal of the highest dilution of serum where a 50% of the cytophatic effect (cpe) is observed relative to noninfected controls. Only samples allowing a clear cpe determination are included. Samples inducing a non cpe-like effect were excluded. When no evident cpe was observed an arbitrary value of 10^1 $TCID_{50}$ below the sensitivity limit (10^2) was assigned. Black lines represent means. Dotted line represents the sensitivity of the assay. The ANOVA test p value for differences among means is indicated. (**C**). Kaplan–Meier plots of BALB/c survival upon transfer with the rMVA ovine immune serum.

In order to confirm these observations a second passive transfer experiment was carried out with a serum pool obtained from a different rMVAGnGc vaccination experiment. Again, the mortality rates were higher and occurred earlier in the rMVAGnGc group than in the control groups (not shown). These data were suggestive of an exacerbating disease effect induced by the serum from animals vaccinated with rMVAGnGc or rMVAGn vaccines. Intriguingly, the extended survival in the rMVA control group was totally unexpected, indicating that the protective effect in the mice was not related to the presence of antiRVFV specific antibodies. In order to check whether the enhanced pathogenic effect of the rMVAGnGc serum was not exclusive of the mouse immune serum, sheep serum pooled from a previous rMVAGnGc vaccination experiment [25] was also used in a similar transfer experiment. The results showed unequivocally an accelerated mortality, with statistical significance ($\chi^2 = 7.740$; df = 2; $p = 0.0209$) in the mice transferred with rMVAGnGc serum with respect to the serum from naive sheep (Figure 6C). Taken together the results observed suggest that the presence of serum anti Gn antibodies may trigger deleterious effects enhancing the infectivity of the virus inoculum.

4. Discussion

We proposed previously that the protective ability of a recombinant MVA vaccine encoding GnGc antigens relied mostly in T-cell immune responses in the absence of a strong in vitro neutralizing antibody response [17]. Apparently, the lack of neutralizing responses could be due to the type of immunity elicited by the vector itself, since the same coding sequence, either expressed by plasmid DNA, subunit vaccine (Gn) or delivered by means of an adenovirus vector eventually elicited stronger neutralizing antibody responses in mice [17,19,26]. In this previous work several MHC class-I restricted peptides from the glycoprotein sequences were identified for their ability to stimulate the secretion of IFNγ by CD8-T cells [17]. Here, our data confirms that BALB/c mice can be also protected upon the RVFV challenge by rMVAGc and, to a lesser extent, by rMVAGn and that this protection can also be achieved in the absence of neutralizing antibodies. According to the role of a cell-mediated immune response, the protection was restricted to a specific genetic background, as shown by the lack of survival upon challenge of 129SvEv mice immunized with the same vaccines (rMVAGn or rMVAGc). The detection of IL-2 and IL-6 supports the induction of cellular responses since both cytokines play a role in T-cell survival and activation. Particularly, Gc-specific T-cell responses may act as a key component in the protection after challenge observed in the rMVA immunized mice, perhaps contributing to the efficient elimination of RVFV infected cells. Our data also point out that the simultaneous expression of both glycoproteins by the MVA vector is an essential requirement for the induction of a protective response in the 129SvEv mouse strain. At this point it could be interesting to explore further how the genetic background determines the efficacy of the immune response and how differences in susceptibility to RVFV challenge may account for the observed differences in efficacy.

One of the most striking findings in this work is the exacerbating effect of some rMVA immune serum in infectivity. This was somewhat unexpected but may help to explain our previous observations in experiments conducted to evaluate the efficacy of the rMVAGnGc vaccine in sheep [25]. An indirect measure of viral replication in the host is the induction of antibody responses to immunogenic epitopes. For RVFV, the most immunogenic epitopes lie in the viral nucleoprotein N. Therefore, detection of antiN serum antibodies reveals the existence of a productive RVFV infection in the host. Earlier antiN antibody detection was observed in the serum from sheep vaccinated with rMVAGnGc when compared to non- and mock vaccinated controls. In addition, the amount of viral RNA detected in blood was higher at early times upon infection than in controls, indicating faster virus replication. We could reproduce here similar results upon the passive transfer of both mouse and sheep serum. One explanation to these findings would be the induction of subneutralizing antibodies able to enhance rather than block virus replication. Antibody dependent enhancement (ADE) has been described in several viral systems, with more detail in flaviviral infections [27–32]. In the case of RVFV it could be suggested that subneutralizing antiGn antibodies could bind to exposed Gn epitopes on the virus particle. In this scenario internalization of virus-antibody immune-complexes would be augmented in cells bearing complement or Fc receptors, increasing virus uptake and pathogenesis. This could explain the increased mortality of mice that were transferred with rMVAGnGc or rMVAGn serum:virus mixtures compared to that of rMVAGc or the MVA control. However, the protection observed in mice receiving the MVA control immune serum is puzzling. A plausible explanation could be that other nonantibody mediated humoral effectors provide some degree of protection although not sufficient to avoid deleterious effects of subneutralizing antibody responses. Thus, MVA or rMVAGc serum transfer would provide such antiviral effect while the transfer of rMVAGnGc or rMVAGn serum would enhance infectivity through subneutralizing antiGn antibodies. Both the classical and alternative pathways of the complement system can be activated upon viral infections and it has been shown that complement system plays an important role in poxvirus immunity [33]. On the other hand, deposition of complement proteins on the surface of enveloped virions enhances uptake by phagocytosis and potentially interferes with receptor interactions, virus entry, and uncoating [34]. Whether this hypothesis is or not true would deserve further experimentation. Nonetheless, it becomes clear that improving the quality of the antibody response of our MVA vaccines would render them more efficacious against a lethal RVFV challenge. Current work is underway to test the ability of novel MVA recombinants using different vector source and stronger promoter sequences for increasing antigen expression and enhancing proper processing of antigens.

5. Conclusions

In conclusion we confirmed the possibility of protecting mice against a lethal RVFV challenge without induction of neutralizing antibody responses, stressing the importance of cell-mediated immune responses in protection. Most importantly, failing in inducing proper neutralizing antibody responses may result in enhanced pathogenesis when the cell mediated immune response is impaired or absent.

Supplementary Materials: The following are available online at http://www.mdpi.com/2076-393X/8/1/82/s1, Table S1: primers used for inverse PCR reaction. Figure S1. Weight loss after passive transfer in mice. Figure S2. Amino acid sequences of eGn and Gc encoded by the recombinant MVAs.

Author Contributions: Conceptualization, A.B. and G.L.; methodology, E.L.-G., S.M., G.L., J.O., B.B. A.B.; formal analysis, E.L.G., G.L., A.B.; writing—original draft preparation, E.L.-G., G.L., A.B.; writing—review and editing, A.B.; supervision, G.L., A.B.; project administration, A.B.; funding acquisition, A.B., B.B. All authors have read and agreed to the published version of the manuscript.

Funding: This work was supported by grants AGL-2011-22485, AGL-2017-83226R from the Spanish Ministry of Science and S2013/ABI-2906, S2018/BAA-4370 from Comunidad de Madrid. ELG was a recipient of a pre-doctoral fellowship program from the Spanish Ministry of Science.

Acknowledgments: We thank Nuria de la Losa for her excellent technical assistance and the animal care staff at Centro de Investigación en Sanidad Animal

Conflicts of Interest: The authors declare no conflict of interest. The funders had no role in the design of the study; in the collection, analyses, or interpretation of data; in the writing of the manuscript, or in the decision to publish the results.

References

1. Pepin, M.; Bouloy, M.; Bird, B.H.; Kemp, A.; Paweska, J. Rift Valley fever virus (Bunyaviridae: Phlebovirus): An update on pathogenesis, molecular epidemiology, vectors, diagnostics and prevention. *Vet. Res.* **2010**, *41*, 61. [CrossRef] [PubMed]
2. Chevalier, V.; Pepin, M.; Plee, L.; Lancelot, R. Rift Valley fever–a threat for Europe? *Euro. Surveill.* **2010**, *15*, 19506. [PubMed]
3. Napp, S.; Chevalier, V.; Busquets, N.; Calistri, P.; Casal, J.; Attia, M.; Elbassal, R.; Hosni, H.; Farrag, H.; Hassan, N.; et al. Understanding the legal trade of cattle and camels and the derived risk of Rift Valley Fever introduction into and transmission within Egypt. *PLoS Negl. Trop. Dis.* **2018**, *12*, e0006143. [CrossRef]
4. Moutailler, S.; Krida, G.; Schaffner, F.; Vazeille, M.; Failloux, A.B. Potential vectors of Rift Valley fever virus in the Mediterranean region. *Vector Borne Zoonotic Dis.* **2008**, *8*, 749–753. [CrossRef]
5. Gomez, C.E.; Najera, J.L.; Krupa, M.; Perdiguero, B.; Esteban, M. MVA and NYVAC as vaccines against emergent infectious diseases and cancer. *Curr. Gene Ther.* **2011**, *11*, 189–217. [CrossRef]
6. Cottingham, M.G.; Carroll, M.W. Recombinant MVA vaccines: Dispelling the myths. *Vaccine* **2013**, *31*, 4247–4251. [CrossRef]
7. Gomez, C.E.; Perdiguero, B.; Garcia-Arriaza, J.; Esteban, M. Clinical applications of attenuated MVA poxvirus strain. *Expert Rev. Vaccines* **2013**, *12*, 1395–1416. [CrossRef]
8. Volz, A.; Fux, R.; Langenmayer, M.C.; Sutter, G. Modified vaccinia virus ankara (MVA)–development as recombinant vaccine and prospects for use in veterinary medicine. *Berl. Munch. Tierarztl. Wochenschr.* **2015**, *128*, 464–472.
9. Bird, B.H.; Nichol, S.T. Breaking the chain: Rift Valley fever virus control via livestock vaccination. *Curr. Opin. Virol.* **2012**, *2*, 315–323. [CrossRef]
10. Besselaar, T.G.; Blackburn, N.K. The synergistic neutralization of Rift Valley fever virus by monoclonal antibodies to the envelope glycoproteins. *Arch. Virol.* **1992**, *125*, 239–250. [CrossRef]
11. Besselaar, T.G.; Blackburn, N.K. The effect of neutralizing monoclonal antibodies on early events in Rift Valley fever virus infectivity. *Res. Virol.* **1994**, *145*, 13–19. [CrossRef]

12. Besselaar, T.G.; Blackburn, N.K.; Meenehan, G.M. Antigenic analysis of Rift Valley fever virus isolates: Monoclonal antibodies distinguish between wild-type and neurotropic virus strains. *Res. Virol.* **1991**, *142*, 469–474. [CrossRef]
13. Suzich, J.A.; Kakach, L.T.; Collett, M.S. Expression strategy of a phlebovirus: Biogenesis of proteins from the Rift Valley fever virus M segment. *J. Virol.* **1990**, *64*, 1549–1555. [CrossRef] [PubMed]
14. Ikegami, T. Molecular biology and genetic diversity of Rift Valley fever virus. *Antiviral Res.* **2012**, *95*, 293–310. [CrossRef]
15. Halldorsson, S.; Li, S.; Li, M.; Harlos, K.; Bowden, T.A.; Huiskonen, J.T. Shielding and activation of a viral membrane fusion protein. *Nat. Commun.* **2018**, *9*, 349. [CrossRef]
16. Allen, E.R.; Krumm, S.A.; Raghwani, J.; Halldorsson, S.; Elliott, A.; Graham, V.A.; Koudriakova, E.; Harlos, K.; Wright, D.; Warimwe, G.M.; et al. A Protective Monoclonal Antibody Targets a Site of Vulnerability on the Surface of Rift Valley Fever Virus. *Cell Rep.* **2018**, *25*, 3750–3758. [CrossRef]
17. Lopez-Gil, E.; Lorenzo, G.; Hevia, E.; Borrego, B.; Eiden, M.; Groschup, M.; Gilbert, S.C.; Brun, A. A Single Immunization with MVA Expressing GnGc Glycoproteins Promotes Epitope-specific CD8+-T Cell Activation and Protects Immune-competent Mice against a Lethal RVFV Infection. *PLoS Negl. Trop. Dis.* **2013**, *7*, e2309. [CrossRef]
18. Lorenzo, G.; Lopez-Gil, E.; Ortego, J.; Brun, A. Efficacy of different DNA and MVA prime-boost vaccination regimens against a Rift Valley fever virus (RVFV) challenge in sheep 12 weeks following vaccination. *Vet. Res.* **2018**, *49*, 21. [CrossRef]
19. Warimwe, G.M.; Lorenzo, G.; Lopez-Gil, E.; Reyes-Sandoval, A.; Cottingham, M.G.; Spencer, A.J.; Collins, K.A.; Dicks, M.D.; Milicic, A.; Lall, A.; et al. Immunogenicity and efficacy of a chimpanzee adenovirus-vectored Rift Valley fever vaccine in mice. *Virol. J.* **2013**, *10*, 349. [CrossRef]
20. Warimwe, G.M.; Gesharisha, J.; Carr, B.V.; Otieno, S.; Otingah, K.; Wright, D.; Charleston, B.; Okoth, E.; Elena, L.G.; Lorenzo, G.; et al. Chimpanzee Adenovirus Vaccine Provides Multispecies Protection against Rift Valley Fever. *Sci. Rep.* **2016**, *6*, 20617. [CrossRef]
21. Malin, A.S.; Huygen, K.; Content, J.; Mackett, M.; Brandt, L.; Andersen, P.; Smith, S.M.; Dockrell, H.M. Vaccinia expression of Mycobacterium tuberculosis-secreted proteins: Tissue plasminogen activator signal sequence enhances expression and immunogenicity of M. tuberculosis Ag85. *Microbes Infect.* **2000**, *2*, 1677–1685. [CrossRef]
22. Jackel, S.; Eiden, M.; Dauber, M.; Balkema-Buschmann, A.; Brun, A.; Groschup, M.H. Generation and application of monoclonal antibodies against Rift Valley fever virus nucleocapsid protein NP and glycoproteins Gn and Gc. *Arch. Virol.* **2014**, *159*, 535–546. [CrossRef]
23. Busquets, N.; Xavier, F.; Martin-Folgar, R.; Lorenzo, G.; Galindo-Cardiel, I.; del Val, B.P.; Rivas, R.; Iglesias, J.; Rodriguez, F.; Solanes, D.; et al. Experimental infection of young adult European breed sheep with Rift Valley fever virus field isolates. *Vector Borne Zoonotic Dis.* **2010**, *10*, 689–696. [CrossRef] [PubMed]
24. Lorenzo, G.; Martin-Folgar, R.; Hevia, E.; Boshra, H.; Brun, A. Protection against lethal Rift Valley fever virus (RVFV) infection in transgenic IFNAR(-/-) mice induced by different DNA vaccination regimens. *Vaccine* **2010**, *28*, 2937–2944. [CrossRef] [PubMed]
25. Busquets, N.; Lorenzo, G.; Lopez-Gil, E.; Rivas, R.; Solanes, D.; Galindo-Cardiel, I.; Abad, F.X.; Rodriguez, F.; Bensaid, A.; Warimwe, G.; et al. Efficacy assessment of an MVA vectored Rift Valley Fever vaccine in lambs. *Antiviral Res.* **2014**, *108*, 165–172. [CrossRef] [PubMed]
26. De Boer, S.M.; Kortekaas, J.; Antonis, A.F.; Kant, J.; van Oploo, J.L.; Rottier, P.J.; Moormann, R.J.; Bosch, B.J. Rift Valley fever virus subunit vaccines confer complete protection against a lethal virus challenge. *Vaccine* **2010**, *28*, 2330–2339. [CrossRef] [PubMed]
27. Beck, Z.; Prohaszka, Z.; Fust, G. Traitors of the immune system-enhancing antibodies in HIV infection: Their possible implication in HIV vaccine development. *Vaccine* **2008**, *26*, 3078–3085. [CrossRef]
28. Hohdatsu, T.; Yamada, M.; Tominaga, R.; Makino, K.; Kida, K.; Koyama, H. Antibody-dependent enhancement of feline infectious peritonitis virus infection in feline alveolar macrophages and human monocyte cell line U937 by serum of cats experimentally or naturally infected with feline coronavirus. *J. Vet. Med. Sci.* **1998**, *60*, 49–55. [CrossRef]
29. Takada, A.; Feldmann, H.; Ksiazek, T.G.; Kawaoka, Y. Antibody-dependent enhancement of Ebola virus infection. *J. Virol.* **2003**, *77*, 7539–7544. [CrossRef]

30. Takada, A.; Kawaoka, Y. Antibody-dependent enhancement of viral infection: Molecular mechanisms and in vivo implications. *Rev. Med. Virol.* **2003**, *13*, 387–398. [CrossRef]
31. Tirado, S.M.; Yoon, K.J. Antibody-dependent enhancement of virus infection and disease. *Viral Immunol.* **2003**, *16*, 69–86. [CrossRef] [PubMed]
32. Wang, S.F.; Tseng, S.P.; Yen, C.H.; Yang, J.Y.; Tsao, C.H.; Shen, C.W.; Chen, K.H.; Liu, F.T.; Liu, W.T.; Chen, Y.M.; et al. Antibody-dependent SARS coronavirus infection is mediated by antibodies against spike proteins. *Biochem. Biophys. Res. Commun.* **2014**, *451*, 208–214. [CrossRef] [PubMed]
33. Price, P.J.; Banki, Z.; Scheideler, A.; Stoiber, H.; Verschoor, A.; Sutter, G.; Lehmann, M.H. Complement component C5 recruits neutrophils in the absence of C3 during respiratory infection with modified vaccinia virus Ankara. *J. Immunol.* **2015**, *194*, 1164–1168. [CrossRef]
34. Sullivan, B.L.; Takefman, D.M.; Spear, G.T. Complement can neutralize HIV-1 plasma virus by a C5-independent mechanism. *Virology* **1998**, *248*, 173–181. [CrossRef] [PubMed]

vaccines

MDPI

Article

Differential Immune Transcriptome and Modulated Signalling Pathways in Rainbow Trout Infected with Viral Haemorrhagic Septicaemia Virus (VHSV) and Its Derivative Non-Virion (NV) Gene Deleted

Blanca Chinchilla [1], Paloma Encinas [2], Julio M. Coll [2] and Eduardo Gomez-Casado [2,*]

[1] Ocular Genomics Institute, Department of Ophthalmology, Massachusetts Eye and Ear Infirmary and Harvard Medical School, Boston, MA 02114, USA; Blanca_chinchillarodriguez@meei.harvard.edu

[2] Department of Biotechnology, National Agricultural and Food Research and Technology Institute (INIA), 28040 Madrid, Spain; paloma.encinas@inia.es (P.E.); juliocoll@inia.es (J.M.C.)

* Correspondence: casado@inia.es; Tel.: +34-913-473-917

Received: 20 December 2019; Accepted: 27 January 2020; Published: 30 January 2020

Abstract: Viral haemorrhagic septicaemia virus (VHSV) is one of the worst viral threats to fish farming. Non-virion (NV) gene-deleted VHSV (dNV-VHSV) has been postulated as an attenuated virus, because the absence of the *NV* gene leads to lower induced pathogenicity. However, little is known about the immune responses driven by dNV-VHSV and the wild-type (wt)-VHSV in the context of infection. Here, we obtained the immune transcriptome profiling in trout infected with dNV-VHSV and wt-VHSV and the pathways involved in immune responses. As general results, dNV-VHSV upregulated more trout immune genes than wt-VHSV (65.6% vs 45.7%, respectively), whereas wt-VHSV maintained more non-regulated genes than dNV-VHSV (45.7% vs 14.6%, respectively). The modulated pathways analysis (Gene-Set Enrichment Analysis, GSEA) showed that, when compared to wt-VHSV infected trout, the dNV-VHSV infected trout upregulated signalling pathways (n = 19) such as RIG-I (retinoic acid-inducible gene-I) like receptor signalling, Toll-like receptor signalling, type II interferon signalling, and nuclear factor kappa B (NF-kappa B) signalling, among others. The results from individual genes and GSEA demonstrated that wt-VHSV impaired the activation at short stages of infection of pro-inflammatory, antiviral, proliferation, and apoptosis pathways, delaying innate humoral response and cellular crosstalk, whereas dNV-VHSV promoted the opposite effects. Therefore, these results might support future studies on using dNV-VHSV as a potential live vaccine.

Keywords: VHSV; non-virion (NV); transcriptome profiling; rainbow trout; immune pathways

1. Introduction

Viral haemorrhagic septicaemia virus (VHSV) belongs to the *Novirhabdovirus* genus, together with infectious haematopoietic necrosis virus (IHNV), snakehead rhabdovirus (SHRV), and hirame rhabdovirus (HIRV). They are all enveloped negative-stranded RNA viruses with a single RNA genome of ~11 Kb [1–3], which encodes five virion proteins (N, P, M, G, and L proteins) and the non-virion (NV) protein that gives the name to the *Novirhabdovirus* genus and differentiates it from other fish rhabdoviruses such as spring viremia carp virus (SVCV). VHSV has been isolated from more than 50 fish species from North America, Asia, and Europe, including 15 farmed [4] and free-living marine fish species [5] like trout, salmon, turbot, and eel, among others. Within a farm, the presence of VHSV infection, even if in only one individual fish, has to be notified to the Office International des Epizooties (OIE, Paris, France) and implies the sacrifice of all the farmed fish, thus leading to serious economic losses [6,7]. The *NV* gene was firstly characterised and named from IHNV genome studies [8]. Some years later, the *NV* gene from VHSV was further characterised by comparative genome studies [9]. Despite the presence of the *NV* gene in the four novirhabdovirus species mentioned above, their NV proteins showed very divergent inter-species sequences [10,11]. Initial studies regarding NV role showed that it was required for the highest efficient replication of IHNV in rainbow trout [12–14] and that of VHSV in olive flounder [13,15] and in *Epithelioma papulosum cyprinid* (EPC) cells [13]. However, NV was not essential for in vitro or in vivo SHRV production in warm-water flatfish [16,17]. Further, in vitro studies using the wild-type (wt) and NV knock-out IHNV or VHSV suggested that NV downregulated the host *ifn1/mx* transcriptional levels during in vitro infection in trout (RTG-2, Rainbow Trout Gonad-2) [18] or EPC cells [15], respectively. The higher levels of IFN-induced *mx* transcript in NV knock-out VHSV vs. wt-VHSV injected flounder found in these studies suggested that NV also interferes with IFN defences in vivo to favour VHSV replication [15]. The early anti-apoptotic role of NV during the first stages of VHSV infection has been also demonstrated [19]. Using recombinant NV protein (rNV) and a trout immune-targeted microarray, we have previously determined not only an anti-apoptotic role for NV, but also a plethora of novel expression changes (mainly downregulated) in genes associated with immune innate and adaptive response (i.e., interferons, MX, tumour necrosis factors, antigen presentation, interleukins) [6]. However, the effects driven by the injection of the rNV protein alone will probably differ from those induced by the NV in the course of VHSV infection. Recently, a microarray study in olive flounder liver infected with VHSV described differential gene expression and gene ontology classification of these genes [20], resulting in a global transcriptome profiling where only a few genes have been classified as immune-related. Gene expression has been also characterised with microarrays in olive flounder infected with a VHSV strain that produces high mortality in this species [21]. In addition, the protection of olive flounder against VHSV was previously assessed by immunization with the *NV* gene-knockout recombinant VHSV, which led to good protection against virulent VHSV [22]. However, the underlying mechanisms of olive flounder protection remain unknown. The aim of this work was to characterise the transcriptomic profiling of immune-related genes in trout infected with the wild-type VHSV (expressing NV) and dNV-VHSV (*NV* gene-deleted) in order to find targeted immune genes and signalling pathways implied in the course of a VHSV infection. This study will contribute to better understand how NV modulates gene expression and how the expression pattern changes in response to dNV-VHSV. The results will help tailoring future vaccines against viral haemorrhagic septicaemia virus and other novirhabdoviruses.

1.1. Viral Haemorrhagic Septicaemia Viruses (VHSV)

Wild type VHSV-23.75 (wt-VHSV) isolated from brown trout [23] (GenBank accession number FN665788) and its derivative *NV* gene-deleted (dNV-VHSV), obtained as previously described [13], were used to infect rainbow trout (*Oncorhynchus mykiss*) by intraperitoneal injection. Both wt- and dNV-VHSV viruses were kindly provided by Dr. Michel Brémont (INRA, France), and further propagated in EPC cells at 14 °C and titrated by the plaque-forming assay (pfu) as previously described [14].

1.2. Virus Dosages and Injection of Fingerling Rainbow Trout

Fingerling rainbow trout (*Oncorhynchus mykiss*) of 6–12 g (approximately 10 cm in length), free of IPNV (Infectious Pancreatic Necrosis Virus) and VHSV antibodies, were obtained from a local fish farm (Los Molinos, Madrid). They were maintained at 14 °C in a 200 L aquarium with tap-dechlorinated carbon-filtered water provided with biological filters and fed with a commercial fish diet. After two weeks of acclimation, fish were separated into seven groups of six trout per group. Due to the non-virion (NV) expression by wt-VHSV, a different replication rate of wt-VHSV and dNV-VHSV in the EPC cell line was established [13], and since the maximum NV expression by wt-VHSV is reached at 48 hpi (hours post-infection), we aimed at establishing the equivalent infectious dosage yielding comparable transcriptomic profile for each virus at 48 hpi. For that, we injected trout intraperitoneally with 100 μL of wt-VHSV (10^4, 10^5 or 35×10^6 pfu), dNV-VHSV (10^4, 10^5 or 35×10^6 pfu) or phosphate-buffered saline (PBS). Each group of injected trout was then released into a 50-L aquarium and maintained at 14 °C. Two days after injection, trout were sacrificed, head kidney and spleen (whole organs) were pooled, and immediately immersed in RNAlater (Ambion, Austin, USA) at 4 °C overnight, before being frozen at −70 °C until further analysis.

1.3. RNA Extraction and cDNA Synthesis

The pooled head kidney and spleen (whole organs) from each individual trout were homogenized using the Tissue Lyser Cell Disruptor (Qiagen Iberia, S.L., Madrid, Spain) for 10 min at 50 Hz with 3 mm glass beads in an RTL buffer (Qiagen Iberia, S.L., Madrid, Spain). RNA was then extracted from the homogenates by using the RNAeasyPlus kit (Qiagen Iberia, S.L., Madrid, Spain) and eluted in RNase-free water. RNA concentrations were estimated by Nanodrop and the presence of 18S and 28S rRNA bands was confirmed by denaturing RNA agarose electrophoresis (Sigma-Aldrich Quimica SA, Madrid, Spain). For qPCR experiments of the nucleoprotein (*N*) and non-virion (*NV*) genes, cDNA synthesis was carried out from RNA (1 µg) by using oligo-dT and PrimeScript^{TM} reverse transcriptase (RR037A TAKARA, Japan) according to the manufacturer's instructions. For microarray experiments, additional RNA quality controls (RNA integrity number, RIN) were performed by NIMGenetics (Madrid, Spain). For each experimental six-trout group, the four trout with best RNA quality (RIN > 7.0) were chosen for microarray hybridisation. cDNA was synthesized by using SuperScript III reverse transcriptase (Invitrogen) and oligo(dT) primer, labelled with Cy3 (GE Healthcare, Spain), and purified with Microcon YM30 (Merck Millipore, Spain).

1.4. Design of Oligo-Microarrays Enriched in Rainbow Trout Immune-Related Genes (Targeted Microarrays)

Oligo-microarrays were enriched in rainbow trout immune-related genes as previously described (immune-targeted microarrays) [6,24,25]. The final 8 × 15K microarray corresponds to Agilent's ID032303 (Gene Expression Omnibus GEO platform submission number GPL14155) and contains 1474 annotated immune-related probes (60-mer) per duplicate. In order to simplify the analysis of results, annotated probes were classified according to the following gene groups: VIG, VHSV-induced genes (number of probes, $n = 22$); IFN, interferons and their receptors ($n = 20$); MX, interferon-inducible proteins mx ($n = 3$); CO, complement components ($n = 6$); IL, interleukins and their receptors ($n = 19$); APM, antigen-presenting machinery genes ($n = 4$); TNFSF, tumour necrosis factor superfamily ($n = 16$); CD, cluster differentiation antigens ($n = 15$); CK, chemokines and their receptors ($n = 32$); CASP, caspases ($n = 3$); and TF, transcription factors ($n = 10$). The trout microarray used for these experiments was previously validated by real-time quantitative PCR (RTqPCR) [24,25]. The number of biological replicas was four. Four chips of eight samples per chip were used and hybridised simultaneously. This home-made rainbow trout oligo-microarray contains more immune-related genes than any other trout microarray available, since it includes all the immune-related genes from the Agilent's EST-derived rainbow trout oligo-microarray (ID16271) [6,24–26].

1.5. Hybridisation and Gene Expression Changes of Trout Transcripts to the Immune-Targeted Microarrays

The labelling of 2 µg of RNA (approximately 50 µg/mL) and hybridisation to the microarrays were performed by NIMGenetics (Madrid, Spain) complying with the Minimum Information about a Microarray Experiment (MIAME) standards [24].

Normalisations were performed by correcting the individual fluorescence in each microarray with the sum of all the fluorescent values according to the formula: fluorescence of each probe/sum of all the probe fluorescence signals per microarray. Raw and normalised data were deposited in GEO [27,28]. After normalisation, outlier values (defined by those fluorescence values above or below mean ± standard deviation per probe) were identified and eliminated from the calculations programmed in Origin Pro 8.6 (OriginLab Corporation, Northampton, MA, USA). Fold-change (FC) for each probe was calculated by the following formula: values of wt-VHSV or dNV-VHSV injected trout/mean of PBS injected trout ($n = 4$). Means and standard deviations of individual folds were calculated for each oligonucleotide probe by the following formula: fluorescent value/mean fluorescent value of the control ($n = 4$). Venn diagrams reflect the percentage of genes which FC value was upregulated, downregulated, and non-regulated for each comparison with these arbitrary criteria previously used [6]: (1) upregulated: FC ≥ 1.5; (2) downregulated: FC ≤ −1.5; and (3) non-regulated (basal) gene expression: −1.5 < FC < 1.5. On the other hand, the heatmap figures reflect the FC for each gene comparison using an arbitrary criteria previously described [6]: (1) non-regulated (basal) gene expression: −1.5 < FC < 1.5 (black); (2) upregulated: 1.5 ≤ FC < 2 (light red box), 2 ≤ FC < 5 (red box), 5 ≤ FC (dark red box); and (3) downregulated: −1.5 ≥ FC > −2 (light green box), −2 ≥ FC > −5 (green box), −5 ≥ FC (dark green box). Differentially expressed gene transcripts were considered significant when FC ≥ 1.5 or FC ≤ −1.5. Negative folds were calculated for those values below 0.66 applying the formula −1/FC. Therefore, FC = 0.66 corresponds to a −1.5 value; FC = 0.5 (more downregulated) corresponds to a −2 value; and FC = 0.2 (even more downregulated) corresponds to a −5 value.

1.6. Quantitative Estimation of Transcripts by Real-Time Quantitative PCR (RTqPCR)

To estimate the wt- or dNV-VHSV replication in rainbow trout head kidney and spleen, both *N* and *NV* transcript levels were estimated by RTqPCR amplification after intraperitoneal injection of the corresponding VHSV, as described in Section 1.2. RNA extraction and cDNA synthesis were carried out as described above. RTqPCR was carried out by mixing 100 ng of cDNA, 0.9 μM of forward primer, 0.9 μM of reverse primer, and Power SYBR Green PCR Master Mix (Life Technologies, Madrid, Spain). The thermal profile was 10 min at 95 °C, followed by 40 cycles of 95 °C for 15 s, and 60 °C for 1 min. For each experiment, the expression level of the analysed genes was calculated using the $2^{-\Delta\Delta Ct}$ relative quantitation method. The Ct for each viral gene was normalised to *β-actin* gene ($\Delta Ct^{gene} = Ct^{gene} - Ct^{\beta\text{-}actin}$), which was used as an internal control due to its low coefficient of variation (CV) among different virus dosages (CV ≤ 3% for 10^4 pfu/trout and 10^5 pfu/trout of wt- and dNV-VHSV; trout injected with 35×10^6 pfu of both viruses showed a CV close to 8%). Means and standard deviations were calculated for each experimental infection by intraperitoneal (ip) injection of either the wt- or dNV-VHSV in trout groups ($n = 6$) with 10^4, 10^5, or 35×10^6 pfu/trout. Primer sequences used were: *β-actin* (accession number AF550583.1) forward 5′CATCACCATCGGCAACGA and reverse 5′GATGTCCACGTCACACTTCAT; nucleoprotein (accession number AJ233396) forward 5′TCTCCGCTCGTCCTCCGTGAG and reverse 5′GTGAGCCCAGAGCCTCTTGTC; and non-virion (*NV*, accession number AJ233396) forward 5′TCAAGGTGACACAGGCAGTCA and reverse 5′CCAGTTCTCTCATGGGCATCAT. Calculated RTqPCR efficiency was 59% for *β-actin*, 45% for *N*, and 43% for *NV* genes. Efficiency was considered to correct the transcript levels obtained by RTqPCR assays.

1.7. Calculations used for Gene Set Enrichment Analysis (GSEA)

In order to explore the possible biological effects of simultaneous and small changes in several related genes, we screened the transcriptional data with the previously described 51 rainbow trout from the immune-related gene-set (GS) collection [25]. The trout GS collection was manually designed from the KEGG (K) and WIKI (W) trout orthologous human pathways (as accessed in 2013), using the trout genes contained in our home-designed microarray. The trout GS collection was then used for analysis by the Gene-Set Enrichment Analysis (GSEA) program [29–31]. Transcriptional data from the dNV-VHSV and wt-VHSV injected trout were analysed by GSEA to assign a normalised enrichment score (NES) for each GS of the collection in each of the three cases [25].

1.8. Ethics Statement

All the animal procedures used in this study were approved by the INIA (National Agricultural and Food Research and Technology Institute) ethical and biosecurity committee (authorization CEEA 2011/022) and performed following the National and European Commission guidelines and regulations on laboratory animals' care. Periodic examinations were performed several times a day during infections so as to euthanize fish with abnormal behaviour. To minimize animal suffering, fingerling rainbow trout were sacrificed by using a lethal dose of tricaine methanesulfonate (MS-222, 50 mg/mL, Sigma, Madrid, Spain).

2. Results and Discussion

2.1. dNV- and wt-VHSV Dosages used for Microarray Analysis

In this work, we have firstly defined the appropriate infectious dosage for wt-VHSV and dNV-VHSV in order to establish the comparative transcriptomic profiling between them. At 48 h post-infection, the RNA transcripts from head kidney and spleen were analysed by RTqPCR to estimate the corresponding viral replication loads based on *N* transcript levels (Figure 1). The trout injected with 10^4 pfu, 10^5 pfu, and 35×10^6 pfu of the wt-VHSV yielded the following *N* (±SD) values: 2.3 ± 1.1, 9.0 ± 4.1, and 348.8 ± 125, respectively (Figure 1). On the other hand, trout injected with 10^4 pfu, 10^5 pfu and 35×10^6 pfu of the dNV-VHSV yielded the following *N* (±SD) values: 0.6 ± 0.2, 1.1 ± 0.4, and 19.3 ± 7.6, respectively (Figure 1). Wild-type-VHSV/dNV-VHSV ratio for *N* transcripts yielded an approximately 18-fold higher replication rate for the wt-VHSV when both viruses were applied at a dose of 35×10^6 pfu/trout dose. However, this proportion was close to 1 when with the dose used was 10^5 pfu for wt-VHSV and 35×10^6 pfu for dNV-VHSV. For this reason, we considered it best to use the latter for the microarray study. Therefore, we compared the transcriptomic profile of trout injected with 10^5 pfu of wt-VHSV (NV presence) (data deposited on GEO GSE37330) and trout injected with a 350-fold more infectious dose (35×10^6 pfu) of dNV-VHSV (NV absence) (data deposited at GEO GSE43285).

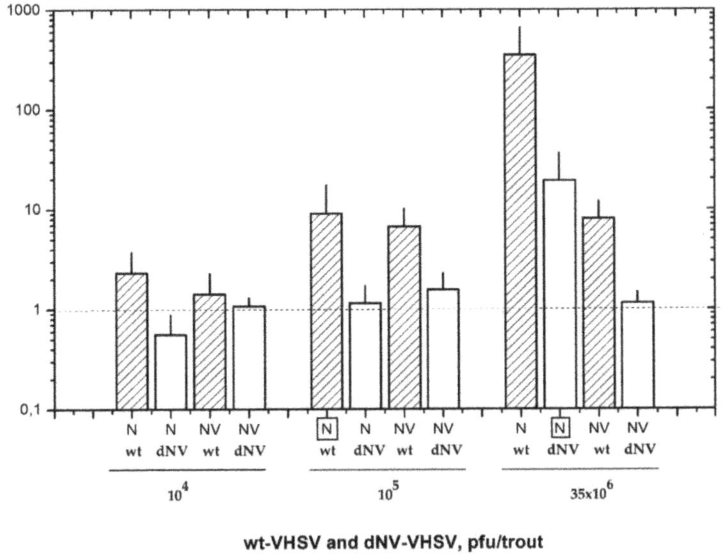

Figure 1. Nucleoprotein (*N*) and non-virion (*NV*) gene expression values (mean ± SD) obtained by RTqPCR of six trout injected with wild-type (wt)-VHSV (hatched bars) and *NV* gene-deleted (dNV)-VHSV (white bars). Animals were injected with three different dosages (10^4, 10^5, and 35×10^6 pfu/trout) of each virus and analysed 48 hpi. The results showed similar nucleoprotein (boxed N) transcript levels of wt-VHSV (10^5 pfu/trout) and dNV-VHSV (35×10^6 pfu/trout), indicating their similar replication levels. Horizontal dotted line corresponds to negative control. VHSV: viral haemorrhagic septicaemia virus.

2.2. Overview of the Expression Profiles Obtained

Normalised FC values of microarray datasets from wt-VHSV (10^5 pfu/trout) and dNV-VHSV (35×10^6 pfu/trout) were classified based on the groups defined for this study (see Section 1.5) and calculated the percentage of upregulated, downregulated and non-regulated genes. Figure 2A shows the upregulated genes between groups (wt-VHSV and dNV-VHSV) with fold changes (FC) ≥ 1.5 in Venn diagrams. The trout injected with dNV-VHSV showed the highest number of upregulated genes (65.6%), followed by those injected with wt-VHSV (45.7%). Probably, the upregulation increase in the dNV-VHSV injected trout was due to the absence of NV. In addition, dNV-VHSV and wt-VHSV shared 25.8% of the upregulated genes, which should be due to other viral proteins rather than NV.

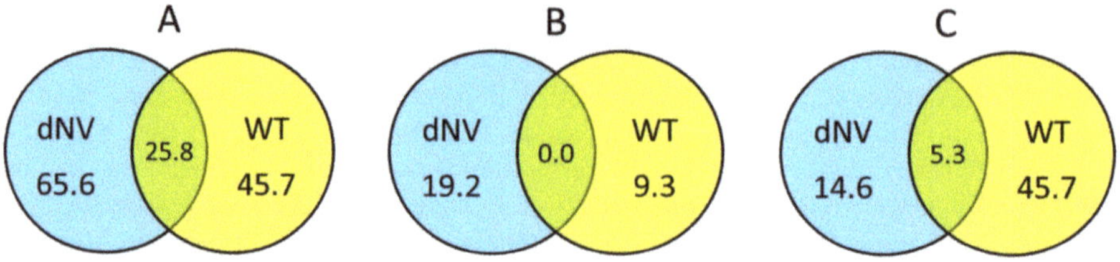

Figure 2. Venn diagrams showing the general transcriptomic relationships between trout injected with dNV-VHSV and wt-VHSV. Numbers indicate the percentage of upregulated (fold change, FC ≥ 1.5, (**A**), downregulated (FC ≤ −1.5, (**B**), and non-regulated (−1.5 < FC < 1.5, (**C**) genes, 48 h after injection with dNV-VHSV and wt-VHSV.

Figure 2B displays Venn diagrams with downregulated genes (FC ≤ −1.5), which indicate that fish infected with dNV-VHSV downregulated more genes than fish infected with wt-VHSV (19.2% vs 9.3%, respectively). On the other hand, dNV-VHSV and wt-VHSV do not have any downregulated genes in common.

When the non-regulated gene transcript levels with folds −1.5 < FC < 1.5 (Figure 2C) were analysed by Venn diagrams, the trout infected with wt-VHSV had the highest number of non-regulated genes (45.7%), followed by dNV-VHSV (14.6%). The Venn diagram also showed that 5.3% of non-regulated genes were shared by wt-VHSV and dNV-VHSV.

2.3. dNV- and wt-VHSV Infection Effects on Trout Immune-Related Genes

A detailed study of the transcriptomic changes driven by wt-VHSV and dNV-VHSV at 48 hpi was conducted. A heatmap was generated with the FC of the genes grouped in the categories described in methods. In addition, individual genes were also correlated with the pathways (KEGG database) [32] in which they participate (Table 1).

Table 1. Pathways related to modulated genes by WT-VHSV and dNV-VHSV. The pathways were obtained from the KEGG database [32]. See also Figures 3 and 4 for correlation with the genes.

(a) Antigen processing and presentation (b) Apoptosis (c) B-cell receptor signalling (d) Chemokine signalling (e) Complement and coagulation cascades	(q) Th1 and Th2 cell differentiation (r) Th17 cell differentiation (s) TLR (Toll-like receptor) signalling (t) TNF (Tumour necrosis factor) signalling (u) Cytokine-cytokine receptor interaction
(f) ErbB (Erb-B2 Receptor Tyrosine Kinase 2) signalling	(v) PI3-Akt (phosphatidylinositol 3-kinase and Protein kinase B) signalling (w) FoxO (Forkhead box O)signalling
(g) IL-17 signalling	(x) Natural killer cell-mediated cytotoxicity
(h) Jak–Stat signalling (Janus kinase-Signal transducer and activator of transcription) (i) MAPK (Mitogen-Activated Protein Kinase) signalling (j) Necroptosis signalling (k) NF-kappa B signalling (Nuclear Factor kappa-light-chain-enhancer of activated B cells)	(y) cAMP (Cyclic adenosine 3′,5′-monophosphate) signalling (z) AMPK (AMP-activated protein kinase) signalling (aa) Cell adhesion molecules (bb) Proteasome (cc) Wnt (wingless-type MMTV integration site family) signalling
(l) NOD-like (nucleotide-binding oligomerization domain-like) receptor signalling	(dd) General transcription factors (ee) Hematopoietic cell lineage (ff) TGFb (Transforming growth factor beta) signalling
(m) p53 signalling (n) Protein processing in endoplasmic reticulum (o) RIG-I-like receptor signalling (p) T-cell receptor signalling	(gg) mTOR (mammalian target of rapamycin) signalling

2.3.1. Cytosolic Sensors

Upon infection, viruses are recognised by host receptors and cytosolic sensors that activate mechanisms (signalling molecules) involved in diverse cellular processes such as the antiviral immune response. The cytosolic sensors studied belong to different gene groups and signalling pathways (Figures 3 and 4, and Table 1, RIG-I-like, and NOD-like signalling). Among the genes involved in these pathways, *tnf*, *ifna*, *irf7*, and *dhx58* and *mavs* (Figure 3, IFN and TNFSF) were upregulated by wt-VHSV and slightly more by dNV-VHSV. *Mavs*, another important cytosolic sensor, was upregulated by dNV-VHSV but non-regulated by wt-VHSV. This fact could be due to the NV expression by wt-VHSV and might indicate that *mavs* would be more functional for starting an appropriate immune response against dNV-VSHV as vaccine virus. Other important signalling molecules are *traf2* and *traf3* (Figure 3, TNFSF), and they are also upregulated by dNV-VHSV and non-regulated by wt-VHSV. These findings also support that dNV-VHSV activates better than wt-VHSV at these stages.

2.3.2. IFN System

We studied different genes belonging to the IFN system and IFN-related group of genes that belong to different signalling pathways (Figure 3, IFN pathways, $n = 14$). Regarding the IFN group of genes (IFN, $n = 20$), wt-VHSV induced the upregulation of the lowest number of genes (35%) compared to dNV-VHSV (85%) (Figure 3, IFN). This fact might be due to an inhibitory effect driven by NV after its expression from wt-VHSV. Among the downregulated and non-regulated (basal) genes, we found *iip30*, *ifng1*, *ifng2*, *iip1*, *iip2*, *ifp58*, *ifp35*, *mavs*, *ifn1*, *ifn2*, and *ifn5* (Figure 3, IFN). On the other hand, the expressions of *dhx58*, *hep*, *ifn3*, *ifna*, *irf1*, *irf7*, and *ifn4* were upregulated by wt-VHSV. Thus, some of them (i.e., *dhx58*, *hep*, *irf7*, *ifn3*) were even more upregulated by dNV-VHSV, probably due to the lack of the NV protein. The NV protein expressed by wt-VHSV induced the non-regulation of *mx2* and *mx3*, whereas *mx1* was slightly upregulated. The results also showed that all *mx* genes were upregulated by dNV-VHSV (Figure 3, MX). Mx proteins are implicated in the antiviral interferon-mediated response. In summary, in contrast to wt-VHSV, dNV-VHSV improved the antiviral immune response based on interferons (and related molecules), which would support its use as a potential live vaccine.

2.3.3. TNF Superfamily and Caspases

This gene group is comprised of molecules with diverse functionality that participate in several signalling pathways ($n = 20$, Figure 3 TNFSF, and Table 1). Most of the 16 TNF superfamily genes (*tnfsf*) studied here were upregulated (75%) by dNV-VHSV, whereas wt-VHSV induced a lower upregulation (50%) of these genes (Figure 3, TNFSF). The *tnfsf* genes upregulated by dNV-VHSV but downregulated or non-regulated by wt-VHSV were *balm*, *tnfd* (decoy), *tnfdr* (decoy receptor), *tnfr*, *tnfsf10*, *tnfsf13*, *tnfsf14*, and *tnfsf6* (Figure 3, TNFSF), which participate in several multipaths (Figure 3, TNFSF, Table 1). The *balm* gene is closely related to *tnfsf13b* (BAFF) and *tnfsf13* (APRIL) genes, and seems to be unique to teleost [33]. The *balm* gene has a constitutive expression in adult trout, mainly in the spleen, lymphocytes, posterior kidney, and anterior kidney and, therefore, *balm* has been assigned an immunological role [33]. The *tnfsf6* (FAS ligand, FASL) and *tnfsf13* (APRIL) genes modulate ligand-induced apoptosis [34]. In addition, *tnfsf10* (or TRAIL) is an inductor of apoptosis acting through *casp3* and *casp8*. Among the upregulated genes induced by wt- and dNV-VHSV injection were *tnfsf14* (stimulator of apoptosis), *tnf* (most important inducer of systemic inflammation), and *ltb1/ltb2* (involved in proliferation, differentiation, survival, and growth). Another member of TNFSF gene group is *tnfaip3* (A20 protein), which is upregulated in trout infected with wt-VHSV and downregulated in those infected with dNV-VHSV. Previous studies showed that A20 inhibited NF-kappa B and apoptosis [35,36] and our results support that dNV-VHSV would promote NF-kappa B signalling in order to set up a successful immune response.

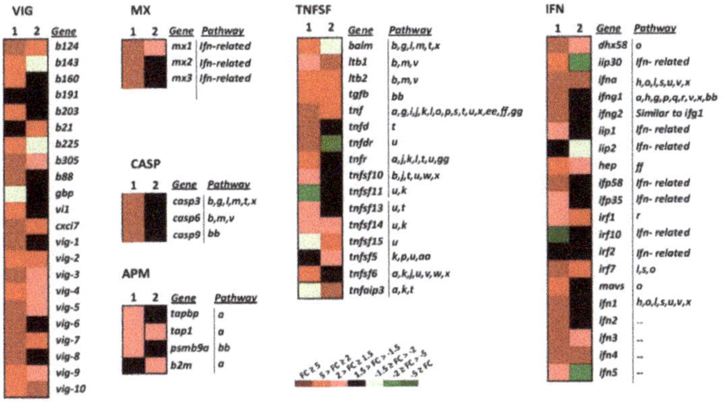

Figure 3. Heatmap showing the transcriptional expression fold changes (FCs) of the selected gene groups VHSV-induced (VIG), myxovirus resistance proteins (MX), caspases (CASP), tumour necrosis factor superfamily (TNFSF), interferon (IFN), and antigen-presenting machinery (APM) induced by dNV-VHSV and wt-VHSV in infected trout. *Gene* denotes names, and the *Pathway* column correlates with Table 1. –, unassigned pathway. Column 1, dNV-VHSV, each box corresponds to the average FC from four trout. Column 2, wt-VHSV, each box corresponds to the average FC from four trout. VIG group: b191 (c-lectin, AF483535), vig-1 (AF076620), vig-2 (AF290477), vig-3 (AF483529), vig-4 (AF483530), vig-5 (clone B17), vig-6 (clone B126), vig-7 (AF483527), vig-8 (clone B68), vig-9 (AF483533), vig-10 (AF483534), b203 (AF483538), b143 (AF483539), b225 (AF483540), b88 (AF483541), b160 (AF483545), b124 (AF483546), b305 (AF483542), cxci7 (VHSV induced protein 7 (vig7)), vi1 (VHSV induced protein 1), gbp (guanylate-binding protein GTPase, b21 (CD9, AF483544)). MX group: mx1 (myxovirus resistance 1), mx2 (myxovirus resistance 2), mx3 (myxovirus resistance 3). CASP group: casp3 (caspase 3), casp6 (caspase 6), casp9 (caspase 9). TNFSF group: balm (BAFF and APRIL-like molecule), ltb1 (lymphotoxin beta 1), ltb2 (lymphotoxin beta 2), tgfb (tumour growth factor beta), tnf (tumour necrosis factor alpha), tnfd (tumour necrosis factor decoy), tnfdr (tumour necrosis factor decoy receptor), tnfr (tumour necrosis factor receptor), tnfsf10 (tumour necrosis factor superfamily 10), tnfsf11 (tumour necrosis factor superfamily 11), tnfsf13 (tumour necrosis factor superfamily 13), tnfsf14 (tumour necrosis factor superfamily 14), tnfsf15 (tumour necrosis factor superfamily 15), tnfsf5 (tumour necrosis factor superfamily 5 (CD40)), tnfsf6 (tumour necrosis factor superfamily 6), tnfaip3 (tumour necrosis factor alpha-induced protein 3). IFN group: dhx58 (RIG-I-like receptor LGP2), iip30 (interferon gamma inducible protein 30), ifna (interferon alpha), ifng1 (interferon gamma 1), ifng2 (interferon gamma 2), iip1 (interferon inducible protein 1), iip2 (interferon inducible protein 2), hep (hepcidin), ifp58 (interferon-induced protein 58), ifp35 (interferon-induced protein 35), irf1 (interferon regulatory factor 1), irf10 (interferon regulatory factor 10), irf2 (interferon regulatory factor 2), irf7 (interferon regulatory factor 7), mavs (mitochondrial antiviral signalling protein), ifn1 (type 1 interferon 1), ifn2 (type 1 interferon 2), ifn3 (type 1 interferon 3), ifn4 (type 1 interferon 4), ifn5 (type 1 interferon 5). APM group: tapbp (tapasin (TAP binding protein)), tap1 (transporter associated with antigen processing 1), psmb9a (proteasome subunit type 9), b2m (beta-2 microglobulin).

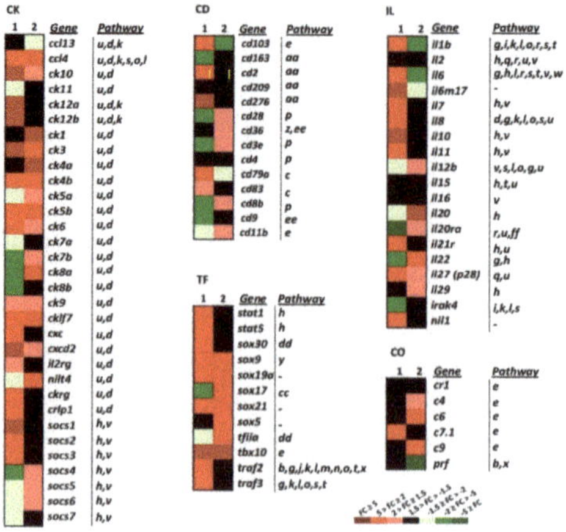

Figure 4. Heatmap showing the transcriptional expression fold changes (FCs) of the selected gene groups cytokines (CK), interleukins (IL), cluster of differentiation antigens (CD), complement (CO) and transcription factor (TF), induced by dNV-VHSV and wt-VHSV. *Gene* denotes names, and the *Pathway* column correlates with Table 1. –, unassigned pathway. Column 1, dNV-VHSV, each box corresponds to the average FC from four trout. Column2, wt-VHSV, each box corresponds to the average FC from four trout. CK group: ccl13 (cc-chemokine 13), ccl4 (cc-chemokine 4), ck10 (cc-chemokine 10), ck11 (cc-chemokine 11), ck12a (cc-chemokine 12a), ck12b (cc-chemokine 12b), ck1 (cc-chemokine 1), ck3 (cc-chemokine 3), ck4a (cc-chemokine 4a), ck4b (cc-chemokine 4b), ck5a (cc-chemokine 5a), ck5b (cc-chemokine 5b), ck6 (cc-chemokine 6), ck7a (cc-chemokine 7a), ck7b (cc-chemokine 7b), ck8a (cc-chemokine 8a), ck8b (cc-chemokine 8b), ck9 (cc-chemokine 9), cklf7 (chemokine-like factor superfamily member 7), cxc (α-chemokines), cxcd2 (cxc d2 chemokine), il2rg (il2 receptor gamma), nilt4 (novel immunoglobulin-like transcript 4 (FM200774.1)), ckrg (cytokine receptor gamma), crlp1 (chemokine receptor-like protein 1 (AJ620468.1)), socs1 (suppressor of cytokine signalling 1), socs2 (suppressor of cytokine signalling 2), socs3 (suppressor of cytokine signalling 3), socs4 (suppressor of cytokine signalling 4), socs5 (suppressor of cytokine signalling 5), socs6 (suppressor of cytokine signalling 6), socs7 (suppressor of cytokine signalling 7). IL group (r means receptor): il1b, il2, il6, il6m17, il7, il8, il10, il12b, il15, il16, il20, il20ra, il21r, il22, il27 (p28 subunit), il29, Irak4 (interleukin-1 receptor-associated kinase 4), nil1 (novel il-1 cytokine family member). CD group: cd103, cd163, cd2, cd209, cd276, cd28, cd36, cd3e (epsilon), cd4, d79a, cd83, cd8b (beta), cd9. CO group: cr1 (complement receptor type 1), c4 (complement component 4), c6 (complement component 6), c7.1 (complement component 7-1), c9 (complement component 9), prf (perforin). TF group: stat1 (signal transducer and activator of transcription 1), stat5 (signal transducer and activator of transcription 5), sox30 (SRY-related HMG box 30 gene family), sox9 (SRY-related HMG box 9 gene family), sox19a (SRY-related HMG box 19a gene family), sox17 (SRY-related HMG box 17 gene family), sox21 (SRY-related HMG box 21 gene family), sox5 (SRY-related HMG box 5 gene family), tfiia (transcription factor IIA), tbx10 (T-box 10 gene).

TNFs have a role as 'double-edged swords' in cellular proliferation, survival, differentiation or apoptosis. Ligands such as APRIL (*tnfsf13* gene), LIGHT (*tnfsf14* gene), RANKL (*tnfsf11* gene), LT-β (*ltb1*, *ltb2* genes), and CD40L (*tnfsf5* gene) bind to receptors with a TRAF-interacting motifs (TIM) domain, leading to the recruitment of TRAF molecules, and the activation of multiple signal transduction pathways such as NF-kappa B, Jun N-terminal kinase (JNK), p38, extracellular signal regulated kinase (ERK), and phosphoinositide-3 kinase (PI3K). On the other hand, ligands such as TNF-α (*tnf* gene), TRAIL (*tnfsf10* gene), FASL (*tnfsf6* gene), and decoy receptor have a dead domain (DD), which ultimately activates apoptosis through caspases. In summary, most of the *tnfsf* genes were upregulated by dNV-VHSV, giving rise to both activation signalling (NF-Kappa B, JNK, etc) and apoptosis signalling pathways.

Regarding the caspase group (Figure 3, CASP, and Table 1), the effector (*casp3, casp6*) and initiator (*casp9*) caspase genes were highly upregulated in the dNV-VHSV infected group while maintained at normal transcription levels in the wt-VHSV infected group. These results suggest that NV expressed by wt-VHSV impairs the upregulation and, consequently, the activation of apoptosis at 48 h post-infection (Figure 3, CASP). Moreover, the upregulation of the *casp* genes by dNV-VHSV promotes the activation of different pathways in which they participate, supporting an appropriate immune response developed by dNV-VHSV.

2.3.4. Antigen Presentation

Among the antigen presenting machinery (APM, $n = 4$) genes studied, TAPASIN (*tapbp*) and proteasome subunit (*psmb9a*) were non-regulated genes, whereas *tap1* and *b2m* were upregulated in wt-VHSV (Figure 3, APM). The APM genes belong to innate and adaptive immune responses. They act within the proteasome for peptide generation (*psmb9a*) and the transport of peptides (*tapbp, tap1*) into the endoplasmic reticulum. MHC (Major histocompatibility complex) class I molecules (together with *b2m*) bind these antigenic peptides to present them to CD8+ T-lymphocytes. Other genes belonging to TNFSF and IFN groups are also implicated in the antigen presentation signalling pathway (Figure 3). Overall, the results indicated that dNV-VHSV favoured the antigen processing and presentation in relation to wt-VHSV.

2.3.5. Cluster of Differentiation: B-Cell, T-Cell, and Cell-to-Cell Interactions

Cluster of differentiation genes (CD) conform a functional heterogeneous group of genes that have been involved in cell adhesion, B-cell receptor signalling, T-cell receptor signalling, complement and coagulation cascades, and hematopoietic markers (Figure 4 CD, and Table 1). In this study, 14 CD genes have been analysed. Downregulated and non-regulated CD genes (CD, $n = 5$ genes, Figure 4 CD) were found in the wt-VHSV dataset. The downregulated genes by wt-VHSV were *cd103* (a marker of dendritic cells) [37] and *cd79a* (associated with membrane-bound immunoglobulin in B-cells). On the other hand, the non-regulated genes in wt-VHSV were *cd2* (implicated in the adhesion T cell-APC through the *CD58* protein), *cd276* (participating in the regulation of the T-cell-mediated immune response), *cd83* (involved in the regulation of antigen presentation) [38], and *cd163* (exclusively expressed in monocytes and macrophages in humans), which was downregulated by dNV-VHSV. Some of the CD markers were found upregulated by dNV-VHSV (*cd103, cd2, cd276, cd279, cd83*) and others upregulated by wt-VHSV (*cd28, cd36, cd3e, cd83, cd11*). This fact might indicate that 48 hpi is a too short time to observe adaptive cellular responses against VHSV.

2.3.6. Cytokines: Chemokines and Interleukins

Among the chemoattractant cytokines or chemokines genes (CK, $n = 32$), 53% were upregulated by wt-VHSV, whereas dNV-VHSV induced the upregulation by 50%. The chemokines showing downregulated or non-regulated fold changes by wt-VHSV were *ccl13, ck11, ck12a, ck12b, ck8b, cxc, ckrg, crlp1*, suppressor of cytokine 1 (*socs1*), *socs2*, *socs3*, and *socs7* (Figure 4, CK). In addition, dNV-VHSV induced the downregulation or non-regulation of the chemokines *ccl13* (basal), *ck1, ck4a, ck5a, ck7a, ck7b, ck8a, ck11, nilt4, socs4*, and *socs5*. Chemokines have different roles in the coordination of the immune response and may promote the activation or inhibition of different pathways (Figure 4 IL, Table 1), and for the most of them their function is unknown on the basis of viral infections.

Previous studies in rainbow trout have shown that recombinant CK1 has an attractant effect for blood leukocytes) [39]. In addition, CK6 is a chemoattractant for mature macrophages from the RTS11 rainbow trout monocyte-macrophage cell line and may also induce interleukin 8 (IL-8), inducible nitric oxide synthase (iNOS), and the CD-18 integrin in these cells, revealing additional immunomodulatory effects [40]. The capacity of trout recombinant CK12 to attract splenocytes has also been reported, establishing that IgM + B cells were one of the target cells recruited [41]. In the present study, CK1, CK6 and CK12 are upregulated by dNV-VHSV in relation to wt-VHSV. Regarding the interleukin genes group (IL, n = 20), the transcriptomic profile obtained after wt-VHSV injection was different from that of dNV-VHSV. Wild-type VHSV downregulated important pleiotropic pro- and anti-inflammatory interleukins such as *il1b*, *il6*, and its related *il6m17* (Figure 4, IL). On the contrary, interleukins *il1*, *il6*, *il6m7*, *il7*, *il8*, *il11*, *il21r*, *il27* and *nil1* were upregulated by dNV-VHSV. These interleukins have a key role in immune pathways (Figure 4 IL, Table 1) and their upregulation are required for an effective immune response followed vaccination, suggesting that dNV-VHSV could be an effective attenuated live vaccine.

2.3.7. General Transcription Factors

This group of genes (TF, n = 10 selected genes, Figure 4) are implicated in important cellular processes and pathways: Jak–Stat signalling (*stat1*, *stat5*), general transcription factors and regulatory elements (*sox* genes), and multipath genes previously mentioned (*traf2*, *traf3*). In the dNV-VHSV-injected trout, all the TF selected genes were upregulated except for *sox5* (non-regulated) and *tfiia* (downregulated). In wt-VHSV, all the genes studied were upregulated except for *traf2*, *traf3*, *sox30*, *stat5* and *stat1*, which were non-upregulated. These data reflected that Jak–Stat signalling pathway is upregulated by dNV-VHSV, which in turn promoted interferon responses leading to an improved antiviral stage.

2.3.8. Complement and VIG Genes

Among complement genes studied (CO, n = 6, Figure 4), the trout injected with dNV-VHSV maintained most of the genes non-regulated and only one was upregulated. It is interesting to note that C9 was upregulated by wt-VHSV, whereas perforin (*prf*) was downregulated by the same virus.

VHSV-induced genes (VIG, n = 22) were firstly identified by subtractive hybridisation performed in a previous work [42]. We found that NV from wt-VHSV inhibited the upregulation of 50% of all *vig* genes (*b143*, *b160*, *b191*, *b203*, *b225*, *b88*, *gbp*, *vi1*, *vig-1*, *vig-6*, *vig-8*) while these genes were upregulated in dNV-VHSV, except for *b191* and *gbp* (Figure 3, VIG). Viperin (*vig1*) is expressed by mitochondria and is an IFN-inducible protein that inhibits the replication of a variety of viruses [43]. In addition, *vig-2* [44], *vig-3*, *vig-4*, *vig5*, and probably *vig-6* are also induced by interferon [42]. On the other hand, *vig-7*, *vig-8*, *vig-9* have chemoattractant function, *vig-9* also has an apoptotic function, and *vig-10* is related to apoptosis and transcription repression [42].

The present study is the first one describing the trout transcriptomic profile driven by dNV-VHSV. There are scarce studies regarding whole gene effects upon VHSV infection in trout, the most relevant to our study is the characterization of the RNA microarray profile in olive flounder liver after VHSV infection by immersion [20]. Regarding the role of immune-related genes, we found that both wt-VHSV and dNV-VHSV induced an upregulation of hepcidin, (a regulator of the iron metabolism that is implicated in inflammatory processes) in trout similar to the results observed in VHSV infected olive flounder. However, the *irf2* gene was found non-regulated in the wt-VHSV injected trout, which differs from the upregulation found in olive flounder .The differences found between trout and olive flounder could be due to the expression profile of immune response genes in spleen/head kidney, which could be slightly different from those in liver.

Another recent study determined the miRNA expression profile after VHSV infection. Among the immunity-associated target genes of 63 differentially expressed miRNA after VHSV infection of olive flounder, the authors described IL (*il1b*, *il8*, *il10*), *mx*, interferon regulatory factors (*irf3*, *irf5*, *irf7*), TNF (*tnfsf*), and heat shock proteins (*hsp10*, *hsp60*, *hsp70*, *hsp90*) [45]. For instance, *mx* mRNA was regulated by one miRNA (pol-miR-1388-5p) only, for which the highest expression was at 0 hpi and the lowest at 72 hpi. At 48 hpi, the *mx* expression was not modulated by this miRNA. Our data in trout showed a non-regulation of *mx* at 48h after wt-VSHV injection, being coincident with those of miRNA in olive flounder. Maybe in the future, a correlation between miRNA and mRNA expression levels could be established in infected VHSV fish, as it has been done for some miRNAs in primary human osteoblasts from healthy individuals [46].

2.4. Modulated Pathways in dNV- and wt-VHSV-Injected Trout using GSEA

To define the impact of dNV-VHSV or wt-VHSV when targeting different pathways or gene sets (GS) in head kidney/spleen, we used the Gene-Set Enrichment Analysis (GSEA) program. Briefly, 51 trout GS collection previously defined [25] were used to obtain normalised enrichment scores (NES). The GS were then classified according to their NES values, as follows: (1) upregulation in dNV-VHSV in relation to wt-VHSV ($n = 19$), and (2) no regulation in dNV-VHSV in relation to wt-VHSV (Figure 5). Among the upregulated GS in dNV-VHSV in relation to wt-VHSV (Figure 5A), higher differences were found in those corresponding to "Protein processing in endoplasmic reticulum", "Regulation of autophagy", and "Autoimmune thyroid disease" (> 2 to 4-fold) (Figure 5A, red lines and symbols). Other GSs which showed lower improvement of upregulations with dNV-VHSV were those implicated in anti-viral interferon networks ("Toll-like receptor signalling pathway", "Toll-like receptor wikipathway", "Type II interferon signalling (IFNG)"), inflammation ("TNFa NF-kappa B signalling", "Cytokine inflammatory response pathway"), recognition of nucleic acids ("Cytosolic DNA sensing pathway", "RIG-I-like receptor signalling"), viral- and bacterial-caused diseases ("Hepatitis C", "Influenza A", "Measles", "Herpes simplex infection", "Epithelial cell *Helicobacter pylori*"), and others ("NF-kappa B signalling pathway", "T cell receptor signalling pathway", "Natural killer cell mediated cytotoxicity-K", "Interleukin 5"). The remaining GSs showed no differences between dNV-VHSV and wt-VHSV (Figure 5B). The "Type II IFN signalling (IFNG)" pathway was one of the top enriched GS found in VHSV survivor zebrafish [47], indicating that both species share similar mechanisms to fight VHSV. Other improved pathways in dNV-VHSV such as "Toll-like receptor signalling", "RIG-I-like receptor signalling", "Natural killer cell-mediated cytotoxicity", "Hepatitis C", and "Influenza A and Measles" were among the most targeted pathways in SVCV zebrafish infections [48]. Finally, "NF-kappa B signalling pathway", "Toll-like receptor wikipathway", "Natural killer cell mediated cytotoxicity", "RIG-I-like receptor signalling", "Autoimmune thyroid disease", "Influenza A", and "Herpes simplex infection" were also modulated in trout when injected with thyroid hormone analogues [25]. All the above-mentioned pathways participated in generating resistance to fish viral infections and underlined the importance that their upregulation by dNV-VHSV might have in case this defective virus is used as a potential attenuated live vaccine.

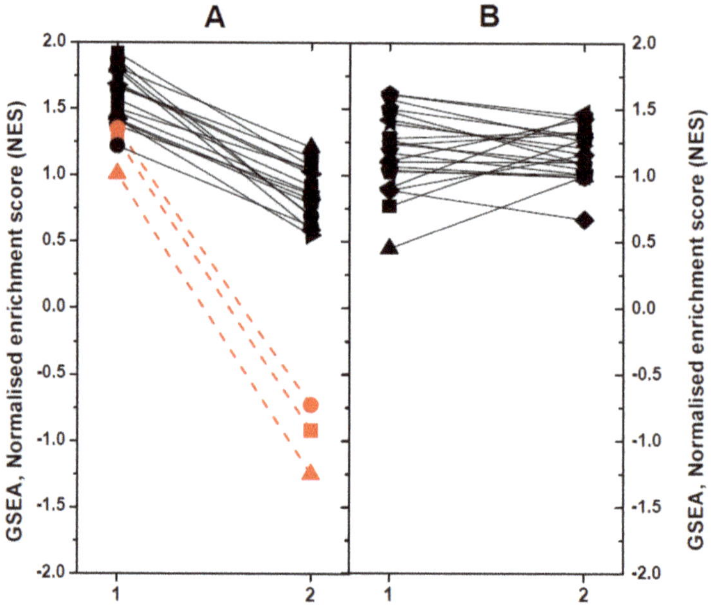

Figure 5. Comparison of significant normalised enrichment scores (NESs) of rainbow trout gene-sets (GSs) by Gene-Set Enrichment Analysis (GSEA). X axis: 1, dNV-VHSV. 2, wt-VHSV. Trout GSs were obtained from the KEGG (-K) and WIKI (-W) pathway databases as described before [25]. For comparative purposes, the NESs calculated by GSEA were represented in a diagram by linking the results obtained with lines. For better clarity, the results were not individually identified by GS. (**A**) GS which show upregulation in dNV-VHSV in relation to wt-VHSV: Toll-like receptor wikipathway-W, Hepatitis C-K, Toll-like receptor signalling pathway-W, RIG-I-like receptor signalling-K, Influenza A-K, Type II interferon signalling (IFNG)-W, Measles-K, NF-kappa B signalling pathway-K, TNFa NF-kappa B signalling-W, Herpes simplex infection-K, Epithelial cell *Helicobacter pylori*-K, T cell receptor signalling pathway-K, Cytosolic DNA sensing pathway-K, Natural killer cell mediated cytotoxicity-K, Interleukin 5-W, Cytokine inflammatory response pathway-W. The most upregulated pathways by dNV-VHSV in relation to wt-VHSV were: Red circle, Autoimmune thyroid disease-K; Red square, Regulation of autophagy-K; and Red triangle, Protein processing in endoplasmic reticulum-K. (**B**) GS which showed no regulation in relation to wt-VHSV: Interferon type I-W, Interferon alpha beta signalling-W, Apoptosis modulation by HSP70-W, B-cell receptor signalling pathway-W, EGFR1 signalling pathway-W, MAPK signalling pathway-K, Interleukin 6-W, Ubiquitin mediated proteolysis-K, TSH signalling pathway-W, Antigen processing and presentation-K, MAPK signalling pathway-W, Interleukin 2-W, HTLV-K, androgen receptor signalling-W, TP53 network signalling-W, AHR pathway-W, Interleukin 3-W, Hematopoietic cell lineages-K, T-cell receptor pathway-W, JAK–STAT signalling pathway-K, PI3K–AKT signalling pathway-K, FGF signalling pathway-W.

3. Conclusions

The results presented in this study support the hypothesis that dNV-VHSV can be considered an attenuated virus and a potential live vaccine, based on the fact that many critical host gene pathways are activated upon infection. On the contrary, NV expressed at first stages of infection by wt-VHSV modulates the expression levels of interferons, VIG, chemokines, CD, transcription factors, and other immune-related genes, leading to an immune unresponsiveness state that interferes with the early innate immune response. Importantly, this work opens new avenues for the use of NV-deleted novirhabdoviruses as a tool to study the regulation of immune pathways in other teleost fish.

Author Contributions: Experimental design, E.G.C. and J.M.C.; Methodology, B.C., P.E., J.M.C., and E.G.C.; Formal analysis, E.G.C.; Original draft preparation, B.C. and E.G.C; Writing—review and editing, B.C., P.E., and E.G.C.; Funding acquisition, J.M.C. and E.G.C. All authors have read and agreed to the published version of the manuscript.

Funding: This research was partially funded by the Ministry of Science, Innovation and Universities of Spain grants AGL2014-51773-C3-3 and AGL2017-85494-C2-2-R, and the APC was funded by Ministry of Science, Innovation and Universities of Spain grant AGL2017-85494-C2-2-R.

Acknowledgments: Authors are in debt to Dr. Rosario Fernández-Godino for her helpful comments.

Conflicts of Interest: Authors declare that they have no conflict of interest.

References

1. Nishizawa, T.; Iida, H.; Takano, R.; Isshiki, T.; Nakajima, K.; Muroga, K. Genetic relatedness among Japanese, American and European isolates of viral hemorrhagic septicemia virus (VHSV) based on partial G and P genes. *Dis. Aquat. Org.* **2002**, *48*, 143–148. [CrossRef] [PubMed]
2. Schutze, H.; Enzmann, P.J.; Kuchling, R.; Mundt, E.; Niemann, H.; Mettenleiter, T.C. Complete genomic sequence of the fish rhabdovirus infectious haematopoietic necrosis virus. *J. Gen. Virol.* **1995**, *76*, 2519–2527. [CrossRef] [PubMed]
3. Schutze, H.; Mundt, E.; Mettenleiter, T.C. Complete genomic sequence of viral hemorrhagic septicemia virus, a fish rhabdovirus. *Virus Genes* **1999**, *19*, 59–65. [CrossRef] [PubMed]
4. Skall, H.F.; Olesen, N.J.; Mellergaard, S. Viral haemorrhagic septicaemia virus in marine fish and its implications for fish farming - a review. *J. Fish Dis.* **2005**, *28*, 509–529. [CrossRef] [PubMed]
5. Brudeseth, B.E.; Evensen, O. Occurrence of viral haemorrhagic septicaemia virus (VHSV) in wild marine fish species in the coastal regions of Norway. *Dis. Aquat. Org.* **2002**, *52*, 21–28. [CrossRef] [PubMed]
6. Chinchilla, B.; Encinas, P.; Estepa, A.; Coll, J.M.; Gomez-Casado, E. Transcriptome analysis of rainbow trout in response to non-virion (NV) protein of viral haemorrhagic septicaemia virus (VHSV). *Appl. Microbiol. Biotechnol.* **2015**, *99*, 1827–1843. [CrossRef]
7. Wahli, T.; Bergmann, S.M. Viral haemorrhagic septicaemia (VHS): Detection, distribution and combat. *Cab. Rev: Persp. Agric. Vet. Sci. Nutr. Nat. Resour.* **2011**, *6*, 1–10. [CrossRef]
8. Kurath, G.; Leong, J.C. Characterization of infectious hematopoietic necrosis virus mRNA species reveals a nonvirion rhabdovirus protein. *J. Virol.* **1985**, *53*, 462–468. [CrossRef]
9. Schutze, H.; Enzmann, P.J.; Mundt, E.; Mettenleiter, T.C. Identification of the non-virion (NV) protein of fish rhabdoviruses viral haemorrhagic septicaemia virus and infectious haematopoietic necrosis virus. *J. Gen. Virol.* **1996**, *77*, 1259–1263. [CrossRef]
10. Einer-Jensen, K.; Ahrens, P.; Lorenzen, N. Parallel phylogenetic analyses using the N, G or Nv gene from a fixed group of VHSV isolates reveal the same overall genetic typing. *Dis. Aquat. Org.* **2005**, *67*, 39–45. [CrossRef]
11. Kurath, G.; Higman, K.H.; Björklund, H.V. Distribution and variation of NV genes in fish rhabdoviruses. *J. Gen. Virol.* **1997**, *78*, 113–117. [CrossRef] [PubMed]
12. Biacchesi, S.; Thoulouze, M.I.; Bearzotti, M.; Yu, Y.X.; Bremont, M. Recovery of NV knockout infectious hematopoietic necrosis virus expressing foreign genes. *J. Virol.* **2000**, *74*, 11247–11253. [CrossRef] [PubMed]
13. Biacchesi, S.; Lamoureux, A.; Merour, E.; Bernard, J.; Bremont, M. Limited interference at the early stage of infection between two recombinant novirhabdoviruses: Viral hemorrhagic septicemia virus and infectious hematopoietic necrosis virus. *J. Virol.* **2010**, *84*, 10038–10050. [CrossRef] [PubMed]
14. Thoulouze, M.I.; Bouguyon, E.; Carpentier, C.; Bremont, M. Essential role of the NV protein of Novirhabdovirus for pathogenicity in rainbow trout. *J. Virol.* **2004**, *78*, 4098–4107. [CrossRef] [PubMed]
15. Kim, M.S.; Kim, K.H. Effects of NV gene knock-out recombinant viral hemorrhagic septicemia virus (VHSV) on Mx gene expression in *Epithelioma papulosum cyprini* (EPC) cells and olive flounder (*Paralichthys olivaceus*). *Fish Shellfish Immunol.* **2012**, *32*, 459–463. [CrossRef]
16. Alonso, M.; Kim, C.H.; Johnson, M.C.; Pressley, M.; Leong, J.A. The NV gene of snakehead rhabdovirus (SHRV) is not required for pathogenesis, and a heterologous glycoprotein can be incorporated into the SHRV envelope. *J. Virol.* **2004**, *78*, 5875–5882. [CrossRef]

17. Johnson, M.C.; Simon, B.E.; Kim, C.H.; Leong, J.A. Production of recombinant snakehead rhabdovirus: The NV protein is not required for viral replication. *J. Virol.* **2000**, *74*, 2343–2350. [CrossRef]
18. Choi, M.K.; Moon, C.H.; Ko, M.S.; Lee, U.H.; Cho, W.J.; Cha, S.J.; Do, J.W.; Heo, G.J.; Jeong, S.G.; Hahm, Y.S.; et al. A nuclear localization of the infectious haematopoietic necrosis virus NV protein is necessary for optimal viral growth. *PLoS ONE* **2011**, *6*, e22362. [CrossRef]
19. Ammayappan, A.; Vakharia, V.N. Nonvirion protein of novirhabdovirus suppresses apoptosis at the early stage of virus infection. *J. Virol.* **2011**, *85*, 8393–8402. [CrossRef]
20. Cho, H.K.; Kim, J.; Moon, J.Y.; Nam, B.H.; Kim, Y.O.; Kim, W.J.; Park, J.Y.; An, C.M.; Cheong, J.; Kong, H.J. Microarray analysis of gene expression in olive flounder liver infected with viral haemorrhagic septicaemia virus (VHSV). *Fish Shellfish Immunol.* **2016**, *49*, 66–78. [CrossRef]
21. Hwang, J.Y.; Kwon, M.G.; Seo, J.S.; Do, J.W.; Park, M.A.; Jung, S.H.; Ahn, S.J. Differentially expressed genes after viral haemorrhagic septicaemia virus infection in olive flounder (Paralichthys olivaceus). *Vet. Microbiol.* **2016**, *193*, 72–82. [CrossRef] [PubMed]
22. Kim, M.S.; Kim, K.H. Protection of olive flounder, Paralichthys olivaceus, against viral hemorrhagic septicemia virus (VHSV) by immunization with NV gene-knockout recombinant VHSV. *Aquaculture* **2011**, *314*, 39–43. [CrossRef]
23. De Kinkelin, P.; LeBerre, M. Isolament d'un rhabdovirus pathogéne de la truite fario (*Salmo trutta L.*,1766). *C R Acad. Sci. Hebd. Seances Acad. Sci. D* **1977**, *284*, 101–104. (in French). [PubMed]
24. Ballesteros, N.A.; Saint-Jean, S.S.; Encinas, P.A.; Perez-Prieto, S.I.; Coll, J.M. Oral immunization of rainbow trout to infectious pancreatic necrosis virus (IPNV) induces different immune gene expression profiles in head kidney and pyloric ceca. *Fish Shellfish Immunol* **2012**, *33*, 174–185. [CrossRef]
25. Quesada-Garcia, A.; Encinas, P.; Valdehita, A.; Baumann, L.; Segner, H.; Coll, J.M.; Navas, J.M. Thyroid active agents T3 and PTU differentially affect immune gene transcripts in the head kidney of rainbow trout (*Oncorhynchus mykiss*). *Aquat. Toxicol.* **2016**, *174*, 159–168. [CrossRef]
26. Salem, M.; Kenney, P.B.; Rexroad, C.E.; Yao, J. Development of a 37 k high-density oligonucleotide microarray: A new tool for functional genome research in rainbow trout. *J. Fish Biol.* **2008**, *72*, 2187–2206. [CrossRef]
27. Gene Expression Omnibus. Available online: https://www.ncbi.nlm.nih.gov/geo/query/acc.cgi?acc=GSE37330 (accessed on 29 January 2020).
28. Gene Expression Omnibus. Available online: http://www.ncbi.nlm.nih.gov/geo/query/acc.cgi?acc=GSE37797 (accessed on 29 January 2020).
29. GSEA - Broad Institute. Available online: http://www.broad.mit.edu/GSEA (accessed on 29 January 2020).
30. Subramanian, A.; Tamayo, P.; Mootha, V.K.; Mukherjee, S.; Ebert, B.L.; Gillette, M.A.; Paulovich, A.; Pomeroy, S.L.; Golub, T.R.; Lander, E.S.; et al. Gene set enrichment analysis: A knowledge-based approach for interpreting genome-wide expression profiles. *Proc. Natl. Acad. Sci. USA* **2005**, *102*, 15545–15550. [CrossRef]
31. Subramanian, A.; Kuehn, H.; Gould, J.; Tamayo, P.; Mesirov, J.P. GSEA-P: A desktop application for Gene Set Enrichment Analysis. *Bioinformatics* **2007**, *23*, 3251–3253. [CrossRef]
32. KEGG: Kyoto Encyclopedia of Genes and Genomes. Available online: http://www.kegg.jp (accessed on 29 January 2020).
33. Glenney, G.W.; Wiens, G.D. Early diversification of the TNF superfamily in teleosts: Genomic characterization and expression analysis. *J. Immunol.* **2007**, *178*, 7955–7973. [CrossRef]
34. Roth, W.; Wagenknecht, B.; Klumpp, A.; Naumann, U.; Hahne, M.; Tschopp, J.; Weller, M. APRIL, a new member of the tumor necrosis factor family, modulates death ligand-induced apoptosis. *Cell Death Differ.* **2001**, *8*, 403–410. [CrossRef]
35. De Valck, D.; Jin, D.Y.; Heyninck, K.; Van de Craen, M.; Contreras, R.; Fiers, W.; Jeang, K.T.; Beyaert, R. The zinc finger protein A20 interacts with a novel anti-apoptotic protein which is cleaved by specific caspases. *Oncogene* **1999**, *18*, 4182–4190. [CrossRef] [PubMed]
36. Kelly, C.; Shields, M.D.; Elborn, J.S.; Schock, B.C. A20 regulation of nuclear factor-kappaB: Perspectives for inflammatory lung disease. *Am. J. Respir. Cell Mol. Biol.* **2011**, *44*, 743–748. [CrossRef] [PubMed]
37. Zelante, T.; Wong, A.Y.; Ping, T.J.; Chen, J.; Sumatoh, H.R.; Vigano, E.; Hong Bing, Y.; Lee, B.; Zolezzi, F.; Fric, J.; et al. CD103(+) Dendritic Cells Control Th17 Cell Function in the Lung. *Cell Rep.* **2015**, *12*, 1789–1801. [CrossRef] [PubMed]

38. Chapoval, A.I.; Ni, J.; Lau, J.S.; Wilcox, R.A.; Flies, D.B.; Liu, D.; Dong, H.; Sica, G.L.; Zhu, G.; Tamada, K.; et al. B7-H3: A costimulatory molecule for T cell activation and IFN-gamma production. *Nat. Immunol.* **2001**, *2*, 269–274. [CrossRef]
39. Dixon, B.; Shum, B.; Adams, E.J.; Magor, K.E.; Hedrick, R.P.; Muir, D.G.; Parham, P. CK-1, a putative chemokine of rainbow trout (*Oncorhynchus mykiss*). *Immunol. Rev.* **1998**, *166*, 341–348. [CrossRef]
40. Montero, J.; Coll, J.; Sevilla, N.; Cuesta, A.; Bols, N.C.; Tafalla, C. Interleukin 8 and CK-6 chemokines specifically attract rainbow trout (*Oncorhynchus mykiss*) RTS11 monocyte-macrophage cells and have variable effects on their immune functions. *Dev. Comp. Immunol.* **2008**, *32*, 1374–1384. [CrossRef]
41. Montero, J.; Ordas, M.C.; Alejo, A.; Gonzalez-Torres, L.; Sevilla, N.; Tafalla, C. CK12, a rainbow trout chemokine with lymphocyte chemo-attractant capacity associated to mucosal tissues. *Mol. Immunol.* **2011**, *48*, 1102–1113. [CrossRef]
42. O'Farrell, C.; Vaghefi, N.; Cantonnet, M.; Buteau, B.; Boudinot, P.; Benmansour, A. Survey of transcript expression in rainbow trout leukocytes reveals a major contribution of interferon-responsive genes in the early response to a rhabdovirus infection. *J. Virol.* **2002**, *76*, 8040–8049. [CrossRef]
43. Seo, J.; Yaneva, Y.R.; Cresswell, P. Viperin: A multifunctional, interferon-inducible protein that regulates virus replication. *Cell Host Microbe* **2011**, *10*, 534–539. [CrossRef]
44. Boudinot, P.; Salhi, S.; Blanco, M.; Benmansour, A. Viral haemorrhagic septicaemia virus induces vig-2, a new interferon-responsive gene in rainbow trout. *Fish Shellfish Immunol.* **2001**, *11*, 383–397. [CrossRef]
45. Najib, A.; Kim, M.S.; Choi, S.H.; Kang, Y.J.; Kim, K.H. Changes in microRNAs expression profile of olive flounder (*Paralichthys olivaceus*) in response to viral hemorrhagic septicemia virus (VHSV) infection. *Fish Shellfish Immunol.* **2016**, *51*, 384–391. [CrossRef] [PubMed]
46. Laxman, N.; Rubin, C.J.; Mallmin, H.; Nilsson, O.; Pastinen, T.; Grundberg, E.; Kindmark, A. Global miRNA expression and correlation with mRNA levels in primary human bone cells. *Rna* **2015**, *21*, 1433–1443. [CrossRef] [PubMed]
47. Estepa, A.; Coll, J. Innate Multigene Family Memories Are Implicated in the Viral-Survivor Zebrafish Phenotype. *PLoS ONE* **2015**, *10*, e0135483. [CrossRef] [PubMed]
48. Encinas, P.; Garcia-Valtanen, P.; Chinchilla, B.; Gomez-Casado, E.; Estepa, A.; Coll, J. Identification of multipath genes differentially expressed in pathway-targeted microarrays in zebrafish infected and surviving spring viremia carp virus (SVCV) suggest preventive drug candidates. *PLoS ONE* **2013**, *8*, e73553. [CrossRef] [PubMed]

vaccines

MDPI

Review

Current Progress of Avian Vaccines Against West Nile Virus

Nereida Jiménez de Oya, Estela Escribano-Romero, Ana-Belén Blázquez, Miguel A. Martín-Acebes and Juan-Carlos Saiz *

Department of Biotechnology, National Agricultural and Food Research and Technology Institute (INIA), 28040 Madrid, Spain; jdeoya@inia.es (N.J.d.O.); eescribano@inia.es (E.E.-R.); blazquez@inia.es (A.-B.B.); martin.mangel@inia.es (M.A.M.-A.)

* Correspondence: jcsaiz@inia.es; Tel.: +34-9-1347-1497

Received: 31 July 2019; Accepted: 19 September 2019; Published: 23 September 2019

Abstract: Birds are the main natural host of West Nile virus (WNV), the worldwide most distributed mosquito-borne flavivirus, but humans and equids can also be sporadic hosts. Many avian species have been reported as susceptible to WNV, particularly corvids. In the case that clinical disease develops in birds, this is due to virus invasion of different organs: liver, spleen, kidney, heart, and mainly the central nervous system, which can lead to death 24–48 h later. Nowadays, vaccines have only been licensed for use in equids; thus, the availability of avian vaccines would benefit bird populations, both domestic and wild ones. Such vaccines could be used in endangered species housed in rehabilitation and wildlife reserves, and in animals located at zoos and other recreational installations, but also in farm birds, and in those that are grown for hunting and restocking activities. Even more, controlling WNV infection in birds can also be useful to prevent its spread and limit outbreaks. So far, different commercial and experimental vaccines (inactivated, attenuated, and recombinant viruses, and subunits and DNA-based candidates) have been evaluated, with various regimens, both in domestic and wild avian species. However, there are still disadvantages that must be overcome before avian vaccination can be implemented, such as its cost-effectiveness for domestic birds since in many species the pathogenicity is low or zero, or the viability of being able to achieve collective immunity in wild birds in freedom. Here, a comprehensive review of what has been done until now in the field of avian vaccines against WNV is presented and discussed.

Keywords: birds; vaccines; West Nile virus; flavivirus; herd immunity

1. Introduction

Currently, the ecology of many pathogens is changing because of climate warming that is driving vector colonization of new geographical niches. This fact, together with human behavior and global trade, puts human and animal health at risk. An example is the (re)emergence of West Nile virus (WNV) that nowadays is the most worldwide distributed mosquito-borne flavivirus [1,2]. Since the introduction of a lineage 1 WNV strain in the US in 1999, the virus quickly spread, causing hundreds of deaths in humans and horses and a very high avian mortality [1,2]. More recently, the strains of lineage 2 colonized and spread throughout Europe, leading to outbreaks among wild birds [3] and being responsible for up to 1.875 human cases, including 115 deaths in 2018 [4].

WNV is a small (about 50 nm of diameter), spherical, enveloped flavivirus (*Flaviviridae* family) whose genome consists of a single-stranded RNA molecule of positive polarity that encodes three structural proteins and seven non-structural proteins [1]. Up to nine distinct genetic lineages of WNV have been described, with lineage 1 and 2 being the most distributed worldwide, although only a single serotype is recognized [1,5].

Birds are the main natural host of West Nile virus, though humans and equids can also be sporadically infected [1,2]. Hundreds of avian species have been reported as susceptible to WNV, particularly corvids (Corvidae), which can develop high levels of viremia [6,7], and are notable virus amplifiers [7–9], being, thus, important actors in the epidemiology of the virus [10–14]. Both domestic and wild avian species are susceptible to WNV infection and, in some cases, develop a WNV-associated disease that can lead to high mortality, as occurred during the US outbreak where crow populations declined alarmingly [14–17].

Currently, there is no antiviral therapy against WNV, and the licensed vaccines are only for use in equids [1,18,19]. The availability of avian vaccines would benefit bird populations, both domestic (like farm birds and those grown for restocking and hunting activities) and wild ones (mainly endangered species housed in rehabilitation and wildlife reserves, and birds located at recreational facilities like zoos). Avian vaccination may also help to prevent outbreaks and spread, mainly if herd immunity can be induced. Here, a comprehensive review of our current knowledge, about experimental avian vaccination with different candidates (inactivated, attenuated, and recombinant viruses, and subunit and DNA-based vaccines) in domestic and wild birds, is presented.

2. WNV Biology

2.1. Genome Organization

The genome of WNV is composed of a single-stranded positive-sense RNA (ssRNA(+)) of about 11 kb in length (Figure 1) [1]. It contains a 5′-cap structure (m(7)GpppAm) that is methylated at the guanine N-7 and the ribose 2′-OH positions of the first transcribed adenine [20] but lacks a 3′ polyA tail. The single open reading frame (ORF) is flanked by two untranslated regions (UTRs) with important functions for viral replication [21]. Remarkably, the 3′ UTR is a key determinant of WNV virulence, which makes it attractive for vaccine design [22]. The ORF is translated into a polyprotein that is co-translational and post-translationally cleaved by viral and cellular proteases. The structural capsid (C) protein is involved in the nucleocapsid formation by association with the genomic RNA, the M is produced by cleavage of the prM, and the E is involved in receptor binding, viral entry, and membrane fusion [23]. The non-structural NS2B is the membrane anchor and the co-activator of the NS3 viral serine protease. The NS1 is secreted and has been related to replication, virulence, immunomodulation, and pathogenesis [24]. The NS5 exhibits the methyltransferase activity required for capping of viral RNA and is also the RNA-dependent RNA polymerase in charge of genome replication [21]. Replication of WNV is associated with intracellular membranes of the Endoplasmic Reticulum (ER) [25]. Accordingly, NS2A, NS2B, NS4A, and NS4B are multipass transmembrane proteins. The ER is the place for viral replication and particle biogenesis. The newly assembled immature particles are produced by budding into the lumen of this organelle and traffic across the secretory pathway. Viral particles maturate towards infectious virions by proteolytic processing of the prM to render the M protein. This cleavage takes place inside the *trans*-Golgi network and is catalyzed by the cellular protease furin [23]. Maturation converts the spiky immature particles [26] into smooth mature virions [27] that are released from the cell by exocytosis.

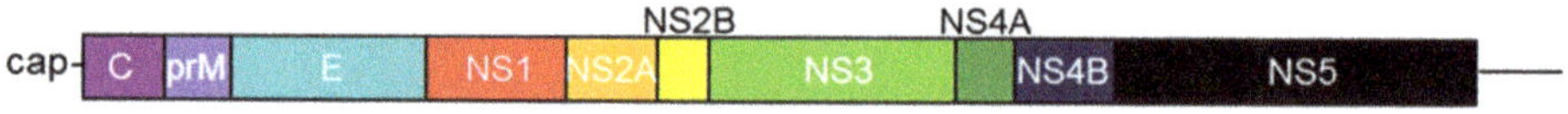

Figure 1. Genome organization. Schematic representation of the WNV (West Nile virus) genome. See text for details.

2.2. Molecular Classification and Phylogeny

WNV is a member of the *Flavivirus* genus, within the *Flaviviridae* family. WNV classification was initially based on cross-neutralization reactions, locating it as a member of the Japanese encephalitis virus (JEV) serocomplex. Later on, the molecular phylogeny analyses supported this antigenic classification and revealed the existence of up to nine distinct genetic lineages of WNV (Figure 2), being lineage 1 and 2 the most worldwide distributed [5]. Lineage 2 was restricted to Africa until recently when it was isolated for the first time in Europe from a goshawk in Hungary in 2004 [28]. Since then, lineage 2 strains have been isolated in mosquitoes, humans, and several domestic and wild birds across the continent [29–31]. In any case, despite this genomic variability, there is only a single WNV serotype described, which could facilitate the development of unique vaccines to protect against all WNV genotypes.

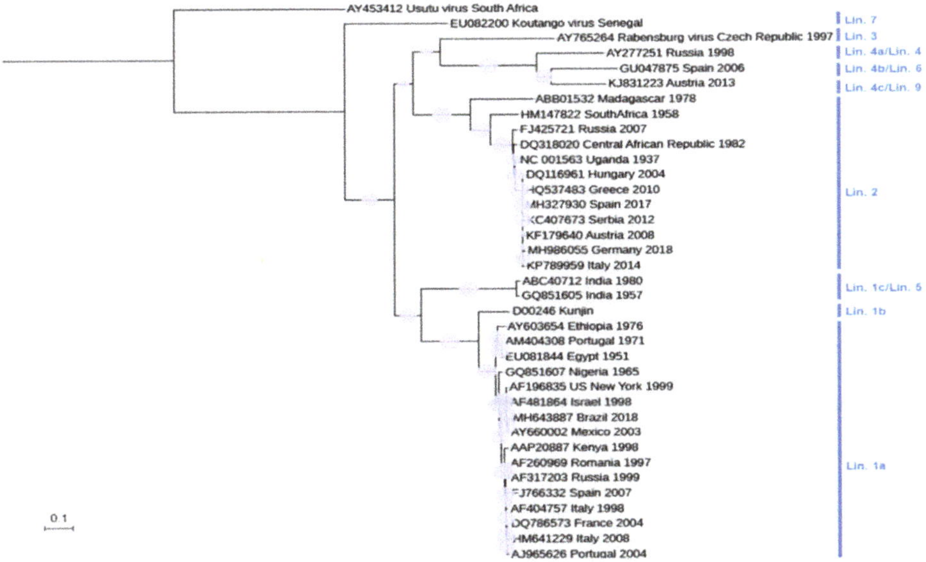

Figure 2. Phylogram, showing the relationships between the WNV strains. The tree is based on the complete nucleotide sequence of NS5 (except for HU2925/06 and MH327930). Multiple alignment was performed using MUSCLE [32], and a maximum likelihood tree was built using W-IQ-TREE [33]. The tree was visualized with iTOL [34]. Usutu virus was included as an outgroup for tree rooting. GenBank accession is indicated for each sequence. The country of origin and year of isolation is displayed when available. Circles size denotes the percentage of replicates in the bootstrap analysis (1000 bootstrap analyses). The scale indicates 0.1 substitutions/site. Phylogenetic lineages (Lin.) are indicated according to [5]. Genetic lineage 8 was not included in the tree because only partial sequence, not including NS5, is available (KJ131502).

2.3. Antigenic Structure

Mature virions are about 50 nm in diameter, and the majority of their surface is occupied by the E glycoprotein (Figure 3A). This external protein shell is composed of 180 copies of E protein arranged as antiparallel homodimers and confers the virions a herringbone T = 3 pseudo-icosahedral symmetry [27]. The E protein is N-glycosylated at Asn 154 in most WNV isolates (Figure 3B). This surface glycoprotein constitutes the major target for neutralizing antibodies, becoming the base of many vaccine candidates [35]. While the lack of glycosylation influences WNV replication in experimentally infected chickens, it does not compromise the induction of antibodies [36]. Notably, the E protein carries both flavivirus cross-reactive and WNV-specific epitopes. The cross-reactivity between WNV and related flaviviruses is the result of the high degree of structural homology between them and can lead to cross-protection but also to adverse effects due to antibody-dependent enhancement of infection [37–40]. This high cross-reactivity also complicates the precise serological diagnosis of flavivirus infections by immunological techniques, such as ELISA, making necessary the use of confirmatory tests, including related flaviviruses, with the neutralization assay as the gold standard [19]. The E glycoprotein is organized into three domains (DI to DIII), DI is an eight-stranded β-barrel, DII contains the conserved fusion loop (residues 98–110), and DIII adopts an immunoglobulin-like fold form (Figure 3B). Antibody epitopes have been identified in all three domains, with the most prominent neutralizing antibodies targeting DIII, making it an interesting candidate for vaccine development [35]. Antibodies against proteins other than the E have also been identified, so that experimentally infected chickens elicited antibodies against prM and NS1 [41,42]. While antibodies against NS1 have been related to protection in mammals [43], results obtained with red-legged partridges (*Alectoris rufa*) suggest that this could not be always the case [44].

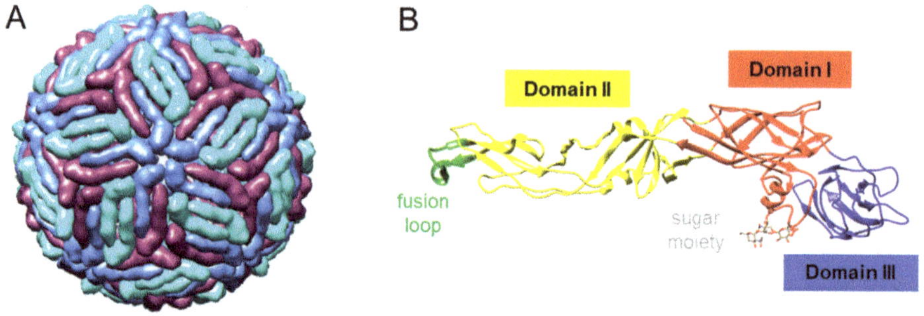

Figure 3. Structure of WNV. (**A**) Cryo-electron microscopy reconstruction of a WNV particle (Protein Data Bank accession 3J0B). E monomers are blue, purple, and turquoise. (**B**) Ribbon diagram of the crystal structure of WNV E glycoprotein (Protein Data Bank accession 2HG0). Domain I is red, domain II is yellow, domain III is blue, and the fusion loop is green. The N-linked sugar moiety of Asn 154 is also displayed. Images were produced using Chimera package [45].

3. Avian Susceptibility

Birds are the main vertebrate hosts for WNV, being commonly infected and frequently developing high levels of viremia [6]. Susceptibility of the avian population to the infection can vary depending on the species, being Corvidae (order Passeriformes) the most susceptible family [46–48], and important virus amplifiers [7–9], that play a key role in the epidemiology of the virus [10–14]. In fact, WNV epidemics in the US were associated with high crow mortality, driving to a significant decrease of native crow species [14–17]. According to the Centers for Disease Control and Prevention (CDC), birds from almost 300 different species have been found dead since 1999 in the US [49]. This avian WNV-associated mortality has been reported around the world in domestic [50–52] and wild birds [11,17,53,54], including endangered species [55,56], as well as in ones adapted to human environments [16].

Differences in pathogenicity, virulence, viremia, the clinical course of the infection, and mortality after experimental infections of birds with WNV strains of either lineage 1 or 2 have been reported [57,58], although no differences have been observed by other authors [8,59].

Main transmission route in birds is by mosquito bites, but other sporadic routes have also been described, such as oral [7,60,61] and bird-to-bird contact [7,13,62–65], suggesting that WNV-infected birds can be a source of contamination in nature [46,64,66].

A great range of viremias has been reported in different species, which may influence viral transmission. Birds that develop viremia greater than 10^6 pfu/mL are usually considered competent reservoirs to spread the virus [67], although, for some vectors, it has been described in the range of 10^4–10^5 pfu/mL [68]. In fact, while in some species (Columbiformes and Galliformes), viremias are quite low, in others (Passeriformes, Charadriiformes, or Strigiformes) are high, making these species more efficient competent hosts for WNV transmission [7]. Viremia can be detected as soon as one day after infection in high susceptible species [7,69–71]. Moreover, WNV has been detected in blood as early as 30–45 min after the bite of infected mosquitoes, suggesting that local replication is not necessary in birds for the primary viremia [72]. Viremia can last up to 7–11 days depending of the avian species [7,59]. Dissemination of the virus to the different tissues has been reported as early as one day after infection in the spleen of crows [73], until 14 days post-infection in kidney and spleen of an American Kestrel (*Falco sparverius*, Falconidae) [7], and even 27 days after infection in the kidney of a horned owl (Strigidae) [74]. WNV can also be detected in oral and fecal swabs from the first day after infection in most of the susceptible species studied with a viral shedding timing that overall reflects that of viremia [8,70,75].

4. Avian Pathology

No clinical signs are observed in most WNV-infected birds, and, when they show up, the most common are lethargy, reluctance to move, ruffled feathers, and lack of appetite with marked body weight losses (Figure 4) [7,8,63,75]. Dehydration [70], intermittent head twitching [70], convulsions [47,76], profuse oral and nasal discharge [77], or reduced fecal output [78] are less common. When a fatal outcome occurs, it happens within the first 24 h after the onset of clinical signs [7,8].

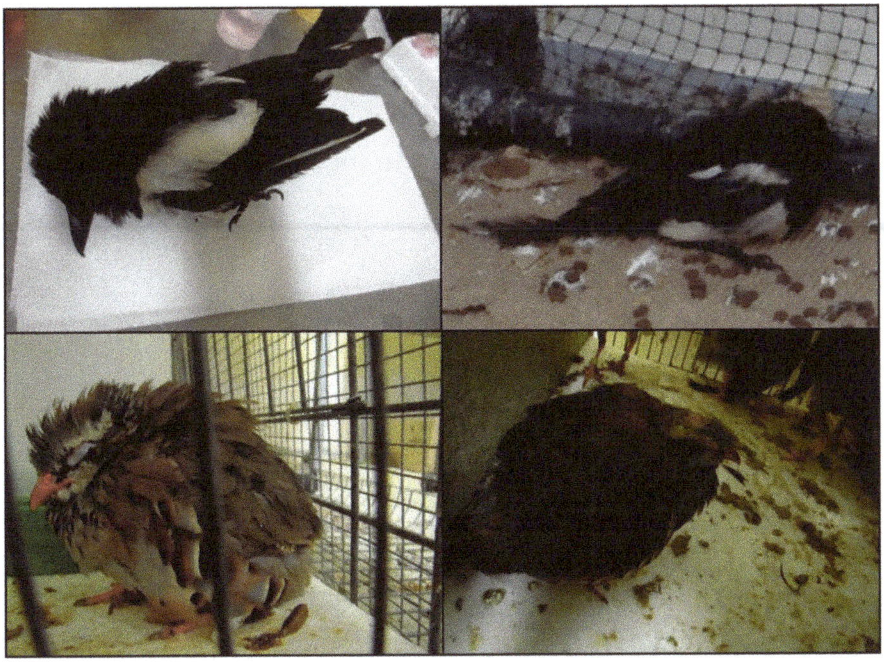

Figure 4. Clinical signs observed in experimentally infected birds. Magpies (upper panel) and partridges (lower panel) experimentally infected with WNV. Birds that die develop high morbidity hours before their death. Evident clinical signs like loss of appetite, ruffled feathers, paralysis, hunchback position, and unresponsiveness are observed in WNV-infected birds from 3 to 8 days post-infection (dpi).

Macroscopic lesions are observed in infected birds between 7 and 10 days after infection, although it can be delayed until 21 days post-infection (dpi) [79], and even become chronic [47]. The most affected organs are the brain, presenting encephalitis with cerebellar involvement, heart, liver, spleen, and kidney [75,80,81]. Lesions, such as diffuse pallor or pale foci in epicardium and myocardium [70], or in the hepatic, splenic, and renal parenchyma [80], as well as hepatomegaly and splenomegaly [58,74,75], have also been reported.

Among the histopathological findings of the affected organs (Figure 5), central nervous system lesions are mainly characterized by hemorrhages in the brain [81–83], mild perivascular cuffs consisting of lymphocytes and plasma cells, scattered individual necrotic neurons, lymphoplasmacytic, and histiocytic meningoencephalitis characterized by gliosis and glial nodules [47,48,59]. The main findings in the heart are lymphoplasmacytic and histiocytic myocarditis with myocardial necrosis, concurrent fibrosis, sometimes with thrombi, hypereosinophilia of cardiomyocytes, myocytolysis, nuclear swelling, pyknosis, loss of striations, myofiber degeneration, and hemorrhages [70,80,84]. Liver lesions include multifocal randomly distributed granulomatous and lymphohistiocytic hepatitis, with mild to moderate coagulative hepatocellular necrosis and deposition of fibrin [75]. The spleen is also affected by WNV infection, where multifocal lymphocytic necrosis occurs characterized by the presence of karyorrhectic nuclear debris [75,81]. Significant histopathological abnormalities present in the kidney are mild multifocal proximal tubular necrosis and mild to moderate lymphoplasmacytic interstitial nephritis that can occasionally be perivascular [70,75,85]. Ocular lesions are also common in WNV-infected birds. These lesions consist of the disarray of the retinal pigmented epithelial cell layer, pectenitis, choroidal or retinal inflammation, cellular necrosis, muscular degeneration in the iris, mild optic neuritis, impaired vision, and even blindness [47,76,86–88]. Other less common described lesions include pancreatitis, pulmonary edema, infiltration of lymphocytes, plasma cells and histiocytes in the intestinal tract, necrotizing mucosal duodenitis, myofiber degeneration with lymphoplasmacytic inflammation, and fibrosis in skeletal muscle [89,90].

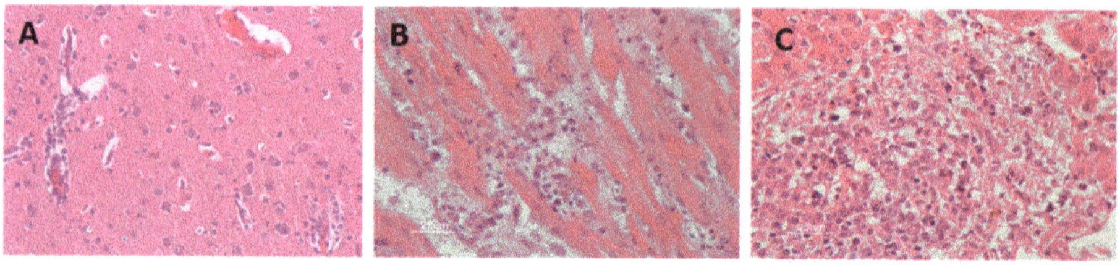

Figure 5. Histopathological findings in WNV-infected red-legged partridge. (**A**) Moderate gliosis, and lymphoplasmacytic and histiocytic perivascular cuffs observed in the brain. (**B**) Extensive myocardial degeneration and necrosis with inflammatory infiltrate composed of lymphocytes, plasma cells, and histiocytes observed in the heart. (**C**) Extensive liver necrosis with predominantly lymphoplasmacytic infiltrate. Images courtesy of Dr. U. Höfle and Dr. V. Gamino.

WNV can persist in the organs of infected birds up to several months [91], thus playing a possible role in viral overwintering and enabling possible new infections through mosquito bites or bird-to-bird transmission [14,92,93].

5. Vaccines

Vaccines to protect humans against certain flaviviruses have been available for long time, such as that against yellow fever virus (YFV) in use since more than 80 years, or that against Japanese encephalitis virus (JEV) approved in 2009, and, thus, it is expected that the same principles could be applied to WNV vaccine development. In fact, several commercial formulations are currently available for equid vaccination, and its effectiveness was demonstrated after immunization of horses, which led to a marked decrease of severe WNV disease (WND) in the following years in the US [94,95]. In many cases, experiments with birds have tested some of these commercially available vaccines approved for use in equids [18,19], such as the formalin-inactivated whole-WNV vaccine originally developed by Fort Dodge (Fort Dodge, IA, USA), which has been commercialized under different names (West Nile-Innovator, Duvaxyn® renamed EQUIP WNV®) [96–104], and was licensed in 2003 and subsequent years (Vetera®), a DNA-based vaccine subsequent formulation expressing the prM and E WNV proteins also from Fort Dodge (West Nile-Innovator DNA equine®) [97,105], which was licensed in 2004 in the US but later removed from the market in 2010, and a recombinant live canarypox virus vaccine (ALVAC®) that expresses the prM/E WNV proteins (Recombitek® Equine West Nile virus in the US, Merial, GA, USA; or Proteq WNV® in Europe) [96,105].

Additionally, experimental prototypes have been assayed, like a chimeric virus based on the yellow fever 17D vaccine strain in which the surface proteins were replaced by that of WNV (ChimeriVax-WN) [106], or a vaccine [64] based on WNV recombinant subviral particles (RSPs) produced by a HeLa-3 cell line stably transfected with a plasmid encoding the signal peptide of the C protein and the prM/E proteins [107]. Several other approaches have used DNA vaccines, like the DNA-plasmid vaccine (pCBWN) [108], also encoding the WNV prM/E proteins [98,105,109–111], and a modified version of it [112]. Another DNA vaccine that codes for the prM/M and E proteins of WNV produced by Aldevron [99], and two DNA-plasmid vaccines expressing the ectodomain of the WNV E protein of lineage 1 or 2 in the modified backbone vector pVax1 were also tested [113]. Likewise, a recombinant protein vaccine originally developed for humans, the WN-80E, consisting of a portion of the WNV envelope protein has been assayed too [114]. All these vaccines, commercial and experimental, have been evaluated in different domestic (Table 2) and wild (Table 1) avian species following different routes of administration and vaccination regimens, resulting in varied outcomes.

The availability of vaccines for use in birds, the natural hosts of the virus, will be highly useful, mostly during outbreaks. These vaccines could be used in birds held in captivity in recreational installations and zoos, in wildlife rehabilitation and endangered species breeding centers, and even in birds grown for restocking or hunting activities that are yearly released by the thousands into the environment in many countries. Even more, some of these vaccines could be also administered during surveillance programs [64].

Table 1. Vaccines tested in wild birds.

Vaccines					Birds Used			Results				Ref.
Type	**Name**	**Route**	**Dose**	**Adjuvant**	**Family**	**Latin Name**	**Common Name**	**Safety Concerns**	**Protection**	**Competence Break**	**Antibodies**	
Chimeric Virus	ChimeriVax-WN	SC	×3	no	Corvidae	*Corvus ossifragus*	Fish crows	yes	NA	no	yes (NAI, L)	[106]
Live Recombinant Vector	Recombitek® Equine West Nile Virus	IM	×1	no	Corvidae	*Aphelocoma californica*	Western scrub-jays	yes	80% vs. 40%	no	yes (L)	[105]
		IM	×2/×3	no	Falconidae	*Falco spp*	Large falcons	yes	100% vs. 50%	yes	yes (L) 2× yes (NAI) 3×	[96]
Inactivated Whole Virus	West Nile - Innovator	IM	×1	MetaStim	Phoenicopteridae	*Phoenicopterus chilensis*	Chilean flamingos	no	NT	NA	no	[101]
		IM	×1	MetaStim	Accipitridae	*Buteo jamaicensis*	Red-tailed hawks	no	NT	NA	no	
		IM	×3	MetaStim	Accipitridae	*Buteo jamaicensis*	Red-tailed hawks	NR	NT	NA	yes*	[100]
		IM	×3	MetaStim	Accipitridae	*Parabuteo unicinctus*	Harris' hawks					
		IM	×3	MetaStim	Accipitridae	*Accipiter cooperii*	Cooper's hawks					
		IM	×3	MetaStim	Accipitridae	*Buteo swainsoni*	Swainson's hawks					
		IM	×3	MetaStim	Accipitridae	*Haliaeetus leucocephalus*	Bald eagle					
		IM	×3	MetaStim	Accipitridae	*Aquila chrysaetos*	Golden eagle					
		IM	×3	MetaStim	Falconidae	*Falco mexicanus*	Prairie falcon					
		IM	×3	MetaStim	Falconidae	*Falco peregrinus*	Peregrine falcon					
		IM	×3	MetaStim	Corvidae	*Corvus corax*	Common raven					
		IM	×3	MetaStim	Cathartidae	*Cathartes aura*	Turkey vultures					
		IM	×3	MetaStim	Strigidae	*Otus kennicottii*	Western screech- owls					
		IM	×3	MetaStim	Strigidae	*Bubo virginianus*	Great horned owls					
		IM	×3	MetaStim	Tytonidae	*Athene cunicularia*	Burrowing owls					
		IM	×3	MetaStim	Tytonidae	*Tyto alba*	Barn owls					
		IM	×2	MetaStim	Corvidae	*Corvus brachyrhynchos*	American crow	NC	11% vs. 0%	no	yes (NAI, L)	[98]
		IM	×2	MetaStim	Spheniscidae	*Spheniscus demersus*	Black-footed penguins	no	NT	NA	yes (NAI)	[102]
		IM	×2	MetaStim	Spheniscidae	*Eudyptula minor*	Little blue penguins	no	NT	NA	yes (NAI)	
		IM	×3	MetaStim	Phasianidae	*Tympanuchus cupido attwateri*	Attwater's prairie chickens	no	NT	NA	yes (NAI)	
		IM	×3	MetaStim	Phoenicopteridae	*Phoenicopterus chilensis*	Chilean flamingos	no	NT	NA	yes (NAI)	
		IM	×2	MetaStim	Phoenicopteridae	*Phoenicopterus ruber*	American flamingos	no	NT	NA	yes (NAI)	
		IM	×2	MetaStim	Spheniscidae	*Spheniscus humboldti*	Humboldt penguins	no	NT	NA	yes (NAI)	[99]
		IM	×2	MetaStim	Spheniscidae	*Spheniscus magellanicus*	Magellanic penguins	no	NT	NA	yes (NAI)	

Table 1. *Cont.*

Vaccines					Birds Used			Results				Ref.
Type	Name	Route	Dose	Adjuvant	Family	Latin Name	Common Name	Safety Concerns	Protection	Competence Break	Antibodies	
		IM	×2	MetaStim	Spheniscidae	*Pygoscelis papua*	Gentoo penguins	no	NT	NA	yes (NAI)	
		IM	×2	MetaStim	Spheniscidae	*Eudyptes chrysocome*	Rockhopper penguins	no	NT	NA	yes (NAI)	
		IM	×3	MetaStim	Gruidae	*Grus canadensis*	Sandhill cranes	no	NA	yes	no	[103]
		IM	×3**	MetaStim	Corvidae	*Aphelocoma insularis*	Island scrub-jays	no	NT	NA	yes (NAI)	[97]
		IM	×2/×3	MetaStim	Falconidae	Falco *spp*	Large falcons	NR	80% (x2)–100% (x3) vs. 50%	no (2x) yes (3x)	yes	[96]***
Recombinant Subunit	RSP-WNV	SC	×1	aluminum hydroxide	Corvidae	*Pica pica*	Eurasian magpies	NR	71% vs. 22%	yes	yes (NAI)	[64]
DNA	West Nile-Innovator DNA equine®	IM	×1	MetaStim	Corvidae	*Aphelocoma insularis*	Island scrub-jays	no	NT	NA	yes (NAI)	[97]
		IM	×1	MetaStim	Corvidae	*Aphelocoma californica*	Western scrub-jays	NR	80% vs. 40%	no	yes (L)	[105]
	pCBWN	OR	×1	sodium alginate	Corvidae	*Corvus ossifragus*	Fish crows	NC	100% vs. 50%	NA	yes (NAI)	[111]
		IM	×1	sodium alginate	Corvidae	*Corvus ossifragus*	Fish crows	NC	no	NA	no	
		IM	×2	no	Corvidae	*Corvus brachyrhynchos*	American crows	NC	44% vs. 0%	no	yes (NAI, L)	[98]
		IM	×2	aluminum phosphate	Corvidae	*Corvus brachyrhynchos*	American crows	NC	60% vs. 0%	no	yes (NAI, L)	
		OR	×4	no	Corvidae	*Corvus brachyrhynchos*	American crows	NC	no	no	no	
		IM	×1	no	Turdidae	*Turdus migratorius*	American robins	NC	NA	yes	no	[109]
		IM	×2	aluminum phosphate	Accipitridae	*Buteo jamaicensis*	Red-tailed hawks	no	NA	NA	yes (NAI, L)	[110]
		IM	×1	no	Corvidae	*Aphelocoma californica*	Western scrub-jays	NR	100% vs. 40%	no	yes (L)	[105]
	pCBWN-Amp C	IM	×2	aluminum phosphate	Cathartidae	*Vultur gryphus*	Andean condors	no	NT	NA	yes (L)	[112]
		IM	×2	aluminum phosphate	Cathartidae	*Gymnogyps californianus*	California condors	no	NT	NA	yes (L)	
	prM/E-Aldevron	IM	×2	aluminum hydroxide	Spheniscidae	*Spheniscus humboldti*	Humboldt penguins	no	NT	NA	yes (NAI)	[99]
		IM	×2	aluminum hydroxide	Spheniscidae	*Spheniscus magellanicus*	Magellanic penguins	no	NT	NA	yes (NAI)	

Table 1. *Cont.*

Vaccines					Birds Used				Results			Ref.
Type	Name	Route	Dose	Adjuvant	Family	Latin Name	Common Name	Safety Concerns	Protection	Competence Break	Antibodies	
		IM	×2	aluminum hydroxide	Spheniscidae	*Pygoscelis papua*	Gentoo penguins	no	NT	NA	yes (NAI)	
		IM	×2	aluminum hydroxide	Spheniscidae	*Eudyptes chrysocome*	Rockhopper penguins	no	NT	NA	yes (NAI)	
	pVax-E-ect-lin.1	IM	×2	no	Falconidae	Falco *spp*	Large falcons	NR	60% vs. 50%	yes	yes (NAI, L)	
	pVax-E-ect-lin.2	IM	×2	no	Falconidae	Falco *spp*	Large falcons	NR	100% vs. 50%	yes	yes (NAI, L)	[113]
	pVax-E-ect-lin.1	IM+EP	×2	no	Falconidae	Falco *spp*	Large falcons	NR	100% vs. 50%	yes	yes (NAI, L)	
	pVax-E-ect-lin.1/ rE-dIII	IM-EP/ SC	×1/×2	no/ISA 70	Falconidae	Falco *spp*	Large falcons	NR	80% vs. 50%	yes	yes (NAI, L)	
Recombinant Protein	WN-80E	IM	×2	ISA 720	Anatidae	*Branta sandvicensis*	Hawaiian Nēnē	no	NT	NA	yes	[114]

* Low number of single species in each group (few seroconversion and low titers with the highest dose tested); ** Whenever possible, as birds were captured and release after each vaccination and eventually recaptured; *** Duvaxyn® commercial formulation used; RSP: recombinant subviral particles; WNV: West Nile virus; SC: subcutaneous; IM: intramuscular; OR: oral; IM+EP: intramuscular + electroporation; NC: not commented; NR: not relevant; NA: not applicable; NT: not tested; NAI: not in all individuals; L: low titer; Break of competence: vaccine lowers viremia levels below the threshold of competence (see text).

5.1. Vaccination in Domestic Birds

The first description of disease and deaths caused by WNV in domestic birds was reported in 1997–1999 in Israel [115], involving hundreds of young geese (*Anser anser*). This species had also been the most affected domestic avian species during virus spread in the US [116]. Symptomatic infections have also been reported in several Psittacine species [90], although experimental infection of birds of these species indicated that they are not very competent [7]. Galliformes, such as chickens (*Gallus gallus domesticus*) and turkeys (*Meleagris gallopavo*), seroconvert but remain asymptomatic. On the other hand, outbreaks among farmed chukar partridges (*Alectoris chukar*) and Impeyan pheasants (*Lophophorus impejanus*) have been reported [52].

After the initial outbreaks in geese in Israel mentioned above [115], both live attenuated and inactivated WNV vaccines have been successfully used there. A live attenuated WNV vaccine was generated by serially passaging a WNV Israeli isolate in a mosquito cell line and selecting an escape mutant using a specific monoclonal antibody [117]. The resulting variant, WN-25A, lost all neuroinvasiveness, while it fully protected geese (20/20) upon a lethal challenge with an Israeli strain isolated from a moribund goose. Later, an attenuated, commercial heterologous flavivirus vaccine derived from Israel turkey meningoencephalitis virus (TMEV) was experimentally tested in laboratory and field settings in geese intra-cranially challenged with WNV two weeks after immunization [115]. The level and duration of protection achieved were quite high and long-lasting (71–93%, 12/17–14/15, protection in laboratory assays, and 39–72%, 9/23–18/25 in the farm ones); however, some goose flocks reacted unfavorably to the vaccination in field trials, showing neurological signs and appreciable mortality. Such undesirable side effects were not observed when they tested a formalin-inactivated WNV strain passaged in suckling mice brains [115]. The same authors reported a 63% (5/8) protection upon intra-cranial challenge when a double dose of this prototype was administered in a single injection and up to 94% (15/16) when a single dose was administered in two injections spaced two weeks apart. Similar studies carried out in farmed goose flocks resulted in 52–80% (13/25–16/20) protection [115]. The efficacy of this vaccine was later evaluated in 829 geese, 298 laboratory-vaccinated, 231 farm-vaccinated, and 300 non-vaccinated, showing 86.58% (258/298), 75.32% (174/231), and 8.33% (25/300) survival rates, respectively, after WNV challenge [118].

Subsequently, an inactivated vaccine was developed using an adapted WNV-Isr98 isolate highly virulent for geese and the PER.C6® cell line platform [119]. When the vaccine was administered with mineral oil as an adjuvant to geese, 91.4% (53/58) survived to the infection, while only 5% (1/20) of the control PER.C6 sham-vaccinated group did. However, the PER.C6-ISR98 candidate did not seem to be sterilizing since, after the challenge, a boost of neutralizing antibodies was detected. In addition, the importance of the use of adjuvants was noted since the administration of the vaccine without adjuvant resulted in 53.3% (32/60) protection [119].

By 2011, the inactivated West Nile-Innovator vaccine was tested for its capability to induce antibodies in chicks and adult thick-billed parrots (*Rhynchopsitta pachyrhyncha*) that received five and three doses with annual boosts along 3 and 7 years, respectively [104]. None of the birds seroconverted after the initial injections, but 2/4 and 3/4 of the chicks developed antibodies 1 and 2 years later, respectively, while only 1/12 and 2/8 of the adults had them 1 and 3 years later, being 6/6 positive after 7 years of annual vaccination. However, as the birds were likely naturally exposed to WNV during the experiment, the interpretation of the results is complicated.

Chimeric vaccines have also been evaluated in domestic birds. So that, an attenuated chimeric vaccine constructed by inserting the prM/E of WNV in dengue virus serotype 4 backbone (WNV/DENV4), and a similar one with a 30-nucleotide deletion in the 3′ non-coding region of DENV4 (WN/DEN4-3′Δ30), which were previously shown to prevent viremia in challenged mice and rhesus macaques [120], were tested in young domestic geese [121]. None of these chimeric vaccines stimulated protective immunity against WNV challenge, and high morbidity rates (3/4 in each group), and a high level of viremia were recorded among vaccinated goose, similar to that in non-vaccinated animals [121].

A different approach was used by testing, in domestic geese, a WNV subunit vaccine that comprised 80% of the E protein (WN-80E) combined with adjuvant and administered twice 4 weeks apart [122]. Using viremia as the clinical endpoint, no virus was detected in the serum of groups of six birds immunized with medium or a high-dose (5 or 10 μg) of the vaccine up to 14 dpi. However, the virus was detected in oral swabs 3–6 dpi in some of the birds, and an increase in antibody titers was observed at 14 dpi, indicating that the vaccine did not induce sterile immunity. Likewise, using a recombinant WNV-E as immunogen to orally (20 μg or 100 μg/dose), or intramuscularly (20 μg/dose), vaccinate Leghorn chickens (*G. gallus domesticus*) three times with a 2-week interval [123], it was shown that, in the birds immunized intramuscularly, the levels of viremia were lower and the total production of WNV E protein-specific IgY was significantly higher than in the animals immunized by the oral route. In this line, a recombinant WNV envelope E (rE) protein produced in insects [124], highly protective in mice [125], was assayed in red-legged partridges. Birds were intramuscularly vaccinated twice at the two-week interval with 10 μg/animal of the rE protein administered with adjuvant, and a control group was similarly sham-immunized. Partridges from both groups were subcutaneously challenged with the NY99 WNV strain [63]. All the rE vaccinated birds (22/22) survived to WNV infection, while 33.3% (6/18) of the sham-immunized partridges succumbed between 3 and 8 dpi, being the mortality rate higher among younger (9 weeks of age at the time of challenge) than among older (13 weeks of age) animals (45.5% vs. 14.3%, respectively). An age-dependent susceptibility had been previously reported in a related species, the chukar partridges, in which 25% mortality was observed in juvenile birds, while no mortality was reported in 14 week-old partridges housed nearby during a WNV outbreak in the US [52], and also in domestic geese [51,126]. Analyses of the humoral immune response elicited by rE vaccinated partridges showed that all animals were ELISA positive after two immunizations [63], similar to what had previously been described in geese and American crows (*Corvus brachyrhynchos*) [98,119]. Again, the immunity elicited by rE vaccinated partridges was not sterilizing, as viremia was detected in 4/22 vaccinated birds 3 dpi, and antibody titers significantly increased after viral challenge to levels similar to those found in non-vaccinated animals. Similar results had been observed after vaccination of geese, red-tailed hawks, and Western scrub-jays (*Aphelocoma californica*) [105,110,119].

Another study tested five different vaccine candidates administered intramuscularly in 47 geese [116]. The prototypes tested were an inactivated whole virus prepared with mineral oil as an adjuvant, three recombinant viruses containing the WNV prM/E (the canarypox viruses ALVAC vCP2017 and vCP2018; and the fowlpox virus vFP2000), and an exogenously produced WNV E protein. Birds were challenged 2 weeks after the booster immunization, except in the last case that was done after 1 week. Since no geese died in the challenged sham-immunized groups and only one developed clinical signs, protection was measured through the following five parameters: clinical pathogenicity index (CPI), plasma virus-positive geese on days 1–4 post-inoculation, plasma virus titers, brain histological lesion rates, and severity scores. The best protection was achieved with the vFP2000 fowlpox virus, which was the one that best scored in the five parameters, followed by the vCP2018 canarypox virus that did it in four, the vCP2017 in three, the E protein in one, and the oil-emulsion WNV in none.

Table 2. Vaccines tested in domestic birds.

Vaccines					Birds			Results				Ref.
Type	Name	Route	Dose	Adjuvant	Family	Latin Name	Common Name	Safety Concerns	Protection	Competence Break	Antibodies	
Live Recombinant Vector	vCP2017	IM	×2	PM	Anatidae	*Anser anser*	Domestic geese	NC	NA	yes	yes (NAI)	[116]
	vCP2018	IM	×2	PM	Anatidae	*Anser anser*	Domestic geese	NC	NA	yes	yes (NAI)	
	vFP2000	IM	×2	PM	Anatidae	*Anser anser*	Domestic geese	NC	NA	yes	yes	
	rAdE	IM	×2	no	Phasianidae	*Coturnix japonica*	Japanese quail	NC	NT	NA	yes	[127]
	rAdNS3	IM	×2	no	Phasianidae	*Coturnix japonica*	Japanese quail	NC	NT	NA	yes (L)	
Live Attenuated Whole Virus	WNI-25A	IP	×1	no	Anatidae	*Anser anser*	Domestic geese	NC	100% vs. 0%	NT	NT	[117]
	TMEV	SC	NC	no	Anatidae	*Anser anser*	Domestic geese	yes	71–93% vs. 0%	NT	NT	[115]
		IM	NC	no	Anatidae	*Anser anser*	Domestic geese	yes	82–93% vs. 0%	NT	NT	
Inactivated Whole Virus	TME-formalin boosted with live TME	SC	NC	oil	Anatidae	*Anser anser*	Domestic geese	no	100% vs. 0%	NT	NT	[115]
		IM	NC	oil	Anatidae	*Anser anser*	Domestic geese	no	100% vs. 0%	NT	NT	
	WNV-formalin inactivated	SC	×2	mineral oil	Anatidae	*Anser anser*	Domestic geese	no	92% vs. 0%	NT	NT	[115]
		IM	×2	mineral oil	Anatidae	*Anser anser*	Domestic geese	no	80% vs. 0%	NT	NT	
		SC	×2	mineral oil	Anatidae	*Anser anser*	Domestic geese	no	75–86% vs. 8%	NT	NT	[118]
	PER.C6-ISR98	SC	×2	mineral oil	Anatidae	*Anser anser*	Domestic geese	no	91.4% vs. 5%	NT	yes (L)	
	West Nile - Innovator	IM	×3*	MetaStim	Psittacidae	*Rhynchopsitta pachyrhyncha*	Thick-billed parrots	NC	NT	NA	yes**	[104]
	WNV-formaldehyde inactivated	IM	×2	mineral oil	Anatidae	*Anser anser*	Domestic geese	NC	NA	no	yes (NAI)	[116]
Recombinant Protein	WN-80E	IM	×2	ISA 720	Anatidae	*Anser anser*	Domestic geese	no	NA	NA	yes (L)	[122]
		IM	×2	no	Anatidae	*Anser anser*	Domestic geese	no	NA	NA	no	
	rE protein	OR	×3	LTK63	Phasianidae	*Gallus gallus*	Domestic chickens	NC	NA	NA	no	[123]
		IM	×3	LTK63	Phasianidae	*Gallus gallus*	Domestic chickens	NC	NA	NA	yes	
	E protein	IM	×2	mineral oil	Anatidae	*Anser anser*	Domestic geese	NC	NA	NA	yes (NAI)	[116]
	rE protein	IM	×3	Specol	Phasianidae	*Alectoris rufa*	Red-legged partridges	no	100% vs. 33%	NA	yes	[63]

* Vaccine administered x3 in the first year followed by yearly boosters (7 years); ** all animal seroconverted 3 (chicks) to 7 (adults) years after annuall boosters; TMEV: Israel turkey meningoencephalitis virus; WNV: West Nile virus; SC: subcutaneous; IM: intramuscular; IP: intraperitoneal; OR: oral; PM: adjuvant provided by the manufacturer; NC: not commented; NA: not applicable; NT: not tested; NAI: not in all individuals; L: low titer; Break of competence: vaccine lowers viremia levels below the threshold of competence (see text).

5.2. Vaccination in Wild Birds

Vaccination of wild species presents associated problems, such as the limited access to individuals, aggravated by the high number of susceptible species described, and environmental safety concerns, especially with attenuated or genetically engineered live virus-based vaccines. However, since, in many of them, WNV-related pathogenesis is not clinically relevant and/or they have a limited, if any, role in virus ecology, most of them do not seem to represent a target for vaccine campaigns implementation. Indeed, most efforts in experimental vaccine development have selected members of the Corvidae family as model, although raptors (Accipitridae and Falconidae), nocturnal bird preys (Strigidae and Tytonidae), and members of other families (Phoenicopteridae, Spheniscidae, Gruidae, Turdidae, Cathartidae, Phasianidae, and Anatidae) have also been used (Table 1). For most of them, WNV-associated mortality has been described [8,74,128], and some have been related to virus spreading and re-introduction in different geographical areas due to their migratory behavior.

The main aim of a vaccine is conferring protection. A single intramuscular dose of the pCBWN DNA vaccine administered to fish crows resulted in 100% (8/8) survival rate in comparison with the 50% recorded in non-vaccinated (5/10), or orally immunized (4/8) birds [111]. However, the same vaccine intramuscularly administered to American crows resulted in 44% (4/9) survival, while none (0/10) of the sham-inoculated birds survived [98]. The same authors reported up to 60% (6/10) increased survival rate when intramuscular immunization was performed with an adjuvant, a lack of protection with the adjuvant alone (0/8), or when the oral route was used (0/10), and a low one (11%, 1/9) when the West Nile-Innovator vaccine was intramuscularly administered [98]. Another study reported that a single intramuscular vaccination of Western scrub-jays with the pCBWN vaccine protected 100% (3/3) of the birds, and that 80% (4/5) of the corvids intramuscularly vaccinated with a single dose of the Fort Dodge West Nile-Innovator DNA equine® vaccine or the Recombitek® Equine West Nile virus formulation also survived to the infection compared to the 40% (2/5) of survival reached by the control group [105]. Dispensation to falcons of the Duvaxyn® inactivated vaccine resulted in 80% (4/5) and 100% (4/4) protection when administered twice or thrice, respectively, and 100% protection with two (5/5) or three doses (4/4) was achieved with the Recombitek® Equine West Nile virus formulation, while only 50% (4/8) survival was recorded in non-vaccinated animals [96]. Two DNA vaccines that express the ectodomain of the E protein of WNV of lineage 1 or 2 also tested in large falcons conferred protection against a WNV challenge and, based on their results with different protocols, the authors indicated that protection was dependent on the lineage, regimen, and way of administration used. Birds intramuscularly immunized with the plasmid, encoding the protein of lineage 2, reached 100% (5/5) survival in comparison to the 60% (3/5) reached by those immunized with that of lineage 1, or the 50% (4/8) showed by non-vaccinated birds [113]. Finally, a single intramuscular dose of an RSP-based vaccine protected magpies (*Pica pica*) as 71.4% (5/7) of the vaccinated birds survived to viral challenge, compared to the 22.2% (2/9) survival rate observed among sham-immunized magpies [64].

Remarkably, in one study [106], vaccination of fish crows with the chimeric ChimeriVax-WN resulted in a high mortality rate upon WNV challenge when compared with non-vaccinated birds (25%, 2/8 and 0%, 0/4, respectively) that was accused to a possible antibody-dependent viral enhancement effect, although such effect has not been observed in nature.

Reduced morbidity and pathogenicity were also observed upon experimental vaccination of wild birds. Thus, a reduced pathology was noted in sandhill cranes (*Grus Canadensis*) vaccinated with the Fort Dodge inactivated vaccine [103], clinical signs alleviations were also reported after administration of three doses of Duvaxyn® or Recombitek® Equine West Nile virus vaccines in large falcons [96], and reduced clinical scores and antigen deposition in their organs upon DNA vaccination were also documented [113]. Likewise, a less pronounced and shorter loss of weight and a lack of clinical signs were described in RSP-vaccinated magpies that survived to viral challenge [64].

5.3. Sterilizing Immunity

As commented above, most of the tested vaccines conferred protection when animals were challenged, but, in none of them, induction of sterilizing immunity was observed, as viral replication could be detected in vaccinated birds, although with the exception of one study performed in vaccinated Western scrub-jays in which no reduction of viral titers was reported [105], those were usually lower in vaccinated than in sham-immunized animals [64,96,98,103,109–111,113]. For instance, viremia was detected in 4/22 rE vaccinated partridges 3 dpi, and antibody titers increased significantly after viral challenge to levels similar to those found in non-vaccinated animals [63].

On the other hand, in many cases [64,96,103,109,113], viremia reached levels below what is considered necessary to be a competent reservoir [7], although, for some vaccines, two [113] or three [96,103] doses were required to achieve it. In this respect, it was reported that for *Culex pipiens* and *Culex quinquefasciatus* [129], two vectors considered key to virus maintenance, these levels must be above 10^5 pfu/mL, although lower viremia levels (around 10^4 pfu/mL) also seemed to be relevant for other vectors, such as *Culex univittatus* or *Culex perexiguus* [68]. Additionally, a boost of antibodies in vaccinated birds was usually observed after viral challenge [64,103,105,110].

5.4. Immunogenicity

Induction of antibodies prior to challenge has not always been detected [101,103,109] and, if so, they are present at low levels [96,100,105,110,112,113], and not in all vaccinated individuals [64,97–100,102,106,110,111,113]. As commented above, humoral immune response priming that induces an enhanced and prominent/lasting antibody production has been described after viral challenge in vaccinated birds [64,103,105,110]. Although an association between antibody induction and protection has been suggested [64,98], sometimes, as no challenge was conducted, this hypothesis could not be confirmed [97,99–102,112,114]. For instance, a non-replicating recombinant adenoviruses, expressing either the WNV envelope (rAdE) or the NS3 (rAdNS3) proteins, was assayed in Japanese quails (*Coturnix japonica*) [127], but, since no challenge was performed, the efficacy of the vaccines was measured in terms of WNV-specific antibodies levels and T cells specific activation, which were both increased in vaccinated birds compared to unvaccinated controls. This antibody response was higher and more robust with the rAdE candidate than with the rAdNS3, probably due to the expression of the entire E protein on the cell surface, thus allowing B cells to bind to any available epitope on the molecule. Even more, vaccination with rAdE triggered the activation of more WNV-specific $CD4^+$ T cells, which would be required to fully activate the WNV primed B cells to produce antibodies. In line with this, vaccines based on DNA and live vectors favor the availability of cytotoxic T lymphocytes (CTLs) epitopes and therefore, should improve protection after viral challenge if T-cell responses are important. One work performed in large falcons compared the efficacy of the inactivated Duvaxyn® and the live vector-based Recombitek® Equine West Nile virus vaccines, showing a slightly better protection of the later one, as mentioned above [96], and, thus, pointing to a protective role of the cellular immune response. However, another study conducted in American crows with the pCBWN and the inactivated West Nile-Innovator vaccines showed the opposite results, as survival rates were 44% (4/9) and 11% (1/9), respectively [98]. Moreover, many vaccines tested included adjuvant, which could favor antigen presentation to T cells and prolong the presence of viral antigens for B cell recognition. So that, the pCBWN vaccine provided microencapsulated in sodium alginate [111], or with aluminum [98,110], increased the survival rates of immunized and challenged American crows when compared with those which received the vaccine alone (44%, 4/9 and 60%, 6/10, respectively) [98]. Aluminum has also been used with DNA [99] and RSP-based vaccines with good results [64].

5.5. Herd Immunity

Horizontal transmission of WNV in experimentally infected birds was early described [7]. This can be due to direct contact or by fecal-oral route since the virus can be detected in cloacal and oral swabs [7,8,61,128] and in feathers of infected birds [8]. Moreover, viremia levels reached in the absence of mosquito-borne transmission can be as high as those obtained by mosquito natural exposure [7]. Several vaccines have demonstrated to be effective in diminishing the risk of this type of transmission as they were able to either shorten [103,110] or reduce viral shedding [96,110,113] and virus presence in feathers [8]. Even more, it has been reported that RSPs vaccination completely broke horizontal transmission, as none (0/4) of the contact birds housed with challenged-vaccinated magpies got infected in contrast to 50% (3/6) that did it when were housed with challenged, unvaccinated cage-mates [64]. These data point to the induction of herd immunity through bird vaccination.

On the other hand, transmission in the absence of mosquito-borne infection has also been reported by the consumption of birds infected with WNV by scavenger species [60,128,130]. Therefore, and even in the absence of sterilizing immunity, reduction of viral load in organs after vaccination is desirable. In fact, reduction of viral load in the organs of challenged falcons vaccinated with commercially available WNV vaccines, such as Duvaxyn®, Recombitek® Equine West Nile virus [96], or with DNA-plasmid vaccines encoding the ectodomain of the E protein, has been reported [113].

5.6. Side Effects and Feasibility

An additional important point that must be taken into account for vaccine implementation is the lack of undesirable side effects. Even though local inflammation at the site of administration has been observed, probably due to hypersensitivity reactions to the vaccines or the natural effect of the adjuvants employed in some DNA-based and RSP-based vaccines [64,113], in most cases, no such side effects have been described. Two commercial Fort Dodge vaccines designed for equids (virus inactivated and DNA) showed no adverse side effects in corvids, cranes, or falcons [96,103,105]. The inactivated formulation has also been assayed in flamingos, hawks, eagles, vultures, owls, penguins, and wild chickens [99–102], showing good safety profiles, although, since no viral challenge was done, the immunopathological effects related to the vaccine during the infection were not evaluated. Moreover, vaccines based on live vectors can provoke adverse effects, such as the unexpected increase in mortality observed in corvids vaccinated with the ChimeriVax-WN [106], the development of necrotic lesions also in corvids [105], the massive local inflammation reported in falcons immunized with the Recombitek® Equine West Nile virus formulation [96], or the neurological signs and appreciable mortality observed in geese vaccinated with the heterologous TMEV-based vaccine candidate [115]. Even more, vaccines should avoid any environmental effects. In this regard, shedding by the fecal-oral route of vaccines based on virus or plasmid was not found in falcons immunized with Recombitek® Equine West Nile virus [96], or with DNA-plasmids vaccines expressing WNV proteins of lineage 1 or 2 [113].

As commented above, the biggest drawback for implementation feasibility of wild bird vaccines is access to the target host. This could be bypassed if herd immunity can be established, preferably by oral vaccination in, for example, feeding stations, which has already been useful for controlling other zoonotic diseases, such as rabies [131]. However, so far, experimental vaccination of birds by the oral route has failed in conferring protection [98,111], and it has not even able to stimulate the production of antibodies. In any case, avian vaccination can be a realistic option in specific situations, such as in birds grown for restocking activities, endangered species in captive breeding projects, wildlife reserves, recreation installations, or during epidemiological surveillance programs.

6. Conclusions

The objective of any vaccine is the induction of protection that, preferably, should be long-lasting and sterilizing, and induce herd immunity. Experimental vaccination with different formulations (attenuated, inactivated, recombinant viruses, and subunits and DNA-based candidates) has been assayed in domestic and wild birds from different species and ages following different routes of administration and regimens, which has resulted in varied outcomes. Even though, due to logistical and ethical concerns, among others, the number of birds included in the studies has generally been rather low, mainly when wild birds were used, the reported data indicate that, overall, vaccination induces humoral and, more probably, cellular responses, and reduces WNV-associated disease, lesions, viremia, viral shedding, and, more significantly, mortality. However, no sterilizing immunity has been observed, induction of antibodies has not always been recorded, and, if detected, it was not always in every bird. Remarkably, when evaluated, no horizontal transmission from challenged-vaccinated birds has been observed, pointing to the induction of herd immunity that would prevent virus maintenance in the environment and, thus, its spread. Nevertheless, the implementation of bird vaccines faces several drawbacks, such as the difficult feasibility of access to the target host, mainly for wild species, as well as the administration route, as oral, the most feasible one, has failed to confer protection. In any case, the availability of effective avian vaccines against WNV would be very helpful, mainly during outbreaks, and therefore, research should go on.

Author Contributions: Conceptualization and resources J.-C.S.; writing—original draft preparation, N.J.d.O., E.E.-R., A.-B.B., M.A.M.-A., J.-C.S.; writing—review and editing, J.-C.S.; funding acquisition, J.-C.S.

Funding: This research was partially funded by Instituto Nacional de Investigación y Tecnología Agraria y Alimentaria, (INIA) grants RTA-2015-00009-00-00 and E-RTA-2017-00003-C02-01, and Comunidad Autónoma de Madrid grant S2018/BAA-4370 (PLATESA2-CM).

Acknowledgments: Authors are in debt to Dr. Ursula Höfle and Dr. Virginia Gamino for kindly providing some of the images.

Conflicts of Interest: The authors declare no conflict of interest.

References

1. Martin-Acebes, M.A.; Saiz, J.C. West Nile virus: A re-emerging pathogen revisited. *World J. Virol.* **2012**, *1*, 51–70. [CrossRef] [PubMed]
2. Munoz, L.S.; Garcia, M.A.; Gordon-Lipkin, E.; Parra, B.; Pardo, C.A. Emerging Viral Infections and Their Impact on the Global Burden of Neurological Disease. *Semin. Neurol.* **2018**, *38*, 163–175. [CrossRef] [PubMed]
3. Zehender, G.; Veo, C.; Ebranati, E.; Carta, V.; Rovida, F.; Percivalle, E.; Moreno, A.; Lelli, D.; Calzolari, M.; Lavazza, A.; et al. Reconstructing the recent West Nile virus lineage 2 epidemic in Europe and Italy using discrete and continuous phylogeography. *PLoS ONE* **2017**, *12*, e0179679. [CrossRef] [PubMed]
4. European Centre for Disease Prevention and Control. Available online: https://ecdc.europa.eu (accessed on 16 September 2019).
5. Pachler, K.; Lebl, K.; Berer, D.; Rudolf, I.; Hubalek, Z.; Nowotny, N. Putative new West Nile virus lineage in Uranotaenia unguiculata mosquitoes, Austria, 2013. *Emerg. Infect. Dis.* **2014**, *20*, 2119–2122. [CrossRef] [PubMed]
6. Hayes, E.B.; Komar, N.; Nasci, R.S.; Montgomery, S.P.; O'Leary, D.R.; Campbell, G.L. Epidemiology and transmission dynamics of West Nile virus disease. *Emerg. Infect. Dis.* **2005**, *11*, 1167–1173. [CrossRef]
7. Komar, N.; Langevin, S.; Hinten, S.; Nemeth, N.; Edwards, E.; Hettler, D.; Davis, B.; Bowen, R.; Bunning, M. Experimental infection of North American birds with the New York 1999 strain of West Nile virus. *Emerg. Infect. Dis.* **2003**, *9*, 311–322. [CrossRef] [PubMed]
8. Jimenez de Oya, N.; Camacho, M.C.; Blazquez, A.B.; Lima-Barbero, J.F.; Saiz, J.C.; Hofle, U.; Escribano-Romero, E. High susceptibility of magpie (*Pica pica*) to experimental infection with lineage 1 and 2 West Nile virus. *PLoS Negl. Trop. Dis.* **2018**, *12*, e0006394. [CrossRef]
9. Lim, S.M.; Brault, A.C.; van Amerongen, G.; Bosco-Lauth, A.M.; Romo, H.; Sewbalaksing, V.D.; Bowen, R.A.; Osterhaus, A.D.; Koraka, P.; Martina, B.E. Susceptibility of Carrion Crows to Experimental Infection with Lineage 1 and 2 West Nile Viruses. *Emerg. Infect. Dis.* **2015**, *21*, 1357–1365. [CrossRef]
10. Eidson, M. "Neon needles" in a haystack: The advantages of passive surveillance for West Nile virus. *Ann. N. Y. Acad. Sci.* **2001**, *951*, 38–53. [CrossRef]
11. Eidson, M.; Komar, N.; Sorhage, F.; Nelson, R.; Talbot, T.; Mostashari, F.; McLean, R. Crow deaths as a sentinel surveillance system for West Nile virus in the northeastern United States, 1999. *Emerg. Infect. Dis.* **2001**, *7*, 615–620. [CrossRef]
12. Eidson, M.; Kramer, L.; Stone, W.; Hagiwara, Y.; Schmit, K. Dead bird surveillance as an early warning system for West Nile virus. *Emerg. Infect. Dis.* **2001**, *7*, 631–635. [CrossRef] [PubMed]

13. Hinton, M.G.; Reisen, W.K.; Wheeler, S.S.; Townsend, A.K. West Nile Virus Activity in a Winter Roost of American Crows (*Corvus brachyrhynchos*): Is Bird-To-Bird Transmission Important in Persistence and Amplification? *J. Med. Entomol.* **2015**, *52*, 683–692. [CrossRef]
14. Reisen, W.K.; Barker, C.M.; Carney, R.; Lothrop, H.D.; Wheeler, S.S.; Wilson, J.L.; Madon, M.B.; Takahashi, R.; Carroll, B.; Garcia, S.; et al. Role of corvids in epidemiology of West Nile virus in southern California. *J. Med. Entomol.* **2006**, *43*, 356–367. [CrossRef]
15. Ernest, H.B.; Woods, L.W.; Hoar, B.R. Pathology associated with West Nile virus infections in the yellow-billed magpie (*Pica nuttalli*): A California endemic bird. *J. Wildl. Dis.* **2010**, *46*, 401–408. [CrossRef] [PubMed]
16. Foss, L.; Padgett, K.; Reisen, W.K.; Kjemtrup, A.; Ogawa, J.; Kramer, V. West Nile Virus-Related Trends in Avian Mortality in California, USA, 2003–2012. *J. Wildl. Dis.* **2015**, *51*, 576–588. [CrossRef] [PubMed]
17. LaDeau, S.L.; Kilpatrick, A.M.; Marra, P.P. West Nile virus emergence and large-scale declines of North American bird populations. *Nature* **2007**, *447*, 710–713. [CrossRef] [PubMed]
18. Beck, C.; Jimenez-Clavero, M.A.; Leblond, A.; Durand, B.; Nowotny, N.; Leparc-Goffart, I.; Zientara, S.; Jourdain, E.; Lecollinet, S. Flaviviruses in Europe: Complex circulation patterns and their consequences for the diagnosis and control of West Nile disease. *Int. J. Environ. Res. Public Health* **2013**, *10*, 6049–6083. [CrossRef]
19. Dauphin, G.; Zientara, S. West Nile virus: Recent trends in diagnosis and vaccine development. *Vaccine* **2007**, *25*, 5563–5576. [CrossRef]
20. Ray, D.; Shah, A.; Tilgner, M.; Guo, Y.; Zhao, Y.; Dong, H.; Deas, T.S.; Zhou, Y.; Li, H.; Shi, P.Y. West Nile virus 5′-cap structure is formed by sequential guanine N-7 and ribose 2′-O methylations by nonstructural protein 5. *J. Virol.* **2006**, *80*, 8362–8370. [CrossRef]
21. Brinton, M.A. Replication cycle and molecular biology of the West Nile virus. *Viruses* **2013**, *6*, 13–53. [CrossRef]
22. Kaiser, J.A.; Wang, T.; Barrett, A.D. Virulence determinants of West Nile virus: How can these be used for vaccine design? *Future Virol.* **2017**, *12*, 283–295. [CrossRef] [PubMed]
23. Mukhopadhyay, S.; Kuhn, R.J.; Rossmann, M.G. A structural perspective of the flavivirus life cycle. *Nat. Rev. Microbiol.* **2005**, *3*, 13–22. [CrossRef] [PubMed]
24. Rastogi, M.; Sharma, N.; Singh, S.K. Flavivirus NS1: A multifaceted enigmatic viral protein. *Virol. J.* **2016**, *13*, 131. [CrossRef] [PubMed]
25. Martin-Acebes, M.A.; Blazquez, A.B.; Jimenez de Oya, N.; Escribano-Romero, E.; Saiz, J.C. West Nile virus replication requires fatty acid synthesis but is independent on phosphatidylinositol-4-phosphate lipids. *PLoS ONE* **2011**, *6*, e24970. [CrossRef] [PubMed]
26. Zhang, Y.; Kaufmann, B.; Chipman, P.R.; Kuhn, R.J.; Rossmann, M.G. Structure of immature West Nile virus. *J. Virol.* **2007**, *81*, 6141–6145. [CrossRef] [PubMed]
27. Mukhopadhyay, S.; Kim, B.S.; Chipman, P.R.; Rossmann, M.G.; Kuhn, R.J. Structure of West Nile virus. *Science* **2003**, *302*, 248. [CrossRef] [PubMed]
28. Bakonyi, T.; Ivanics, E.; Erdelyi, K.; Ursu, K.; Ferenczi, E.; Weissenbock, H.; Nowotny, N. Lineage 1 and 2 strains of encephalitic West Nile virus, central Europe. *Emerg. Infect. Dis.* **2006**, *12*, 618–623. [CrossRef]
29. Erdelyi, K.; Ursu, K.; Ferenczi, E.; Szeredi, L.; Ratz, F.; Skare, J.; Bakonyi, T. Clinical and pathologic features of lineage 2 West Nile virus infections in birds of prey in Hungary. *Vector Borne Zoonotic Dis.* **2007**, *7*, 181–188. [CrossRef] [PubMed]
30. Petrovic, T.; Blazquez, A.B.; Lupulovic, D.; Lazic, G.; Escribano-Romero, E.; Fabijan, D.; Kapetanov, M.; Lazic, S.; Saiz, J. Monitoring West Nile virus (WNV) infection in wild birds in Serbia during 2012: First isolation and characterisation of WNV strains from Serbia. *Euron. Surveill.* **2013**, *18*, 20622. [CrossRef]
31. Savini, G.; Capelli, G.; Monaco, F.; Polci, A.; Russo, F.; Di Gennaro, A.; Marini, V.; Teodori, L.; Montarsi, F.; Pinoni, C.; et al. Evidence of West Nile virus lineage 2 circulation in Northern Italy. *Vet. Microbiol.* **2012**, *158*, 267–273. [CrossRef]
32. Edgar, R.C. MUSCLE: Multiple sequence alignment with high accuracy and high throughput. *Nucleic Acids Res.* **2004**, *32*, 1792–1797. [CrossRef] [PubMed]
33. Trifinopoulos, J.; Nguyen, L.T.; von Haeseler, A.; Minh, B.Q. W-IQ-TREE: A fast online phylogenetic tool for maximum likelihood analysis. *Nucleic Acids Res.* **2016**, *44*, W232–W235. [CrossRef] [PubMed]
34. Letunic, I.; Bork, P. Interactive Tree Of Life (iTOL) v4: Recent updates and new developments. *Nucleic Acids Res.* **2019**, *47*, W256–W259. [CrossRef] [PubMed]

35. Austin, S.K.; Dowd, K.A. B cell response and mechanisms of antibody protection to West Nile virus. *Viruses* **2014**, *6*, 1015–1036. [CrossRef] [PubMed]
36. Totani, M.; Yoshii, K.; Kariwa, H.; Takashima, I. Glycosylation of the envelope protein of West Nile Virus affects its replication in chicks. *Avian Dis.* **2011**, *55*, 561–568. [CrossRef] [PubMed]
37. Heinz, F.X.; Stiasny, K. Flaviviruses and flavivirus vaccines. *Vaccine* **2012**, *30*, 4301–4306. [CrossRef] [PubMed]
38. Lobigs, M.; Diamond, M.S. Feasibility of cross-protective vaccination against flaviviruses of the Japanese encephalitis serocomplex. *Expert Rev. Vaccines* **2012**, *11*, 177–187. [CrossRef]
39. Halstead, S.B. Pathogenic Exploitation of Fc Activity. In *Antibody Fc Linking Adaptive and Innate Immunity*; Ackerman, M., Ed.; Academic Press: Cambridge, MA, USA, 2014; pp. 333–350.
40. Mehlhop, E.; Ansarah-Sobrinho, C.; Johnson, S.; Engle, M.; Fremont, D.H.; Pierson, T.C.; Diamond, M.S. Complement protein C1q inhibits antibody-dependent enhancement of flavivirus infection in an IgG subclass-specific manner. *Cell Host Microbe* **2007**, *2*, 417–426. [CrossRef]
41. Hirota, J.; Shimizu, S. A new competitive ELISA detects West Nile virus infection using monoclonal antibodies against the precursor-membrane protein of West Nile virus. *J. Virol. Methods* **2013**, *188*, 132–138. [CrossRef]
42. Oceguera, L.F., 3rd; Patiris, P.J.; Chiles, R.E.; Busch, M.P.; Tobler, L.H.; Hanson, C.V. Flavivirus serology by Western blot analysis. *Am. J. Trop. Med. Hyg.* **2007**, *77*, 159–163. [CrossRef]
43. Chung, K.M.; Nybakken, G.E.; Thompson, B.S.; Engle, M.J.; Marri, A.; Fremont, D.H.; Diamond, M.S. Antibodies against West Nile Virus nonstructural protein NS1 prevent lethal infection through Fc gamma receptor-dependent and -independent mechanisms. *J. Virol.* **2006**, *80*, 1340–1351. [CrossRef] [PubMed]
44. Rebollo, B.; Llorente, F.; Perez-Ramirez, E.; Sarraseca, J.; Gallardo, C.; Risalde, M.A.; Hofle, U.; Figuerola, J.; Soriguer, R.C.; Venteo, A.; et al. Absence of protection from West Nile virus disease and adverse effects in red legged partridges after non-structural NS1 protein administration. *Comp. Immunol. Microbiol. Infect. Dis.* **2018**, *56*, 30–33. [CrossRef] [PubMed]
45. Pettersen, E.F.; Goddard, T.D.; Huang, C.C.; Couch, G.S.; Greenblatt, D.M.; Meng, E.C.; Ferrin, T.E. UCSF Chimera—A visualization system for exploratory research and analysis. *J. Comput. Chem.* **2004**, *25*, 1605–1612. [CrossRef] [PubMed]
46. Benzarti, E.; Linden, A.; Desmecht, D.; Garigliany, M. Mosquito-borne epornitic flaviviruses: An update and review. *J. Gen. Virol.* **2019**, *100*, 119–132. [CrossRef] [PubMed]
47. Gamino, V.; Hofle, U. Pathology and tissue tropism of natural West Nile virus infection in birds: A review. *Vet. Res.* **2013**, *44*, 39. [CrossRef]
48. Nemeth, N.M.; Thomsen, B.V.; Spraker, T.R.; Benson, J.M.; Bosco-Lauth, A.M.; Oesterle, P.T.; Bright, J.M.; Muth, J.P.; Campbell, T.W.; Gidlewski, T.L.; et al. Clinical and pathologic responses of American crows (*Corvus brachyrhynchos*) and fish crows (*C ossifragus*) to experimental West Nile virus infection. *Vet. Pathol.* **2011**, *48*, 1061–1074. [CrossRef] [PubMed]
49. Centers for Disease Control and Prevention. Species of Dead Birds in Which West Nile Virus Has Been Detected, United States, 1999–2016; Centers for Disease Control and Prevention. Available online: https://www.cdc.gov/westnile/dead-birds/index.html# (accessed on 23 September 2019).
50. Eckstrand, C.D.; Woods, L.W.; Diab, S.S.; Crossley, B.M.; Giannitti, F. Diagnostic exercise: High mortality in a flock of chukar partridge chicks (*Alectoris chukar*) in California. *Vet. Pathol.* **2015**, *52*, 189–192. [CrossRef]
51. Swayne, D.E.; Beck, J.R.; Smith, C.S.; Shieh, W.J.; Zaki, S.R. Fatal encephalitis and myocarditis in young domestic geese (*Anser anser domesticus*) caused by West Nile virus. *Emerg. Infect. Dis.* **2001**, *7*, 751–753. [CrossRef]
52. Wunschmann, A.; Ziegler, A. West Nile virus-associated mortality events in domestic Chukar partridges (Alectoris chukar) and domestic Impeyan pheasants (*Lophophorus impeyanus*). *Avian Dis.* **2006**, *50*, 456–459. [CrossRef]
53. Ludwig, G.V.; Calle, P.P.; Mangiafico, J.A.; Raphael, B.L.; Danner, D.K.; Hile, J.A.; Clippinger, T.L.; Smith, J.F.; Cook, R.A.; McNamara, T. An outbreak of West Nile virus in a New York City captive wildlife population. *Am. J. Trop. Med. Hyg.* **2002**, *67*, 67–75. [CrossRef]
54. Ward, M.R.; Stallknecht, D.E.; Willis, J.; Conroy, M.J.; Davidson, W.R. Wild bird mortality and West Nile virus surveillance: Biases associated with detection, reporting, and carcass persistence. *J. Wildl. Dis.* **2006**, *42*, 92–106. [CrossRef] [PubMed]

55. Jimenez-Clavero, M.A.; Sotelo, E.; Fernandez-Pinero, J.; Llorente, F.; Blanco, J.M.; Rodriguez-Ramos, J.; Perez-Ramirez, E.; Hofle, U. West Nile virus in golden eagles, Spain, 2007. *Emerg. Infect. Dis.* **2008**, *14*, 1489–1491. [CrossRef] [PubMed]
56. Yaremych, S.A.; Warner, R.E.; Mankin, P.C.; Brawn, J.D.; Raim, A.; Novak, R. West Nile virus and high death rate in American crows. *Emerg. Infect. Dis.* **2004**, *10*, 709–711. [CrossRef] [PubMed]
57. Brault, A.C.; Langevin, S.A.; Bowen, R.A.; Panella, N.A.; Biggerstaff, B.J.; Miller, B.R.; Komar, N. Differential virulence of West Nile strains for American crows. *Emerg. Infect. Dis.* **2004**, *10*, 2161–2168. [CrossRef] [PubMed]
58. Perez-Ramirez, E.; Llorente, F.; Del Amo, J.; Nowotny, N.; Jimenez-Clavero, M.A. Susceptibility and role as competent host of the red-legged partridge after infection with lineage 1 and 2 West Nile virus isolates of Mediterranean and Central European origin. *Vet. Microbiol.* **2018**, *222*, 39–45. [CrossRef] [PubMed]
59. Ziegler, U.; Angenvoort, J.; Fischer, D.; Fast, C.; Eiden, M.; Rodriguez, A.V.; Revilla-Fernandez, S.; Nowotny, N.; de la Fuente, J.G.; Lierz, M.; et al. Pathogenesis of West Nile virus lineage 1 and 2 in experimentally infected large falcons. *Vet. Microbiol.* **2013**, *161*, 263–273. [CrossRef] [PubMed]
60. Garmendia, A.E.; Van Kruiningen, H.J.; French, R.A.; Anderson, J.F.; Andreadis, T.G.; Kumar, A.; West, A.B. Recovery and identification of West Nile virus from a hawk in winter. *J. Clin. Microbiol.* **2000**, *38*, 3110–3111. [PubMed]
61. Nemeth, N.M.; Hahn, D.C.; Gould, D.H.; Bowen, R.A. Experimental West Nile virus infection in Eastern Screech Owls (*Megascops asio*). *Avian Dis.* **2006**, *50*, 252–258. [CrossRef]
62. Banet-Noach, C.; Simanov, L.; Malkinson, M. Direct (non-vector) transmission of West Nile virus in geese. *Avian Pathol. J. WVPA* **2003**, *32*, 489–494. [CrossRef]
63. Escribano-Romero, E.; Gamino, V.; Merino-Ramos, T.; Blazquez, A.B.; Martin-Acebes, M.A.; de Oya, N.J.; Gutierrez-Guzman, A.V.; Escribano, J.M.; Hofle, U.; Saiz, J.C. Protection of red-legged partridges (*Alectoris rufa*) against West Nile virus (WNV) infection after immunization with WNV recombinant envelope protein E (rE). *Vaccine* **2013**, *31*, 4523–4527. [CrossRef]
64. Jimenez de Oya, N.; Escribano-Romero, E.; Camacho, M.C.; Blazquez, A.B.; Martin-Acebes, M.A.; Hofle, U.; Saiz, J.C. A Recombinant Subviral Particle-Based Vaccine Protects Magpie (*Pica pica*) Against West Nile Virus Infection. *Front. Microbiol.* **2019**, *10*, 1133. [CrossRef] [PubMed]
65. Langevin, S.A.; Bunning, M.; Davis, B.; Komar, N. Experimental infection of chickens as candidate sentinels for West Nile virus. *Emerg. Infect. Dis.* **2001**, *7*, 726–729. [CrossRef] [PubMed]
66. Reisen, W.K. Ecology of West Nile virus in North America. *Viruses* **2013**, *5*, 2079–2105. [CrossRef] [PubMed]
67. Tolsa, M.J.; Garcia-Pena, G.E.; Rico-Chavez, O.; Roche, B.; Suzan, G. Macroecology of birds potentially susceptible to West Nile virus. *Proc. Biol. Sci.* **2018**, *285*. [CrossRef] [PubMed]
68. Jupp, P.G.; McIntosh, B.M. Quantitative experiments on the vector capability of Culex (*Culex*) *univittatus* Theobald with West Nile and Sindbis viruses. *J. Med. Entomol.* **1970**, *7*, 371–373. [CrossRef] [PubMed]
69. Hofmeister, E.K.; Dusek, R.J.; Fassbinder-Orth, C.; Owen, B.; Franson, J.C. Susceptibility and Antibody Response of Vesper Sparrows (*Pooecetes Gramineus*) to West Nile Virus: A Potential Amplification Host in Sagebrush-Grassland Habitat. *J. Wildl. Dis.* **2016**, *52*, 345–353. [CrossRef] [PubMed]
70. Nemeth, N.M.; Bosco-Lauth, A.M.; Williams, L.M.; Bowen, R.A.; Brown, J.D. West Nile Virus Infection in Ruffed Grouse (*Bonasa umbellus*): Experimental Infection and Protective Effects of Vaccination. *Vet. Pathol.* **2017**, *54*, 901–911. [CrossRef]
71. Reisen, W.K.; Hahn, D.C. Comparison of immune responses of brown-headed cowbird and related blackbirds to West Nile and other mosquito-borne encephalitis viruses. *J. Wildl. Dis.* **2007**, *43*, 439–449. [CrossRef]
72. Reisen, W.K.; Fang, Y.; Martinez, V. Is nonviremic transmission of West Nile virus by Culex mosquitoes (Diptera: Culicidae) nonviremic? *J. Med. Entomol.* **2007**, *44*, 299–302. [CrossRef]
73. Weingartl, H.M.; Neufeld, J.L.; Copps, J.; Marszal, P. Experimental West Nile virus infection in blue jays (*Cyanocitta cristata*) and crows (*Corvus brachyrhynchos*). *Vet. Pathol.* **2004**, *41*, 362–370. [CrossRef]
74. Nemeth, N.; Gould, D.; Bowen, R.; Komar, N. Natural and experimental West Nile virus infection in five raptor species. *J. Wildl. Dis.* **2006**, *42*, 1–13. [CrossRef]
75. Hofmeister, E.K.; Lund, M.; Shearn Bochsler, V. West Nile Virus Infection in American Singer Canaries: An Experimental Model in a Highly Susceptible Avian Species. *Vet. Pathol.* **2018**, *55*, 531–538. [CrossRef]
76. Stockman, J.; Hawkins, M.G.; Burns, R.E.; Fang, Y.; Brault, A.C.; Lowenstine, L.J. West Nile virus infection in a green-winged macaw (*Ara chloropterus*). *Avian Dis.* **2010**, *54*, 164–169. [CrossRef]

77. Clark, L.; Hall, J.; McLean, R.; Dunbar, M.; Klenk, K.; Bowen, R.; Smeraski, C.A. Susceptibility of greater sage-grouse to experimental infection with West Nile virus. *J. Wildl. Dis.* **2006**, *42*, 14–22. [CrossRef]
78. Hofmeister, E.K.; Dusek, R.J.; Brand, C.J. Surveillance Potential of Non-Native Hawaiian Birds for Detection of West Nile Virus. *Am. J. Trop. Med. Hyg.* **2015**, *93*, 701–708. [CrossRef]
79. Senne, D.A.; Pedersen, J.C.; Hutto, D.L.; Taylor, W.D.; Schmitt, B.J.; Panigrahy, B. Pathogenicity of West Nile virus in chickens. *Avian Dis.* **2000**, *44*, 642–649. [CrossRef]
80. Gamino, V.; Escribano-Romero, E.; Blazquez, A.B.; Gutierrez-Guzman, A.V.; Martin-Acebes, M.A.; Saiz, J.C.; Hofle, U. Experimental North American West Nile Virus Infection in the Red-legged Partridge (*Alectoris rufa*). *Vet. Pathol.* **2016**, *53*, 585–593. [CrossRef]
81. Steele, K.E.; Linn, M.J.; Schoepp, R.J.; Komar, N.; Geisbert, T.W.; Manduca, R.M.; Calle, P.P.; Raphael, B.L.; Clippinger, T.L.; Larsen, T.; et al. Pathology of fatal West Nile virus infections in native and exotic birds during the 1999 outbreak in New York City, New York. *Vet. Pathol.* **2000**, *37*, 208–224. [CrossRef]
82. Gancz, A.Y.; Smith, D.A.; Barker, I.K.; Lindsay, R.; Hunter, B. Pathology and tissue distribution of West Nile virus in North American owls (family: Strigidae). *Avian Pathol. J. WVPA* **2006**, *35*, 17–29. [CrossRef]
83. Hubalek, Z.; Kosina, M.; Rudolf, I.; Mendel, J.; Strakova, P.; Tomesek, M. Mortality of Goshawks (*Accipiter gentilis*) Due to West Nile Virus Lineage 2. *Vector Borne Zoonotic Dis.* **2018**, *18*, 624–627. [CrossRef]
84. Busquets, N.; Bertran, K.; Costa, T.P.; Rivas, R.; de la Fuente, J.G.; Villalba, R.; Solanes, D.; Bensaid, A.; Majo, N.; Pages, N. Experimental West Nile virus infection in Gyr-Saker hybrid falcons. *Vector Borne Zoonotic Dis.* **2012**, *12*, 482–489. [CrossRef]
85. Hirata, A.; Yonemaru, K.; Kubo, M.; Murakami, M.; Sakai, H.; Yanai, T.; Masegi, T. Frequent development of inflammatory lesions and lymphoid foci in the kidneys of Japanese wild crows (*Corvus macrorhynchos* and *Corvus corone*) as a result of the entry of causal agents via the renal portal blood. *J. Vet. Med. Sci.* **2010**, *72*, 327–332. [CrossRef]
86. Gamino, V.; Escribano-Romero, E.; Gutierrez-Guzman, A.V.; Blazquez, A.B.; Saiz, J.C.; Hofle, U. Oculopathologic findings in flavivirus-infected gallinaceous birds. *Vet. Pathol.* **2014**, *51*, 1113–1116. [CrossRef]
87. Pauli, A.M.; Cruz-Martinez, L.A.; Ponder, J.B.; Redig, P.T.; Glaser, A.L.; Klauss, G.; Schoster, J.V.; Wunschmann, A. Ophthalmologic and oculopathologic findings in red-tailed hawks and Cooper's hawks with naturally acquired West Nile virus infection. *J. Am. Vet. Med. Assoc.* **2007**, *231*, 1240–1248. [CrossRef]
88. Wunschmann, A.; Armien, A.G.; Khatri, M.; Martinez, L.C.; Willette, M.; Glaser, A.; Alvarez, J.; Redig, P. Ocular Lesions in Red-Tailed Hawks (*Buteo jamaicensis*) With Naturally Acquired West Nile Disease. *Vet. Pathol.* **2017**, *54*, 277–287. [CrossRef]
89. Ellis, A.E.; Mead, D.G.; Allison, A.B.; Stallknecht, D.E.; Howerth, E.W. Pathology and epidemiology of natural West Nile viral infection of raptors in Georgia. *J. Wildl. Dis.* **2007**, *43*, 214–223. [CrossRef]
90. Palmieri, C.; Franca, M.; Uzal, F.; Anderson, M.; Barr, B.; Woods, L.; Moore, J.; Woolcock, P.; Shivaprasad, H.L. Pathology and immunohistochemical findings of West Nile virus infection in Psittaciformes. *Vet. Pathol.* **2011**, *48*, 975–984. [CrossRef]
91. Wheeler, S.S.; Langevin, S.A.; Brault, A.C.; Woods, L.; Carroll, B.D.; Reisen, W.K. Detection of persistent West Nile virus RNA in experimentally and naturally infected avian hosts. *Am. J. Trop. Med. Hyg.* **2012**, *87*, 559–564. [CrossRef]
92. Nemeth, N.; Young, G.; Ndaluka, C.; Bielefeldt-Ohmann, H.; Komar, N.; Bowen, R. Persistent West Nile virus infection in the house sparrow (*Passer domesticus*). *Arch. Virol.* **2009**, *154*, 783–789. [CrossRef]
93. Wheeler, S.S.; Vineyard, M.P.; Woods, L.W.; Reisen, W.K. Dynamics of West Nile virus persistence in House Sparrows (*Passer domesticus*). *PLoS Negl. Trop. Dis.* **2012**, *6*, e1860. [CrossRef]
94. Gardner, I.A.; Wong, S.J.; Ferraro, G.L.; Balasuriya, U.B.; Hullinger, P.J.; Wilson, W.D.; Shi, P.Y.; MacLachlan, N.J. Incidence and effects of West Nile virus infection in vaccinated and unvaccinated horses in California. *Vet. Res.* **2007**, *38*, 109–116. [CrossRef]
95. Iyer, A.V.; Kousoulas, K.G. A review of vaccine approaches for West Nile virus. *Int. J. Environ. Res. Public Health* **2013**, *10*, 4200–4223. [CrossRef]
96. Angenvoort, J.; Fischer, D.; Fast, C.; Ziegler, U.; Eiden, M.; de la Fuente, J.G.; Lierz, M.; Groschup, M.H. Limited efficacy of West Nile virus vaccines in large falcons (Falco spp.). *Vet. Res.* **2014**, *45*, 41. [CrossRef]

97. Boyce, W.M.; Vickers, W.; Morrison, S.A.; Sillett, T.S.; Caldwell, L.; Wheeler, S.S.; Barker, C.M.; Cummings, R.; Reisen, W.K. Surveillance for West Nile virus and vaccination of free-ranging island scrub-jays (*Aphelocoma insularis*) on Santa Cruz Island, California. *Vector Borne Zoonotic Dis.* **2011**, *11*, 1063–1068. [CrossRef]
98. Bunning, M.L.; Fox, P.E.; Bowen, R.A.; Komar, N.; Chang, G.J.; Speaker, T.J.; Stephens, M.R.; Nemeth, N.; Panella, N.A.; Langevin, S.A.; et al. DNA vaccination of the American crow (*Corvus brachyrhynchos*) provides partial protection against lethal challenge with West Nile virus. *Avian Dis.* **2007**, *51*, 573–577. [CrossRef]
99. Davis, M.R.; Langan, J.N.; Johnson, Y.J.; Ritchie, B.W.; Van Bonn, W. West Nile virus seroconversion in penguins after vaccination with a killed virus vaccine or a DNA vaccine. *J. Zoo Wildl. Med.* **2008**, *39*, 582–589. [CrossRef]
100. Johnson, S. Avian titer development against West Nile virus after extralabel use of an equine vaccine. *J. Zoo Wildl. Med.* **2005**, *36*, 257–264. [CrossRef]
101. Nusbaum, K.E.; Wright, J.C.; Johnston, W.B.; Allison, A.B.; Hilton, C.D.; Staggs, L.A.; Stallknecht, D.E.; Shelnutt, J.L. Absence of humoral response in flamingos and red-tailed hawks to experimental vaccination with a killed West Nile virus vaccine. *Avian Dis.* **2003**, *47*, 750–752. [CrossRef]
102. Okeson, D.M.; Llizo, S.Y.; Miller, C.L.; Glaser, A.L. Antibody response of five bird species after vaccination with a killed West Nile virus vaccine. *J. Zoo Wildl. Med.* **2007**, *38*, 240–244. [CrossRef]
103. Olsen, G.H.; Miller, K.J.; Docherty, D.E.; Bochsler, V.S.; Sileo, L. Pathogenicity of West Nile virus and response to vaccination in sandhill cranes (*Grus canadensis*) using a killed vaccine. *J. Zoo Wildl. Med.* **2009**, *40*, 263–271. [CrossRef]
104. Glavis, J.; Larsen, R.S.; Lamberski, N.; Gaffney, P.; Gardner, I. Evaluation of antibody response to vaccination against West Nile virus in thick billed parrots (*Rhynchopsitta pachyrhyncha*). *J. Zoo Wildl. Med.* **2011**, *42*, 495–498. [CrossRef]
105. Wheeler, S.S.; Langevin, S.; Woods, L.; Carroll, B.D.; Vickers, W.; Morrison, S.A.; Chang, G.J.; Reisen, W.K.; Boyce, W.M. Efficacy of three vaccines in protecting Western Scrub-Jays (*Aphelocoma californica*) from experimental infection with West Nile virus: Implications for vaccination of Island Scrub-Jays (*Aphelocoma insularis*). *Vector Borne Zoonotic Dis.* **2011**, *11*, 1069–1080. [CrossRef]
106. Langevin, S.A.; Arroyo, J.; Monath, T.P.; Komar, N. Host-range restriction of chimeric yellow fever-West Nile vaccine in fish crows (*Corvus ossifragus*). *Am. J. Trop. Med. Hyg.* **2003**, *69*, 78–80. [CrossRef]
107. Merino-Ramos, T.; Blazquez, A.B.; Escribano-Romero, E.; Canas-Arranz, R.; Sobrino, F.; Saiz, J.C.; Martin-Acebes, M.A. Protection of a single dose West Nile virus recombinant subviral particle vaccine against lineage 1 or 2 strains and analysis of the cross-reactivity with Usutu virus. *PLoS ONE* **2014**, *9*, e108056. [CrossRef]
108. Davis, B.S.; Chang, G.J.; Cropp, B.; Roehrig, J.T.; Martin, D.A.; Mitchell, C.J.; Bowen, R.; Bunning, M.L. West Nile virus recombinant DNA vaccine protects mouse and horse from virus challenge and expresses in vitro a noninfectious recombinant antigen that can be used in enzyme-linked immunosorbent assays. *J. Virol.* **2001**, *75*, 4040–4047. [CrossRef]
109. Kilpatrick, A.M.; Dupuis, A.P.; Chang, G.J.; Kramer, L.D. DNA vaccination of American robins (*Turdus migratorius*) against West Nile virus. *Vector Borne Zoonotic Dis.* **2010**, *10*, 377–380. [CrossRef]
110. Redig, P.T.; Tully, T.N.; Ritchie, B.W.; Roy, A.F.; Baudena, M.A.; Chang, G.J. Effect of West Nile virus DNA-plasmid vaccination on response to live virus challenge in red-tailed hawks (*Buteo jamaicensis*). *Am. J. Vet. Res.* **2011**, *72*, 1065–1070. [CrossRef]
111. Turell, M.J.; Bunning, M.; Ludwig, G.V.; Ortman, B.; Chang, J.; Speaker, T.; Spielman, A.; McLean, R.; Komar, N.; Gates, R.; et al. DNA vaccine for West Nile virus infection in fish crows (*Corvus ossifragus*). *Emerg. Infect. Dis.* **2003**, *9*, 1077–1081. [CrossRef]
112. Chang, G.J.; Davis, B.S.; Stringfield, C.; Lutz, C. Prospective immunization of the endangered California condors (*Gymnogyps californianus*) protects this species from lethal West Nile virus infection. *Vaccine* **2007**, *25*, 2325–2330. [CrossRef]
113. Fischer, D.; Angenvoort, J.; Ziegler, U.; Fast, C.; Maier, K.; Chabierski, S.; Eiden, M.; Ulbert, S.; Groschup, M.H.; Lierz, M. DNA vaccines encoding the envelope protein of West Nile virus lineages 1 or 2 administered intramuscularly, via electroporation and with recombinant virus protein induce partial protection in large falcons (Falco spp.). *Vet. Res.* **2015**, *46*, 87. [CrossRef]

114. Jarvi, S.I.; Hu, D.; Misajon, K.; Coller, B.A.; Wong, T.; Lieberman, M.M. Vaccination of captive nene (*Branta sandvicensis*) against West Nile virus using a protein-based vaccine (WN-80E). *J. Wildl. Dis.* **2013**, *49*, 152–156. [CrossRef]
115. Malkinson, M.; Banet, C.; Khinich, Y.; Samina, I.; Pokamunski, S.; Weisman, Y. Use of live and inactivated vaccines in the control of West Nile fever in domestic geese. *Ann. N. Y. Acad. Sci.* **2001**, *951*, 255–261. [CrossRef]
116. Sa, E.S.M.; Ellis, A.; Karaca, K.; Minke, J.; Nordgren, R.; Wu, S.; Swayne, D.E. Domestic goose as a model for West Nile virus vaccine efficacy. *Vaccine* **2013**, *31*, 1045–1050. [CrossRef]
117. Lustig, S.; Olshevsky, U.; Ben-Nathan, D.; Lachmi, B.E.; Malkinson, M.; Kobiler, D.; Halevy, M. A live attenuated West Nile virus strain as a potential veterinary vaccine. *Viral Immunol.* **2000**, *13*, 401–410. [CrossRef]
118. Samina, I.; Khinich, Y.; Simanov, M.; Malkinson, M. An inactivated West Nile virus vaccine for domestic geese-efficacy study and a summary of 4 years of field application. *Vaccine* **2005**, *23*, 4955–4958. [CrossRef]
119. Samina, I.; Havenga, M.; Koudstaal, W.; Khinich, Y.; Koldijk, M.; Malkinson, M.; Simanov, M.; Perl, S.; Gijsbers, L.; Weverling, G.J.; et al. Safety and efficacy in geese of a PER.C6-based inactivated West Nile virus vaccine. *Vaccine* **2007**, *25*, 8338–8345. [CrossRef]
120. Pletnev, A.G.; Claire, M.S.; Elkins, R.; Speicher, J.; Murphy, B.R.; Chanock, R.M. Molecularly engineered live-attenuated chimeric West Nile/dengue virus vaccines protect rhesus monkeys from West Nile virus. *Virology* **2003**, *314*, 190–195. [CrossRef]
121. Pletnev, A.G.; Swayne, D.E.; Speicher, J.; Rumyantsev, A.A.; Murphy, B.R. Chimeric West Nile/dengue virus vaccine candidate: Preclinical evaluation in mice, geese and monkeys for safety and immunogenicity. *Vaccine* **2006**, *24*, 6392–6404. [CrossRef]
122. Jarvi, S.I.; Lieberman, M.M.; Hofmeister, E.; Nerurkar, V.R.; Wong, T.; Weeks-Levy, C. Protective efficacy of a recombinant subunit West Nile virus vaccine in domestic geese (*Anser anser*). *Vaccine* **2008**, *26*, 5338–5344. [CrossRef]
123. Fassbinder-Orth, C.A.; Hofmeister, E.K.; Weeks-Levy, C.; Karasov, W.H. Oral and parenteral immunization of chickens (*Gallus gallus*) against West Nile virus with recombinant envelope protein. *Avian Dis.* **2009**, *53*, 502–509. [CrossRef]
124. Alonso-Padilla, J.; Jimenez de Oya, N.; Blazquez, A.B.; Loza-Rubio, E.; Escribano, J.M.; Saiz, J.C.; Escribano-Romero, E. Evaluation of an enzyme-linked immunosorbent assay for detection of West Nile virus infection based on a recombinant envelope protein produced in *Trichoplusia ni* larvae. *J. Virol. Methods* **2010**, *166*, 37–41. [CrossRef]
125. Alonso-Padilla, J.; de Oya, N.J.; Blazquez, A.B.; Escribano-Romero, E.; Escribano, J.M.; Saiz, J.C. Recombinant West Nile virus envelope protein E and domain III expressed in insect larvae protects mice against West Nile disease. *Vaccine* **2011**, *29*, 1830–1835. [CrossRef]
126. Austin, R.J.; Whiting, T.L.; Anderson, R.A.; Drebot, M.A. An outbreak of West Nile virus-associated disease in domestic geese (*Anser anser domesticus*) upon initial introduction to a geographic region, with evidence of bird to bird transmission. *Can. Vet. J.* **2004**, *45*, 117–123.
127. Young, J.A.; Jefferies, W. Towards the conservation of endangered avian species: A recombinant West Nile Virus vaccine results in increased humoral and cellular immune responses in Japanese Quail (*Coturnix japonica*). *PLoS ONE* **2013**, *8*, e67137. [CrossRef]
128. Komar, N. West Nile virus: Epidemiology and ecology in North America. *Adv. Virus Res.* **2003**, *61*, 185–234.
129. Sardelis, M.R.; Turell, M.J.; Dohm, D.J.; O'Guinn, M.L. Vector competence of selected North American *Culex* and *Coquillettidia* mosquitoes for West Nile virus. *Emerg. Infect. Dis.* **2001**, *7*, 1018–1022. [CrossRef]
130. McLean, R.G.; Ubico, S.R.; Docherty, D.E.; Hansen, W.R.; Sileo, L.; McNamara, T.S. West Nile virus transmission and ecology in birds. *Ann. N. Y. Acad. Sci.* **2001**, *951*, 54–57. [CrossRef]
131. Hanlon, C.A.; Niezgoda, M.; Morrill, P.; Rupprecht, C.E. Oral efficacy of an attenuated rabies virus vaccine in skunks and raccoons. *J. Wildl. Dis.* **2002**, *38*, 420–427. [CrossRef]

MDPI
St. Alban-Anlage 66
4052 Basel
Switzerland
Tel. +41 61 683 77 34
Fax +41 61 302 89 18
www.mdpi.com

Vaccines Editorial Office
E-mail: vaccines@mdpi.com
www.mdpi.com/journal/vaccines

www.ingramcontent.com/pod-product-compliance
Lightning Source LLC
LaVergne TN
LVHW070630100526
838202LV00012B/772
9783039436231